Praise for

THE PARKINSON'S PLAN

"Both of us are athletes, Air Force Academy graduates, physicians, veterans of Afghanistan, and mothers. We were diagnosed with Parkinson's in our 40s. Parkinson's is not an 'old man's disease.' It affects all of us. *The Parkinson's Plan* tells us why, how to slow it, treat it, and prevent this terrible disease."

—Dr. Jana Kokkonen Reed and Dr. Sara Whittingham,
both Lieutenant Colonels, U.S. Air Force (retired)

"I was a kid when I lived at Camp Lejeune. I had no idea the water was contaminated with TCE—or that it would contribute to my Parkinson's diagnosis at 36. Learning that years later gave me answers, but it also gave me purpose. *The Parkinson's Plan* turns stories like mine into action—to prevent the next generation from living out the same story."

—Brian Grant, former NBA player and founder,
Brian Grant Foundation

"We lost Robin to a disease we couldn't see coming—Lewy body dementia—but what we're learning now is that many of these brain diseases, including Parkinson's, may not be random. *The Parkinson's Plan* shines a light on the toxic exposures—like pesticides and industrial chemicals—that are harming our brains."

—Susan Schneider Williams, artist and advocate for
Lewy body dementia awareness and research

"For too long we've been passive in our approach to eradicating Parkinson's. In compelling terms, this fascinating book gives us a message of hopefulness—and urgency—that there is a clear path forward."

—Davis Phinney, Olympic medalist and founder,
Davis Phinney Foundation

"My mother battled dementia with Lewy bodies—the second most common form of dementia. These conditions have causes—and *The Parkinson's Plan* uncovers them, offering 25 proven ways to lower your risk."

—Max Lugavere, *New York Times* best-selling author of
Genius Foods and host of The Genius Life podcast

"In *The Parkinson's Plan*, Drs. Okun and Dorsey lay out a vision that takes on Parkinson's with a team approach—where everyone plays a role and every action matters."

—Kirk Gibson, two-time World Series Champion and founder
of the Kirk Gibson Foundation for Parkinson's

"*The Parkinson's Plan* is a call to action, empowering those living with PD and the broader community to advocate for solving the enigma of what exactly causes PD and for the prevention of known environmental toxins fueled by a true sense of urgency."   —Dr. Soania Mathur, cofounder of PD Avengers

"*The Parkinson's Plan* is an essential resource—not just for understanding the science, but for humanizing the experience and making prevention and better care accessible to all."

—Omotola Thomas, founder, Parkinson's Africa

"*The Parkinson's Plan* is a blueprint of hope for those of us living with the disease. It is a must read for all those who envision a future without Parkinson's and want a roadmap to the cure."

—Allie Signorelli, young onset Parkinson's patient and advocate

"Drs. Dorsey and Okun have taken on the important and necessary job of outlining a PLAN that can slow the progression of Parkinson's for those who already have it and prevent it for those who never want it."

—Dr. Karen Jaffe, founder, InMotion™

"This book is a must read for anyone who is interested in this field."

—Dr. Maria De León, best-selling author of *Parkinson's Diva*

"*The Parkinson's Plan* is the kind of resource I wish every family had."
—Jimmy Choi, Parkinson's advocate, athlete, and speaker

"*The Parkinson's Plan* meets people like me with honesty, dignity, and direction."
—Denise Coley, retired tech executive and advocate
for awareness, inclusiveness, and equity

"Parkinson's affected my father, and the evidence is increasingly clear not only that the incidence of this disease is rising but that it may be *preventable*."
—Dr. Justin C. McArthur, professor and director,
Johns Hopkins Department of Neurology

"*The Parkinson's Plan* is written for real people—individuals, families, and entire communities—trying to move together through something complex."
—Christian McBride, nine-time Grammy-winning jazz musician

"For me, this fight is personal—my father lives with this disease, and my grandmother and my wife's father also had Parkinson's. I've seen firsthand the power of having a plan, a purpose, and hope. This book lays out a bold, actionable strategy to move forward and fight back—just like my dad has chosen to do every single day."   —Congressman C. Scott Franklin

"Over one million Americans—including many that are close to us—are living with Parkinson's disease. We can no longer afford to wait. We must have a plan, and we must have action. *The Parkinson's Plan* is an important and timely step forward—a powerful guide that lays out how we can take control, accelerate research, and improve care for everyone facing this disease."   —Congressman Cliff Stearns

"*The Parkinson's Plan* provides a proactive guide for people living with Parkinson's and their loved ones, empowering them to turn hope into action, and action into lasting change."
—John L. Lehr, President and CEO of the Parkinson's Foundation

"*The Parkinson's Plan* is accessible to all—individuals, communities, schools, foundations, and governments."   —Edmond J. Safra Foundation

"*The Parkinson's Plan* links groundbreaking science with urgent questions of prevention, risk, and action."
—Helen Matthews, CEO of Cure Parkinson's, London

"Every three years, the global Parkinson's community assembles for the World Parkinson Congress. *The Parkinson's Plan* challenges us to think about a world where such a gathering is no longer necessary because Parkinson's begins to fade away.
—Eli Pollard, Executive Director, World Parkinson Coalition

"*The Parkinson's Plan* offers a new path forward that empowers people with Parkinson's to live well today while driving progress in prevention, care, and research for tomorrow."
—Dr. Josefa Domingos, President, Parkinson's Europe

"*The Parkinson's Plan* is a powerful resource for the entire Parkinson's community."
—Leslie Chambers, President and CEO, American
Parkinson Disease Association

"Read it, share it, and help light the way to a future without Parkinson's disease."
—Andrea Merriam, CEO, Parkinson and Movement Disorder Alliance

"*The Parkinson's Plan* is a powerful tool in the fight to knock Parkinson's out for good."   —Ryan Cotton, CEO, Rock Steady Boxing

"*The Parkinson's Plan* supports the shift from reaction to prevention, from passive patients to empowered individuals."
—Prof. Bastiaan R. Bloem, director, Radboudumc Center of Expertise
for Parkinson's and Movement Disorders and cofounder, ParkinsonNet

"*The Parkinson's Plan* is an evidence-based call to action, outlining how smart policies, cleaner environments, and redirected investments can turn the tide on one of the fastest-growing neurological diseases of our time."

—Dr. Alberto Espay, author of *Brain Fables*

"*The Parkinson's Plan* speaks to the urgent need to put patients at the center of care, to reduce stigma, and to prevent the disease for all."

—Dr. Indu Subramanian, UCLA

"For 25 years, we have been detailing the likely environmental causes— from pesticides to air pollution—of Parkinson's and other brain diseases. This book conveys this research through compelling stories and lays down a path for preventing Parkinson's for all of us."

—Dr. Deborah Cory-Slechta, University of Rochester

"This book is essential reading for *everyone*."

—Professor Shen-Yang Lim, Chair, Asian-Oceanian Section, International Parkinson and Movement Disorder Society

"Veterans are disproportionately affected by Parkinson's disease—often due to toxic exposures that went unrecognized for far too long. *The Parkinson's Plan* powerfully brings these connections to light."

—Dr. John Duda, National Director, VA Parkinson's Disease Research, Education and Clinical Centers

"A compelling read for clinicians, researchers, and advocates alike. Here's to 0-10-100!"   —Dr. Anthony Lang, University of Toronto

"Drs. Dorsey and Okun present a comprehensive strategy emphasizing avoidance of environmental toxins and adoption of healthy lifestyles for prevention, along with emerging disease-modifying therapies."

—Dr. Eric Topol, author of *Super Agers*

"For decades, powerful industries have used manufactured doubt to delay action on dangerous chemicals—just as Big Tobacco once did. *The Parkinson's Plan* pulls back the curtain on how that same playbook is now costing us lives and brain health."

—Dr. David Michaels, author of *Doubt Is Their Product* and
The Triumph of Doubt

"A must-read for anyone who believes prevention should start with the truth."   —Ken Cook, President, Environmental Working Group

"*The Parkinson's Plan* is a courageous, eye-opening book that challenges the status quo and gives voice to the many who have suffered in silence."

—Jerry Ensminger, retired U.S. Marine Corps Master Sergeant

"This is one of the most compelling arguments I've ever read for why prevention—not treatment—must be the future of medicine."

—Dr. Bruce Lanphear, Simon Fraser University, Canada

"*The Parkinson's Plan* is a game-changing resource for anyone who cares about brain health, root causes, and real prevention."

—Dhru Purohit, host, The Dhru Purohit Podcast

"*The Parkinson's Plan* puts power back where it belongs: in the hands of patients, families, and a movement demanding change."

—Brian Wallach, cofounder, I AM ALS

"*The Parkinson's Plan* offers a bold vision filled with stories and backed by science that applies across the entire spectrum of parkinsonian disorders."

—Dr. Kristophe Diaz, Executive Director and
Chief Science Officer, CurePSP

"*The Parkinson's Plan* presents a blueprint for what prevention in action looks like."

—Alan Tisch, CEO and cofounder, Atria Health and Research Institute

"*The Parkinson's Plan* is an important step in our shared journey towards answers."   —Andrea Goodman, CEO, I AM ALS

"This is an invaluable guide to protect yourself and your children from unthinkable neurological diseases."
—Tim Green, former NFL player, practicing attorney, and
New York Times best-selling author

"*The Parkinson's Plan* is more than a roadmap for managing disease—it's a manifesto for preventing it."
—Dr. David Dodick, Chief Medical and Science Officer,
Atria Health and Research Institute

"My 13-year-old daughter developed brain cancer after exposures in her community to a degreasing chemical known to cause cancer. Eighty children in our town have been diagnosed with cancer. If it was your child, you would want to learn why. If you don't want your child to get cancer, if you don't want to develop cancer yourself or get Parkinson's, read *The Parkinson's Plan*."   —Kari Rhinehart, cofounder and Director, If It Was Your Child

THE
PARKINSON'S
PLAN

A NEW PATH TO
PREVENTION AND TREATMENT

RAY DORSEY, MD, MBA

MICHAEL S. OKUN, MD

PA

PUBLICAFFAIRS

New York

PublicAffairs
Hachette Book Group
1290 Avenue of the Americas, New York, NY 10104
www.publicaffairsbooks.com
@Public_Affairs

Printed in the United States of America

First Edition: August 2025

Published by PublicAffairs, an imprint of Hachette Book Group, Inc. The PublicAffairs name and logo is a registered trademark of the Hachette Book Group.

The Hachette Speakers Bureau provides a wide range of authors for speaking events. To find out more, go to www.hachettespeakersbureau.com or email HachetteSpeakers@hbgusa.com.

PublicAffairs books may be purchased in bulk for business, educational, or promotional use. For more information, please contact your local bookseller or the Hachette Book Group Special Markets Department at special.markets@hbgusa.com.

The publisher is not responsible for websites (or their content) that are not owned by the publisher.

Illustrations and photographs created and provided by authors unless otherwise noted.

Print book interior design by Amy Quinn.

Library of Congress Cataloging-in-Publication Data has been applied for.

ISBNs: 9781541705388 (hardcover), 9781541705401 (ebook)

LSC-H

Printing 3, 2025

CONTENTS

PART 4: NAVIGATE

CONCLUSION

*To the PD Avengers, who will change the course of
Parkinson's for all of us and for all time*

NOTE TO READERS

Dozens of individuals have shared their stories with us and you. In most cases, these amazing individuals have agreed to have their names shared. In some cases, we have changed their names and identities to protect their privacy. We are thankful to all.

GLOSSARY

alpha-synuclein—A small protein found in nerve cells that is misfolded (assembled improperly) in Parkinson's disease.

Alzheimer's disease—A brain disease that commonly affects memory, mood, and behavior.

animal model—The use of a laboratory animal to mimic a disease. The animal model is used to learn about the disease and to test new treatments.

biomarker—Chemicals, often in the blood or spinal fluid, that can be used to measure a disease. Cholesterol is a biomarker of heart disease, for example.

deep brain stimulation (DBS)—A surgical treatment for Parkinson's disease in which wire electrodes are inserted into the brain and connected to a battery-powered device to reduce symptoms and improve function.

dopamine—A chemical produced by some nerve cells that allows them to communicate with one another. In Parkinson's disease, many of the nerve cells that produce dopamine are lost.

dopamine pump—A device that can be inserted into the intestine or under the skin to provide a more continuous flow of levodopa.

gene editing—Altering DNA, often to prevent or treat a disease.

gene therapy—Inserting normal genes to replace or enhance missing or defective ones.

growth factors—Chemicals that help (brain) cells grow, develop, and survive. Scientists squirt growth factors on the brain like we put Miracle-Gro® on plants.

HIV/AIDS—The human immunodeficiency virus (HIV) attacks the immune system and at advanced stages can cause people to have the acquired immunodeficiency syndrome (AIDS).

homeostasis—The stable balance that your body and brain maintain. Your body tries to keep this balance as a way to fight off disease.

incidence—The number of new cases of a disease during a particular period (e.g., a year).

Lewy bodies—Clumps of a misfolded protein (alpha-synuclein) that are found in the brains of most individuals with Parkinson's disease.

microbiome—All the microorganisms (e.g., bacteria) living in a particular environment, such as the gut.

mitochondria—The energy-producing parts of cells, which are often damaged in Parkinson's disease.

MRI—Magnetic resonance imaging creates pictures of the brain and body using a large magnet and radio waves.

nanoparticles—Very tiny particles that are invisible to the human eye and slip easily into the brain. Nanoparticles can help deliver drugs to the brain.

neuron—A nerve cell.

organoid—A three-dimensional mini-brain in a dish that is usually made from growing stem cells.

particulate matter—Tiny pieces of dirt and soot that are suspended in the air. The smallest are less than one-thirtieth the width of a hair and may be an important risk factor for Parkinson's and Alzheimer's diseases.

perchloroethylene (PCE)—A chemical, closely related to trichloroethylene, that is widely used in degreasing and dry-cleaning.

PET scan—A sophisticated imaging test that reveals the chemicals in your brain.

prevalence—The proportion of individuals having a disease at any point in time (e.g., today).

proteins—Large molecules that carry out the functions of a cell.

RNAi therapy—Treatment that interferes with or destroys the instructions that genes give to make different proteins. It can be a "silencing therapy" for Parkinson's disease.

substantia nigra—Latin for "black substance"; the black area of the brain where nerve cells that produce dopamine are lost in Parkinson's disease.

Superfund—A US federal program that allows for cleanup of the most toxic sites in the country, often at the cost of the responsible parties.

toxicant—A synthetic (human-made) chemical that is harmful to health.

toxin—A naturally occurring substance that is hazardous to health. For example, some plants produce toxins that protect them from being eaten by insects.

trichloroethylene (TCE)—A common chemical that has been used to dry-clean clothes, decaffeinate coffee, and degrease metal.

vaccine—A medicine used to stimulate the body's own immune response against a disease. Vaccines have been typically aimed at infectious diseases (like Covid-19) but may also help treat diseases such as Parkinson's.

ABBREVIATIONS

AI   Artificial intelligence

ALS   Amyotrophic lateral sclerosis, a neurological disorder that leads to weakness; also known as Lou Gehrig's disease in the United States or motor neuron disease in the United Kingdom.

DBS   Deep brain stimulation

DDT   Dichloro-diphenyl-trichloroethane, one of the first modern synthetic pesticides

EPA   US Environmental Protection Agency

FDA   US Food and Drug Administration

NIH   US National Institutes of Health

PCE   Perchloroethylene

TCE   Trichloroethylene

WHO   World Health Organization

FOREWORD

For us, Parkinson's is personal.

For Gus, Parkinson's has affected multiple generations. My parents' families emigrated from Greece in the early twentieth century. Both families settled in Tarpon Springs, Florida, known as the "Sponge Capital of the World." When my dad was an infant, his family moved to western Pennsylvania, where my dad's dad worked at local steel mills for forty years.

At an early age, my dad, Michael Bilirakis, sold newspapers and worked every night until 1:00 a.m. as an usher at the local movie theater. After graduating high school, my dad worked at local steel mills before serving in the US Air Force during the Korean War. Following his service, he attended the University of Pittsburgh and received a degree in chemical engineering while working forty-eight hours a week at Westinghouse. He then moved back to Florida and graduated with a JD from the University of Florida. He ultimately returned to Tarpon Springs, resided near a Superfund site, practiced law, and served in the US Congress for twenty-four years. Michael Bilirakis lived the American dream until Parkinson's robbed him of his retirement.

Like our father, my brother Emmanuel attended the University of Florida. He became a successful family practice doctor serving those in need in our community. He was diagnosed with Parkinson's in his forties and died at age sixty-one. Parkinson's robbed him of his life.

For Jennifer, the disease was a shock and a surprise. I explained away my earliest symptoms as everything but Parkinson's—like the stress of this new job in Congress, walking tens of thousands of steps around the Capitol, or just simply getting older. I couldn't believe someone like me could get a disease like this. But in 2022, when my clenching toes and shuffling gait progressed and a tremor in my voice emerged, I sought medical advice and was diagnosed at age fifty-four with Parkinson's disease. On World Parkinson's Day in 2023, I shared that diagnosis publicly.

Unfortunately, my symptoms progressed much faster than expected. My doctors revisited their diagnosis and changed it to a different parkinsonian disorder—progressive supranuclear palsy (PSP)—a kind of Parkinson's on steroids. PSP has robbed me of my speech. But it has not taken away my voice, a voice that I am determined to use to help end these terrible diseases.

Both of us realized that our efforts to address these awful conditions required a plan. And surprisingly, the federal government did not have one. Every six minutes, an American is diagnosed with Parkinson's; yet we had no plan. Every day, one hundred Americans die from the disease, but we had no plan. Every year, the country spends $50 billion on Parkinson's and still no plan.

So with our wonderful colleague, Congressman Paul Tonko from New York, and great supporters in the Senate and beyond, we drafted the National Plan to End Parkinson's Act. The bill directs the secretary of the Department of Health and Human Services to work with experts from the public and private sector to develop a national plan to prevent and to cure Parkinson's disease. On December 14, 2023, the US House of Representatives passed the bipartisan bill 407–9. Six months later, the Senate passed it unanimously. With our families and us at his side, President Joe Biden signed the bill into law.

Like this book, the plan calls for us to **prevent** the disease, **amplify** the voices of patients and caregivers, and **navigate** the frontier of new treatments. However, one element was still missing, and that was to **learn** why people are developing these diseases in record numbers. Unlike many other conditions, like seizures and strokes, which date to biblical times, these diseases are relatively new. The first major description of Parkinson's disease did not happen until 1817. ALS, which causes paralysis, was first observed in 1869. PSP was not described until 1964, just sixty years ago. Dementia with Lewy bodies, another parkinsonian disorder that affected the late actor Robin Williams, was not noticed until 1976. All these diseases are increasingly common. Why?

To answer that question, we have drafted the Healthy Brains Act. The bill instructs the director of the National Institutes of Health to establish research, training, and education programs to identify the underlying environmental causes of neurodegenerative diseases. We have spent a generation studying the genetics of many different diseases, which has advanced our understanding of these conditions. Investigating the environmental causes is long overdue.

The heritability of many of these diseases is modest or low. Most people, like Jennifer, do not have a family history of the disease. They do not carry a genetic risk factor. The prevalences of these diseases vary by geography, and clusters abound. Many are tied to chemicals in our food, water, and air. And many victims, including our families, have lived near polluted sites.

We need to learn why for three reasons. First, the initial step to curing any disease is to determine its cause. This approach has helped us cure hepatitis C and stomach ulcers. Second, once we know its cause, we can slow its progression or at least prevent it from getting worse. This has worked with Covid-19, where early treatment decreases the risk of hospitalization, and with many cancers, where early detection can save lives. Third, and perhaps most powerfully, when we learn why, we can prevent diseases. Textbooks are filled with diseases that no longer exist (e.g., smallpox), are very rare (e.g., polio), or may even one day disappear (e.g., HIV). This all happened because we learned why. And it will happen again for Parkinson's, PSP, and many other brain diseases, but only if we identify and eliminate their root causes.

Parkinsonian disorders do not respect political party or national boundaries. They affect all of us—our neighbors, our friends, and our families.

We have experienced far too much of these diseases. To prevent and end this suffering, we helped pass a bill that calls for a national plan. Ray and Michael, two compassionate and thoughtful neurologists, have now taken the first step toward providing one.

Congressman Gus Bilirakis
Congresswoman Jennifer Wexton
October 28, 2024

INTRODUCTION

It takes as much energy to wish as it does to plan.

—Eleanor Roosevelt

ATHLETICS, MILITARY SERVICE, MEDICINE, AND PARKINSON'S DISEASE
have connected the lives of Jana Reed and Sara Whittingham. Thirty years
ago, as young, talented, ambitious cadets, they met on the US Air Force
Academy's idyllic track at the foot of the Rocky Mountains in Colorado
Springs. Jana was from the California coastal town of San Luis Obispo,
and Sara came from Steamboat Springs, Colorado. Jana, who was a year
older, was a hurdler and long jumper for the Academy, while Sara ran long
distances. Both women majored in biochemistry and were accepted to top
medical schools, Jana at Georgetown and Sara at Tulane. Jana's ability to
navigate obstacles made emergency medicine a natural fit, and Sara's stamina
sent her into anesthesiology. After completing their medical training, they
served throughout the United States and around the world, including in
Afghanistan.

In 2016, Jana noticed something strange. When she propped up her feet,
her left toes would shake. She thought it was a leftover symptom from an

1

old injury, so, like many physicians, she just blew it off. However, over the next two years, while she was working nights in the emergency room, other symptoms began to emerge, and nurses started to notice. They came to her, almost apologetically, with their concerns. One whispered, "I noticed your arm was really shaking when you put on your gown." Another sidelined her and said, "Hey! I noticed you are moving really slow and stiff. Are you injured?" One more said, "You're walking funny, like shuffling. Are you OK?" The nurses were not the only ones concerned. Her friends thought she was sad because her face seldom produced a smile.

Jana blamed fatigue, exhaustion, and menopause. Anything but Parkinson's. Eventually, she saw a neurologist via telemedicine who diagnosed her with the disabling disease. She was forty-seven. Jana decided to stop working shifts in the emergency department because she was concerned that her slowness and stiffness wouldn't let her keep up with the unpredictable pace. And she worried about making a mistake. She started working in a smaller clinic, which hasn't been as satisfying, and because she has had less training there, she finds it stressful.

At about the same time that nurses were becoming worried about Jana, Sara's health caught the eye of a surgeon—her husband, Dr. John Langell. One day John told her, "Your arm's shaking." Sara thought that this was strange. "Why would I have a one-sided resting arm tremor?" The physician did what many people do. She googled it. Two terrifying words kept coming up: Parkinson's disease.

Neurologists later confirmed Sara's diagnosis. She was forty-six. Looking back, Sara realized that her symptoms may have begun five years earlier. A recent triathlon had taken her two hours longer to complete even though she had trained harder than ever. Sara soon became anxious and depressed and gained thirty pounds.

Following their shared diagnosis, the two classmates reconnected. The resilient pair were both stunned by the news, struggling with the diagnosis, falling out of shape, and seeking answers. But they helped each other. Jana completed intense physical therapy following a hamstring injury and was able to exercise again. She even had a new walking partner, a black Lab named Apollo. Sara also learned the benefits of exercise and participated in a clinical trial involving cycling. Soon the mother of two was back on the road to health and determined to return to racing form.

Today, Jana, fifty, cares for her husband, a Navy brat who has brain cancer. She is thinking about retiring from medicine, as her disability is increasing, but she still serves in the California Air National Guard. Sara lives with her family in Aurora, Ohio, and continues to work as an anesthesiologist. She is also helping raise $1 million to study the ability of exercise to alleviate the symptoms of Parkinson's.[1]

Jana and Sara were both in their forties, fit, active, and in the prime of their careers when Parkinson's knocked at the door. How could they both be diagnosed at such a young age? Why did it happen to them in the same month? Why, as they discovered, has it also affected some of their fellow Air Force Academy classmates?

THE DISEASE

Two hundred years before Jana's and Sara's diagnoses, a sixty-one-year-old surgeon witnessed something unusual on the crowded streets of London. There, through the London fog, Dr. James Parkinson saw old men with a tremor, stooped posture, and shuffling gait. In 1817, he wrote "An Essay on the Shaking Palsy" about a disease that had yet to be classified in the medical literature.[2]

In addition to its classic features, which also include stiffness, Parkinson's disease produces a wide range of symptoms, including constipation, urinary urgency, loss of smell, sleep disturbances, decreased facial expression, depression, anxiety, fatigue, drooling, pain, and impaired thinking. The brains of individuals with Parkinson's display a loss of nerve cells, especially in a part of the brain called the substantia nigra. These nerve cells produce a chemical called dopamine. In addition to this loss, the remaining nerve cells are cluttered with garbage bags (named Lewy bodies) that are stuffed with a misfolded or abnormally assembled protein called alpha-synuclein.

Dr. Parkinson described six individuals (five were men; one was not identified) with the novel condition, and their ages ranged from over fifty to seventy-two.[2] In short, Dr. Parkinson's patients were nothing like Jana or Sara.

Dr. Parkinson had little to offer his patients in 1817, but today Parkinson's disease is treatable. Exercise, as Sara has discovered, is quite helpful.[3]

Medications, especially one called levodopa, which is converted to dopamine, can produce a dramatic response, even an "awakening," in most individuals. For the right patients, surgical treatments may be effective. For example, deep brain stimulation (DBS) alleviates symptoms and reduces the side effects of medications. The surgery involves inserting wire electrodes deep into the brain and passing electrical current through them from a battery-powered generator placed under the skin. However, the effects of levodopa and DBS wane over time, both have complications, and neither slows the relentless march of the disease.

In the early stages of Parkinson's, people can function at remarkably high levels. Individuals with Parkinson's disease have walked in space, earned PhDs, practiced law and medicine, conducted research, acted, played professional sports, served in Congress, and led the Catholic Church. However, over time, Parkinson's takes a heavy toll on almost all, including family and friends. Parkinson's, according to Michael J. Fox, "sucks."[4]

A NEW MODEL

Dr. Parkinson was puzzled and concerned by what he observed. He was not sure where the disease began, but he naturally thought that its roots were in the brain. He was likely wrong. In 2003, a brilliant German pathologist, Dr. Heiko Braak, postulated something truly remarkable.[5] Under the microscope, he saw Lewy bodies (the garbage bags full of the misfolded protein) first in the nerve that goes to the intestines (called the vagus nerve) or in the brain's smell center. He concluded that Parkinson's began not in the brain but rather in the gut or maybe even the nose. He knew that polio, which paralyzed children and adults, entered the nervous system via the gut and thought that Parkinson's might do the same.

In 2019, a Danish physician, Dr. Per Borghammer, expanded upon Braak's model and wrote that the disease had two forms: one that begins in the gut ("body-first") and one that starts in the nose ("brain-first").[6] As we shall see, these models have powerful implications for what may be causing the disease.

Jana and Sara learned all about the classic symptoms of Parkinson's in medical school. They knew about the loss of dopamine-producing nerve cells in the substantia nigra. They were familiar with the medical and surgical treatments for the condition. They were also taught that Parkinson's was an old

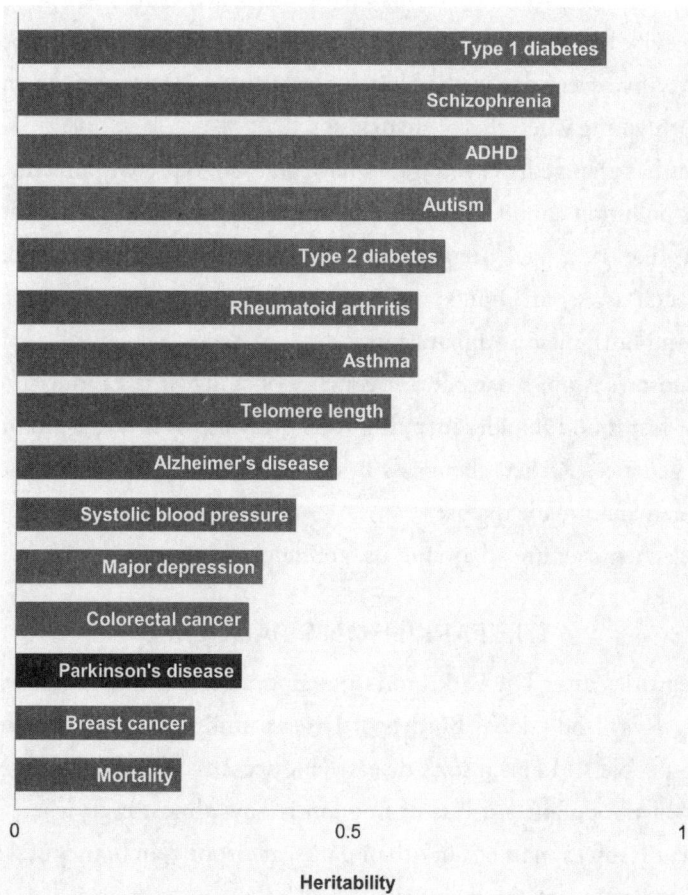

Figure 1. Heritability estimates of different diseases. Courtesy of Dr. Bastiaan Bloem; modified from the source.[7]

man's disease. However, Jana and Sara were women in their forties when they were diagnosed, and their earliest symptoms began years before then. What had changed in the two hundred years since Dr. Parkinson's original essay?

Genes do not change (much) in two hundred years. Jana does carry a mutation in a gene that can cause Parkinson's, but Parkinson's is among the least heritable of all major diseases (**Figure 1**).[7] While diseases like schizophrenia and type 1 diabetes run in families, only about 15% of individuals with Parkinson's have a family history of the disease.[7-9] The vast majority (85%) of individuals do not have any known genetic cause or even a genetic risk factor for the disease.[7-10]

Longevity has certainly increased since 1817. Ten thousand baby boomers turn sixty-five every day in the United States alone. However, Jana and Sara were both young when they were diagnosed.

What has changed? As you might have guessed, our environment. Industrial air pollution engulfed nineteenth-century London, and Jana, Sara, and veterans like them have been exposed to new toxicants. These include defoliants, such as Agent Orange in Vietnam, degreasing chemicals in the Air Force, and burn pits in Afghanistan.

Parkinson's is not a natural consequence of aging. It is an unnatural one. It is not just found in older men. It affects everyone. It is not predominantly due to genetics. Rather, chemicals in our food, water, and air have created this largely man-made disease.

These chemicals are all around us, and none are necessary.

THE PARKINSON'S PANDEMIC

Two centuries after Dr. Parkinson's description of six individuals with the shaking palsy, the Global Burden of Disease study estimated that over six million people had Parkinson's disease (**Figure 2**).[11] What started out as an oddity on the polluted streets of London is now almost everywhere. It can be seen at farmer's markets, in urban parks, at airports, in houses of worship, and on the streets of any major city.

The Parkinson's pandemic is growing fast. Dr. Allison Willis, a professor and Parkinson's expert at the University of Pennsylvania, recently estimated that the number of new cases of Parkinson's in the United States was 90,000 annually, or a staggering 50% higher than previous estimates.[14] Last year, the Global Burden of Disease study calculated that 11.8 million people already had the disease, almost double what they had published just six years earlier.[12]

The Parkinson's pandemic has transformed what was likely an uncommon disease in ancient times into a disturbingly common one today. Seizures, strokes, and migraines have been described for centuries if not millennia. However, ancient Chinese, Egyptian, and Indian descriptions of Parkinson's disease are few.[15-17] And while previous pandemics (e.g., smallpox, influenza) were due to infectious viruses, a new class of "vectors," including

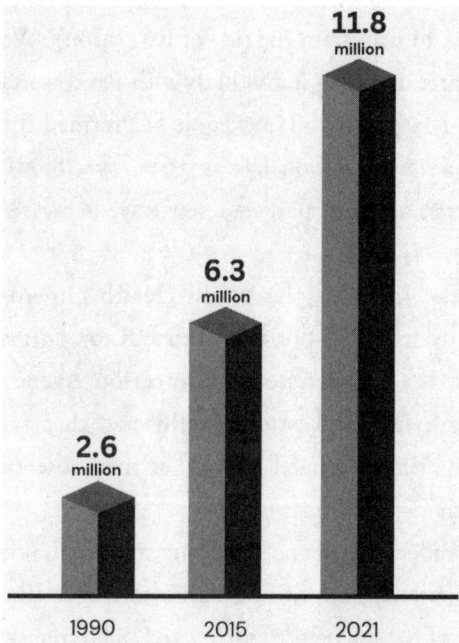

Figure 2. Estimated number of people with Parkinson's disease globally, 1990–2021.[12,13]

pesticides in our food, industrial solvents in our water, and pollution in our air, is responsible for the rise of Parkinson's. These toxicants have spread from the industrialized West to almost every part of the world.[18,19]

If Parkinson's were just due to increasing longevity, the proportion of individuals affected, adjusted for age, would be uniform. For example, the percentage of older adults with the disease in Toronto, Canada, would be the same as in Nairobi, Kenya. But it isn't. Consistent with its links to the environment, the prevalence of Parkinson's is *five* times higher in industrialized countries like Canada than in sub-Saharan Africa.[20] Parkinson's is also rising fastest in countries undergoing rapid industrialization and experiencing spreading pollution. The prevalence of Parkinson's in China, for instance, has more than doubled in just one generation.[11]

UNANSWERED QUESTIONS

In 2020, at the height of the Covid-19 pandemic, we, along with our friends and colleagues, Drs. Todd Sherer from the Michael J. Fox Foundation and Bastiaan Bloem from Radboud University in the Netherlands, wrote *Ending Parkinson's Disease*. In it, we called for activism, similar to the March of

Dimes for polio or Act Up for HIV, to help stem the tide of Parkinson's. We were humbled when a year later, three amazing individuals with Parkinson's disease, Larry Gifford, Dr. Soania Mathur, and Tim Hague Sr., formed the PD Avengers. The global grassroots organization has amassed over 8,000 members from one hundred countries and has sparked a new wave of awareness and activism.[21]

This activism has made progress. In 2022, the World Health Organization identified Parkinson's as a priority and outlined six steps to address global disparities.[22] In 2024, the US Environmental Protection Agency banned two chemicals (trichloroethylene and perchloroethylene) that are strongly associated with Parkinson's disease after finding that they pose an "unreasonable risk to human health."[23,24]

Finally, in 2024, President Joe Biden signed the Dr. Emmanuel Bilirakis and Honorable Jennifer Wexton National Plan to End Parkinson's Act. The bipartisan bill passed the US House of Representatives 407–9 and unanimously passed the Senate. It was named after the late brother of Florida Congressman Gus Bilirakis and Congresswoman Jennifer Wexton. Congresswoman Wexton has courageously served with a rare parkinsonian disorder called progressive supranuclear palsy, or PSP. The bill, for the first time, requires the federal government to develop a plan to prevent and end Parkinson's disease.

While the progress over the last few years has been palpable, we have encountered countless disturbing stories of dry cleaners, farmers, and Marines with Parkinson's. We have visited dozens of the country's most contaminated sites, from the Marine Corps Base Camp Lejeune in North Carolina to a fifteen-mile-wide polluted site underneath Phoenix, Arizona.[25] We have traveled to communities across the country to see the effects of contaminated drinking water and polluted air on individuals, families, and communities. In many instances, those most directly affected are no longer with us. Hundreds of wonderful people have invited us into their homes, firehouses, gyms, community centers, hotels, hospitals, and conference rooms to discuss their experiences with Parkinson's. We will share many of their stories with you. We hope that they engender empathy, anger, and action.

In these encounters, we are constantly peppered with questions. Why do I have Parkinson's? Why did I get the disease, but my family members or coworkers didn't? Are my children at risk? What can I do to protect them? Can I slow the progression of Parkinson's? Why is paraquat, a weed killer linked to Parkinson's, still sprayed on US farms? Why did China ban it but not the United States? Why didn't we know about its health risks? Those struggling with the disease ask how they can access better care. Caregivers, crying—often quietly—for help, want to know what the future holds. Can my loved one receive care at home? Can I get respite care? Is a nursing home inevitable? All ask where the long-promised new treatments are. Are surgical treatments getting better? Can vaccines help Parkinson's? Stem cells? Gene editing? How do we find a cure?

In short, they are calling for a plan.

THE PLAN

This book answers many of these questions and provides a detailed plan to address the Parkinson's pandemic. The plan has four steps:

1. **Prevent**—We must prevent the preventable. The first step to addressing any crisis is to contain it. Right now, we are fueling the rise of Parkinson's with continued and increased use of toxic chemicals that pollute our food, water, and air. For most individuals, the disease is preventable and the suffering avoidable. We will offer the "Parkinson's 25"—twenty-five straightforward actions that you can take in your everyday life to reduce your risk of Parkinson's. If you already have Parkinson's, these actions could possibly slow its progression. They apply to everyone everywhere, from the very young, as the seeds of Parkinson's are often planted early, to those approaching the end of life.

2. **Learn**—We must learn why people develop Parkinson's disease. In concluding his essay, Dr. Parkinson hoped that future scientists and doctors who "humanely employ anatomical examination in detecting the causes and nature of diseases" could direct their attention "particularly to this malady" and in doing so identify relief and a cure.[2] The first step toward curing a disease is to identify its cause, or in the case of Parkinson's, causes. For Parkinson's, its origins

may be in the nose and the gut where chemicals are inhaled and ingested. Whatever the steps that lead to the start, spread, and progression of Parkinson's, we will call for more research to define the "why." When we know the causes of a disease, we can prevent it, slow it, and, in some cases, cure it.

3. **Amplify**—We must amplify the voices of patients and caregivers. For those already afflicted, we need to pivot and dedicate greater efforts to adequately support and treat them. That includes both those living with the disease and those who care for them. For too long, care has been fragmented and focused on a doctor's office. Care needs to be integrated and centered on the needs of individuals. We need to create a universe of services where the patient is the sun. In *The Parkinson's Plan*, we will highlight successes in different regions of the world and discuss how these victories can be extended to reach nearly everyone fighting Parkinson's.

4. **Navigate**—We must navigate the frontier of new treatments. We need novel approaches, and the two of us do not have all the answers. So we interviewed a few dozen of the world's leading Parkinson's experts to identify the most promising therapeutic areas and share their answers with you in this book. In providing a framework to understand the latest research, we hope to prioritize the areas that hold the most promise for alleviating the suffering experienced by so many. We will outline a path for near-, mid-, and long-term treatment options that are inclusive of everyone, both those with the disease and those at risk.

Finally, every good plan needs bold goals. We call ours **0-10-100**. By 2035, we will see a 0% rise in new cases (the incidence) of Parkinson's, a tenfold increase in research funding and in the percentage devoted toward prevention, and universal, or 100%, access to levodopa.

WHO WE ARE

Both of us have devoted our professional lives to reducing the burden of brain diseases. With his colleagues, Ray predicted and mapped the rise of

Parkinson's.[26] He has cared for patients in five states and on six continents via telemedicine and was among the first to use smartphones and smartwatches to measure the disease. He previously directed the Parkinson's disease division at Johns Hopkins and organized the first-ever symposium on the brain and the environment in 2024.

For the past decade, Ray has been pursuing the root causes of Parkinson's disease, so much so that some think he is obsessed. He may be. Now whenever he sees someone walking with Parkinson's on the Erie Canal or at the airport, he becomes upset. He sees their present and future suffering and thinks it is all unnecessary and avoidable. He will tell you why.

Michael is one of the most published researchers in Parkinson's disease. He is a pioneer and world expert in its surgical treatment and author of several books on the subject. He has developed novel care models and chaired the department of neurology at the University of Florida. He cofounded and now leads the Norman Fixel Institute for Neurological Diseases as a distinguished professor.

For the last fifteen years as the medical director and advisor of the Parkinson's Foundation, Michael has probably answered more questions from patients and families than anyone else. He has heard their curiosity, frustration, and desperation. In response, he has questioned the way we deliver care, pursue knowledge, and develop treatments. He will share his answers with you.

Together, Ray and Michael have published over 1,000 papers, cared for 10,000 individuals with the disease, and educated millions about the condition. Yet, on the most fundamental measures, we have failed.

Parkinson's is now the world's fastest-growing neurodegenerative disease. It has risen to become the fourteenth leading cause of death in the United States. Millions still go undiagnosed and untreated with no access to care or medication. Millions more—and their families—suffer with a terrible disease with little hope. And despite billions of dollars in research funding, no major therapeutic breakthroughs have materialized this century.

We have failed enough, and we have seen enough. Most Parkinson's is preventable. And it must end. So together we have developed a plan to help stop the suffering. By preventing the disease, we aim to make Parkinson's increasingly rare. By learning why, we will eliminate the root causes of the disease, slow the rate of progression, and accelerate the development of treatments. By amplifying the voices of patients and caregivers, we will reduce the disease burden for the twelve million already affected and their loved ones. And by navigating the therapeutic frontier, we will slow disease progression and alleviate suffering for individuals at all stages of the disease.

For too long, Parkinson's has been fundamentally misunderstood. The majority of the public, and even many scientists, still view the disease as an inevitable consequence of aging. In their eyes, the disease simply reflects increasing longevity and the unfortunate consequence of genetics. They believe little can be done to prevent the rise of this pandemic. They are mistaken.

We are in the midst of a contest either to stem the tide of Parkinson's or to allow its rise. Few recognize that we are in that competition, and, consequently, we are losing. We need to open our eyes, think differently, and change course.

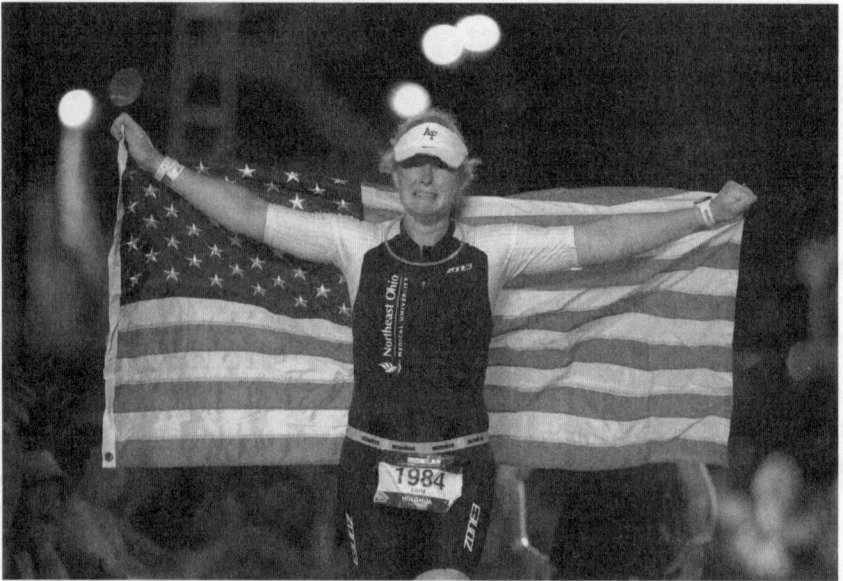

Figure 3. Photograph of Dr. Sara Whittingham after completing the 2023 Ironman Triathlon. Photo by Christian Petersen/Getty Images.

Three years after her diagnosis of Parkinson's, Sara was ready for a contest of her own. She applied for and received an invitation to compete at the Ironman Triathlon in Kailua-Kona, Hawaii. There she swam 2.4 miles in the Pacific Ocean, biked 112 miles in the mountains, and ran 26.2 miles on the roads. Waiting at the finish line were her husband, her two daughters, and her former Air Force Academy teammate Jana, who presented Sara with a US flag from their earlier deployment in Afghanistan (**Figure 3**).[27,28]

If Sara can complete an Ironman three years after developing Parkinson's, what can we do in ten years to address it? Let's create a plan and find out.

PART 1

———

PREVENT

1

PESTICIDES IN OUR FOOD, FARMS, AND FIELDS

History's what people are trying to hide from you,
not what they're trying to show you. You search
for it in the same way you sift through a landfill:
for evidence of what people want to bury.

—Hilary Mantel, historical novelist

In January 1945, a century after Dr. Parkinson's essay, a forty-three-year-old pathologist encountered an entirely new disease on the opposite side of the world. Dr. Harry M. Zimmerman, a Yale-trained physician who would later help found the Albert Einstein College of Medicine, sailed into Guam. On the island 3,800 miles west of Honolulu, he was part of US Naval Medical Research Unit No. 2. His charge was to investigate "diseases of military importance" on the newly recaptured island, which had fallen under harsh Japanese occupation during World War II. Malaria, hepatitis, and other infectious diseases, which threatened American troops in the Pacific theater, were supposed to be his focus.[1]

Instead, he saw something new. The indigenous population of Guam, the Chamorro, thought to have sailed to the Mariana Islands from the Philippines and Singapore 3,500 years earlier, were presenting at astonishing rates with a novel illness.[2]

On the island, which was now teeming with 200,000 US service members, Zimmerman first observed the unmistakable signs of malnourishment, including peeling hands (insufficient niacin) and swollen hearts (deficiency in thiamine). But later, on his sixty-third autopsy on the island, the pathologist evaluated a forty-two-year-old man whose tongue was shriveled and arms and legs wasted. Zimmerman suspected that the man had been suffering from amyotrophic lateral sclerosis (ALS), which was confirmed after examining the man's hardened spinal cord.[1]

About ten days later, Zimmerman performed another autopsy on a thirty-eight-year-old man with ALS. As one of the rising stars in the new field of neuropathology, Zimmerman certainly knew about ALS. American baseball legend and former New York Yankee Lou Gehrig had just died from the condition five years earlier. However, the paralytic illness was rare, affecting less than 1 out of every 10,000 Americans. On Guam, Zimmerman was seeing far more cases in the morgue and in the clinics than that. Subsequent researchers found that the Chamorro, and only the Chamorro, were developing the disease at fifty to one hundred times the rates seen in the United States or other parts of the world.[3]

However, ALS was not the only neurological disease that the growing number of doctors on the island were encountering. They were seeing Chamorro women and men with "pill rolling" tremors, masklike faces, stooped postures, and shuffling gaits. In short, they looked like they had Parkinson's, but with a twist. They were also demented. "They became forgetful. . . . They would lose their way, not find their way home. They couldn't remember the names of their children."[1]

Initially, scientists thought that the disease, which ran in families, had to be genetic. However, no mutation was found.[4] Next, they thought it had to be infectious, but no virus was identified. Then biological factors were considered: vitamin deficiencies, prions (misfolded brain proteins), and hormone imbalances.[5] All were unsatisfactory explanations. Eventually, they turned to the diet.

Researchers began to suspect that food might be to blame.[6] Four hours after bombing Pearl Harbor, the Japanese had attacked and quickly gained control of Guam, which had become a US territory following the Spanish-American War. Over 1,000 local residents died during the Japanese occupation, which was marked by forced labor and food shortages.[7-10] Many lost their fruit and vegetable farms and access to their preferred fishing spots. Consequently, they had to rely more on ancient and, in some cases, less desirable food sources. Among these was the cycad seed.

The seeds derive from a small palm tree–like plant that dates back to the time of dinosaurs. The natives on the island knew that these seeds, with a tough outer coat, were dangerous when eaten raw. So they carefully prepared the seeds over one to three weeks. The preparation process, observed by the anthropologist Marjorie Whiting, included cutting the seeds open, thoroughly washing them, and even testing the toxicity of the wash before they were used to make flour for tortillas. According to Whiting, all the Chamorro knew about "the toxic properties of the plant. Dogs and chickens repeatedly die if they drink the wash water. Preparation is laborious. Directions vary but soaking is required for 'several' days with 'frequent' changes of water."[1]

However, during the Japanese occupation, such careful preparation was not possible. According to a brilliant 1990 *New Yorker* essay, "During the war, with countless families scavenging the forest, Guamanians ate more cycad seeds than at any other period in this century and, being on the run, were more likely to detoxify the seeds incompletely."[1]

In 1987, Dr. Peter Spencer, now a neurotoxicologist at Oregon Health & Science University, showed that the cycad seeds contained a naturally occurring, fat-loving toxin called BMAA (beta-N-methylamino-L-alanine). He was concerned about its toxic properties, so he fed a concentrated amount of the toxin to monkeys. One month later, they developed a "stooped posture, unkempt coat, tremor" and other symptoms. Longer exposure led to "periods of immobility with an expressionless face and blank stare, a crouched

posture and a bradykinetic (slow), shuffling" gait, all symptoms of a parkinsonian disorder.[11]

However, the dose given to the monkeys was large and more than humans
would likely have consumed. To receive an equivalent dose of BMAA,
"[humans] would need to eat massive amounts of cycad seeds on a daily
basis because the processed flour was low in BMAA."[6] If the flour alone
was insufficient to explain the rise of this disease, maybe there was another
possibility.

Humans were not the only ones who ate cycad seeds. Flying foxes, a close
relative of bats and an animal native to Guam, devour cycad seeds at night.
Because the toxin dissolves in fat and not water, flying foxes cannot readily
eliminate the chemical through their urine. Instead, they accumulate the
BMAA toxin in their fat.[6] The concentration of BMAA in flying foxes is one
hundred times what is present in the seed itself.[12]

The Chamorro people prized the flying foxes as a delicacy and enjoyed
the meat boiled in coconut milk.[6] As BMAA moves through the food chain,

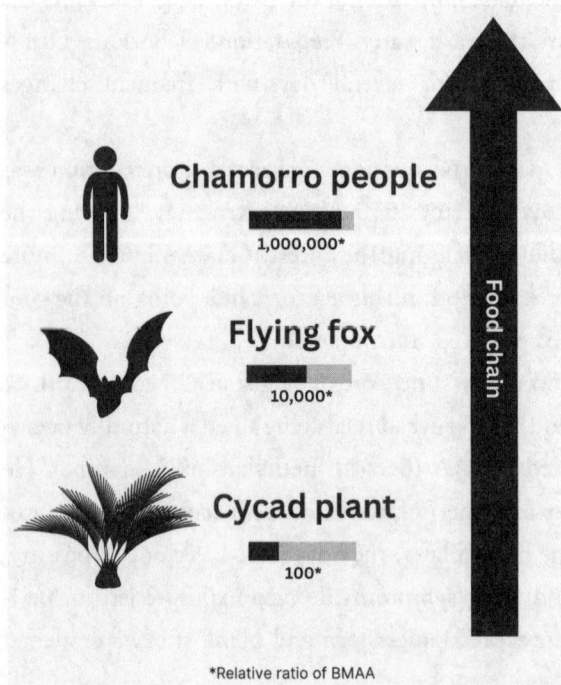

Chamorro people

1,000,000*

Flying fox

10,000*

Cycad plant

100*

Food chain

*Relative ratio of BMAA

Figure 1. Process of biomagnification of BMAA.
Created by the authors.
Ratios estimated based on
data from original study.[6]

it becomes concentrated through a process known as biomagnification (**Figure 1**).[12] The Chamorro people were consuming extremely large amounts of the toxin, as evidenced by the high levels found in the brains of individuals who died of ALS on Guam.[13]

Commercial hunting with guns led to the near extinction of the flying foxes. Twenty years after they began disappearing, so did cases of ALS.[6] Parkinsonian disorders began fading soon thereafter and had ended by 2000. By 2012, the "only Chamorros who suffered were elderly, with most exhibiting symptoms of dementia." Canadian neurologist Dr. John Steele later reported, "We are quite certain no one born after 1951 has developed the disease or is at risk of developing it."[14,15]

The case of the Chamorro people holds important lessons for us today. First, diseases do not just happen. They happen for a reason. It is the job of physicians and scientists to figure out why. Second, chemicals in the environment can be responsible for brain diseases, including parkinsonian disorders. Third, some of these toxins may be "natural," while others, as we shall see, are synthetic or man-made. Fourth, there is a lag between the time of exposure and the development of the disease. The lag can be years or decades, and the relevant exposure can happen at an early age. For example, some Chamorro who later emigrated from Guam to California developed parkinsonian disorders, well after their earlier exposure to the cycad seeds and flying foxes had ended.[16] However, none of their California-born children did. Finally, and most importantly, diseases like Parkinson's, ALS, or Alzheimer's are "not a natural or inevitable consequence of aging." They are preventable.[15]

While the Chamorro suffered the consequences of a natural toxin in their food, individuals with Parkinson's across the world have felt the effects of different chemicals: natural and man-made pesticides.

GOT MILK?

In the late 1970s, the Pineapple Growers Association in Hawaii argued that a dangerous pesticide called heptachlor (related to DDT [dichloro-diphenyl-trichloroethane]) was essential to protecting their cash crop, and the growers successfully gained an exemption to use it. After the pineapples had been harvested, some of their green leafy tops (called the "chop") were fed to dairy cows on the island. Like BMAA, this chemical dissolves in fat, and cows concentrated it in their fat and their milk. Dairies in Oahu were soon found to have unsafe levels of the pesticide. Milk was eventually removed from stores and schools, but for some, it was too late.[17]

In the lab, heptachlor damages the energy-producing parts of cells (called mitochondria) and leads to death of dopamine-producing nerve cells.[18] In Hawaii, researchers found that high milk consumers had a greater risk of Parkinson's disease.[19] Under the microscope, they found that Hawaiians who had consumed the most milk had the fewest number of nerve cells in the part of the brain known to be affected by Parkinson's. Finally, compared to individuals who consumed little milk, the milk lovers were more likely to have the remnants of the pesticide heptachlor in their brains.[17,20,21]

Cows are not the only animals to concentrate or store pesticides like heptachlor in their milk. Humans do the same. In China, nursing women have high concentrations of pesticide residues in their breast milk.[22] So do women in Brazil, Ethiopia, and Uganda. To our knowledge, no one is following their children to see whether they develop Parkinson's decades later.

"IN THE NORWEGIAN SPIRIT"

In 2002, Dr. Stein Nilsen, a scientist at the Norwegian Defence Research Establishment, was diagnosed with Parkinson's disease. As for many others, his symptoms began with a tremor in his right hand. Unlike most, Stein was young—just thirty-nine years old. The mathematician wanted to figure out what caused the disease. He said, "What did I experience that others did not?"

In some cases, early-onset Parkinson's disease may be due to genetic causes, but in most, like Stein's case, the environment may be the primary culprit.[23] Twelve years earlier, Stein had experienced something few mathematicians have. Three thousand miles away in southern Lebanon, Stein served as part of a UN peacekeeping force. For years Norway has contributed about nine hundred soldiers to the United Nations Interim Force in Lebanon because, according to Stein, "Flying around the world trying to make peace . . . is in the Norwegian spirit."

As a twenty-seven-year-old second lieutenant in the Army, his job was to monitor troops coming into and out of Lebanon over the Khardela Bridge. He was stationed at Outpost 4-18, where he and three fellow soldiers were responsible for a 24/7 watch. The four soldiers took turns sleeping in their bunker, which was just big enough to hold four beds.

In addition to the danger from mortar rounds being fired over their heads, the soldiers had to battle bugs. Among them were scorpions, spiders, and venomous centipedes. Stein said, "I was stung by a scorpion on Sunday, April 14, 1991. One scorpion, but it actually stung me twice . . . about a second apart." That was more than enough for him. The soldiers ramped up their countermeasures, which included an aerosolized insect-killing spray called Shell Tox. To keep the bugs out, they sprayed their poorly ventilated bunker on a weekly basis. It worked. However, Stein likely breathed in a significant amount of the insect-killing spray, which contained a class of pesticides called pyrethrins. These are naturally occurring pesticides derived from chrysanthemum flowers ("mums") and can be inhaled or ingested to devastating effect.[24]

You don't have to be a gardener or serve in southern Lebanon to be exposed to such chemicals. Pyrethrins and their more toxic synthetic derivatives (pyrethroids) are found in numerous products, including flea collars, pet shampoos, foggers, and bug sprays.[24,25] Infrequent, low-dose exposures may be safe. However, frequent exposure to these pesticides and their synthetic forms harms the nervous systems of insects and humans.[26]

Determining the exact cause of an individual's Parkinson's is difficult, but numerous studies have linked pesticide exposure to the disease.[27–30] Today, Stein (**Figure 2**) is petitioning the Army for compensation. He still lives in Norway and enjoys visiting his family in the seaside town of Harstad, located north of the Arctic Circle, where he grew up. Snow persists well into spring, and Stein's late father always aimed to have the backyard cleared by May 21 in time to celebrate Stein's mother's birthday. Stein has made adjustments to accommodate his Parkinson's, explaining that he has removed everything in his life that he felt dragged him down, including his television, which he hasn't used in twenty years. He says, "Parkinson's is pretty bad, but you usually get time to right some wrongs."

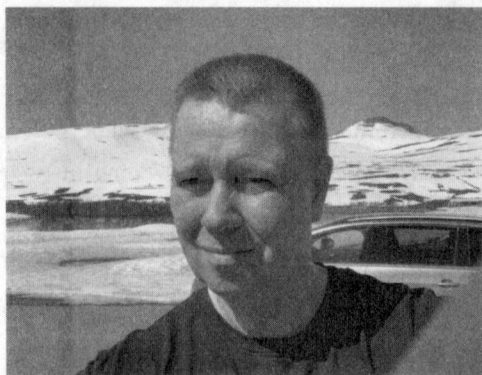

Figure 2. Dr. Stein Nilsen crossing the Arctic Circle around June 2020. Photo courtesy of Dr. Stein Nilsen.

A DOCTOR AND A PATIENT

Pyrethrins are not the only naturally occurring pesticide linked to Parkinson's. In 2000, Dr. Tim Greenamyre, a neurologist and Parkinson's researcher, and his colleagues at Emory University studied another pesticide called rotenone, which they suspected was triggering the disease. Rotenone is produced by many tropical plants in the Caribbean, South America, Southeast Asia, and Southwest Pacific islands. For centuries, extracts from these plants have been used to kill fish.[31] In the 1990s, rotenone, which also exterminates insects including head lice, was one of the most commonly used pesticides in US homes.[32] It is also used in agriculture, and residues of the pesticide have been found on lettuce and tomatoes and even in baby food.[31]

The brain is an energy-guzzling organ. Although it accounts for only 2% of a person's body weight, it consumes 20% of the body's energy production.[33] Nerve cells (or neurons) burn three-quarters of this energy, and those that produce dopamine in the substantia nigra are among the most demanding.[34,35] These poorly insulated nerve cells have a million connections and, if stretched out, would reach four meters (thirteen feet) in length.[36,37] To meet their power demands, they are full of energy-producing engines called mitochondria.

Greenamyre wondered whether rotenone, which damages mitochondria, might produce Parkinson's, so he injected the chemical into the bloodstream of rats. Twenty-five rats were exposed to the chemical for one to five or more weeks, and their brains were examined. Twelve exposed to rotenone (at various doses) had loss of dopamine-producing nerve cells in the substantia nigra, the part of the brain affected in Parkinson's. Other parts of the brain were largely spared. None of the rats in a placebo group had such a loss.[38]

The exposed rats also had slowed movements and hunched postures. Additionally, "seven animals developed severe rigidity, and three animals had shaking of one or more paws that was reminiscent of rest tremor."[38]

Greenamyre concluded, "These results indicate that chronic exposure to a common pesticide can reproduce the anatomical, neurochemical, behavioral, and neuropathological features of [Parkinson's disease]."[38] His team believed that other chemicals, whether natural or man-made, that damage mitochondria could also contribute. They concluded that exposure to these chemicals "through diet, drinking water, or other environmental factors" could "underlie most cases of typical . . . Parkinson's disease."[38]

Eleven years after Greenamyre's experiments in rats, researchers, led by Dr. Caroline Tanner, now at the University of California, San Francisco, found that exposure to rotenone was associated with Parkinson's among humans. A 2011 landmark study examined farmers and other pesticide applicators and found that those exposed to rotenone had a 150% increased risk of Parkinson's.[28]

The route of exposure, at least for rotenone, may be important. In his studies, Greenamyre and his team injected rotenone directly into the bloodstream of rats and observed that rotenone "seems to have little toxicity when administered orally."[38] In Tanner's study with farmers, their primary means of exposure may have been inhalation from spraying the pesticide.

Sixteen years after his landmark study, Greenamyre, who cares for patients with Parkinson's, began noticing concerning symptoms of his own. According to a recent profile in *Science*, "He couldn't smell things. He was constipated. He was shouting and kicking in his sleep. His left arm didn't swing when he walked."[39] In 2021, he approached a fellow neurologist to confirm what he had suspected: he had Parkinson's disease.[39]

Dr. Greenamyre (**Figure 3**), who is now at the University of Pittsburgh, wonders whether his research with rotenone and similar chemicals may have caused his disease. "Because we didn't know as much, we weren't as careful. And I got exposed to things, and particularly rotenone, quite a bit."[39] Today,

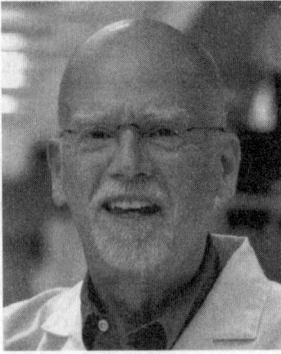

Figure 3. Photograph of Dr. Tim Greenamyre.

Greenamyre still sees patients with Parkinson's and is working to identify other likely environmental causes. He says, "I look forward to a future when we can prevent these toxic encounters and mitigate them if they do occur."

ONE SUMMER IN TEXAS

Dr. Greenamyre's fate is the rare case of someone who was exposed to a Parkinson's-inducing pesticide in the lab. Far more common is exposure in the field. Steve Phillips was a Southern California native who lived to surf in his hometown of Long Beach in the 1960s. When his older brother married into a cotton-growing family in West Texas, a teenage Steve jumped at the chance to earn some money and spend a summer farming. In the summer of 1969, the seventeen-year-old left his surfboard and headed to Pep, Texas, population seven.

There, he had a "chance to make a ton of money." But the price would be high. With no formal training or proper protection, Steve was responsible for mixing chemicals, including the pesticide paraquat. He would load the toxic weed killer into fifty-five-gallon drums that were placed on the back of a tractor. Steve did not wear gloves, goggles, or a respirator. He did not have an enclosed cab, air filters, or air conditioning. Instead, he wore a Dodger blue baseball cap and a red bandana, a gift from his brother to keep the dust out of his nose. He rode the open tractor around one-mile-square tracts enclosed by barbed wire fences. As he drove, he sprayed the cotton plants, and depending on the wind, the pesticide would blow back onto him.

Steve sprayed every weekday for the entire summer. When his fifty-five-gallon tank ran dry, a refueling truck would replenish it. Each day, he would finish a square mile, but even with five to six tractors running, it took weeks to spray all the fields. As soon as they finished, they would begin again.

Flush with cash, Steve returned to Southern California and resumed surfing and listening to rock and roll. In the 1970s, his favorite station was KMET, and his favorite DJ was, by coincidence, "Paraquat" Kelley. Patrick Kelley got his famous nickname by reporting on the news of the day, including the US-supported spraying of paraquat on marijuana and poppy fields in Mexico. Following the use of Agent Orange in Vietnam, the United States provided aircrafts and $30 million in aid to douse marijuana fields in Mexico with the weed killer paraquat.[40,41] Steve would often watch the planes spraying crops when he drove his beloved yellow Volkswagen Microbus to surf in Baja California.

The intent was to destroy the crop, but some of the pesticide-laced plants still made their way into the United States. One study found that over 20% of marijuana samples from the southwestern United States were contaminated with paraquat.[40–43] Steve's beloved DJ reported on the news about the potential lung toxicity from smoking the laced weed.

After studying organization management in college, Steve had a successful career as a leadership consultant. He was looking forward to a healthy and productive retirement until 2008, when, while hosting a dinner for executives in Saint Thomas in the Caribbean, the fifty-seven-year-old could not make his left hand work. Like US Air Force veteran Jana, he looked for alternative explanations, including the couple of drinks he had while sailing earlier in the day, stress, and fatigue. However, he soon noticed that his left foot would occasionally stick to the floor and that his left arm did not swing much when he was walking. He saw a neurologist and was diagnosed with Parkinson's. He was completely unaware that the disease might be related to his activities in the summer of 1969. That changed, however, in 2015 when he started reading the emerging research linking paraquat to the disease.

Four years earlier, Dr. Caroline Tanner, a neurologist and an epidemiologist, and her colleagues in Northern California had conducted a study that highlighted the risks.[28] Tanner was interested in determining whether farmworkers, like Steve, who worked with pesticides known to damage mitochondria, were more likely to develop Parkinson's. To do so, she examined over one hundred farmers and their spouses from Iowa and North Carolina who were diagnosed with Parkinson's, and she compared them to agricultural workers without the disease. Tanner asked both about their exposure to different pesticides. Like those who worked with rotenone, those who worked with paraquat were also 150% more likely to have had Parkinson's.

After reading some of the research, Steve says, "I got pissed off." He wondered whether his disability was due to his summer job in West Texas. He recalls seeing some danger signs on the bottles of the chemicals he would use but, like many teenagers, was not overly concerned.

His parkinsonian symptoms progressed, and three years ago he traveled to see Dr. Michael Okun (one of the book's authors) and Dr. Kelly Foote at the University of Florida to have deep brain stimulation surgery. The surgery has been "a great thing" for Steve, but Parkinson's has changed his plans for retirement. He and his wife, Angelina, had bought thirty-six acres of land in Sámara, Costa Rica, where they were planning to live the life of "beach bums." While he still travels down to Costa Rica, where there are no Parkinson's specialists, he spends most of his life in the United States, dividing his time between Asheville, North Carolina, and San Francisco.

Today, Steve is an active member of the PD Avengers (www.PDavengers .com), a global grassroots organization aimed at ending the disease. He previously led its pesticide action committee and is urging the United States to ban paraquat and protect others from developing this debilitating disease. He says, "There is continuing and mounting evidence that [chemicals in] our food, water, and air are the true causal elements of Parkinson's disease and that Parkinson's disease is entirely avoidable."

MANUFACTURED IGNORANCE

In addition to cotton, paraquat is sprayed on fields of corn, soybeans, and grapes throughout the United States (**Figure 4**). Over the last five years (for which data are available), use of paraquat has doubled. In 2018, a record fifteen million pounds of the weed killer were used in the United States alone.[44] Despite producing the weed killer, England bans the use of paraquat

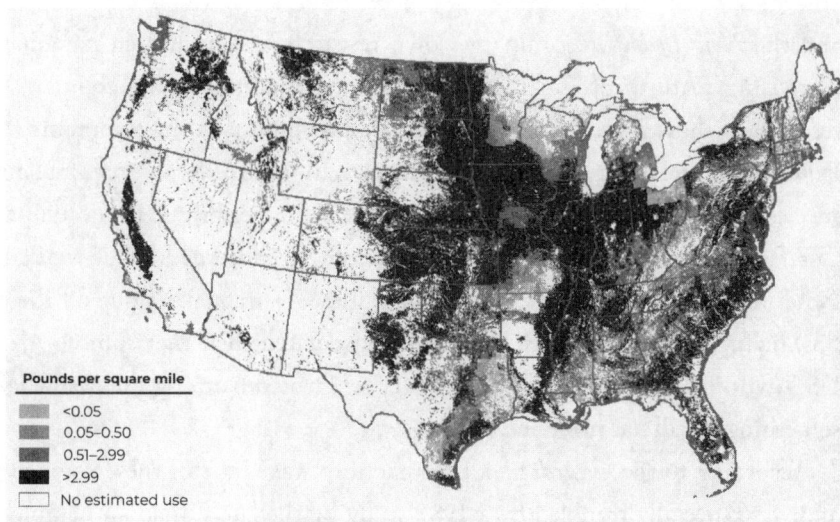

Figure 4. Preliminary estimated agricultural use of paraquat in the United States, 2018, which includes "more extensive estimates of pesticide use not reported in surveys." Map created by the US Geological Survey.[44]

in its own country but exports it to Brazil, Mexico, and the United States.[45] Over fifty countries, including China, have banned the chemical, which has been used to commit suicide and homicide.[46–48]

Paraquat is associated with a substantially higher risk of Parkinson's in humans.[38,49] Laboratory animals exposed to paraquat have reduced mobility and manifest the features of the disease in their brains.[50] The chemical damages the mitochondria, which we know are impaired in Parkinson's.[51,52] In fruit flies, paraquat can lead to misfolding of the protein alpha-synuclein, which is the pathological hallmark of the disease.[53] Multiple researchers from around the world have replicated many of these findings.[54–57] In short, we have everything but a randomized controlled trial, which would not be feasible or ethical, to show that paraquat causes Parkinson's disease. However, the most damning evidence comes not from academics but apparently from the company itself.[45,58]

Countless farmers have filed lawsuits against the weed killer's manufacturer.[45] As part of those lawsuits, the producer has had to disclose internal documents dating back to the 1950s regarding its "blockbuster" product.[45] According to documents reviewed in investigative reports from the *Guardian* and the *New Lede*, the company's own research has implicated paraquat as causing features of Parkinson's in laboratory animals. The company's researchers showed that large doses of paraquat produced the symptoms of Parkinson's, including a stiff gait and tremors, in three different mammalian species: rats, mice, and rabbits.[45] These studies were performed in the 1960s.

Fifty years ago, regulators became increasingly concerned about workers "who might inadvertently lick small quantities of paraquat residue off their lips, or inhale paraquat mist."[45] Rumors circulated then that some in the US Environmental Protection Agency (EPA) favored banning the pesticide, something it still has not done.[45]

According to the *Guardian*, a manufacturer was aware of these concerns and was especially troubled by a 1987 study by the late Canadian neurologist Dr. André Barbeau and his colleagues. The researchers were concerned that environmental factors might be contributing to Parkinson's. They reasoned that if such factors were important, then the prevalence of the disease would not be uniform but would vary, for example, depending on the use of different chemicals. They were right.

They began their investigation in the rural regions of the province of Quebec. They first found "marked variability in the prevalence rate of Parkinson's disease . . . between the various rural regions." According to their analyses, one region that contained the "Garden of Quebec" consistently had the highest rates of Parkinson's. The region was almost exclusively agricultural and was a large supplier of vegetables and apples for the province and beyond. The region was also "by far, the largest consumer of pesticides," including ones like paraquat. The team found a near perfect correlation between pesticide use and the prevalence of Parkinson's.[59]

The "extraordinarily high correlation" concerned a manufacturer of paraquat, and an internal company memo warned that paraquat could, like asbestos, become a huge legal liability.[45] However, rather than withdrawing its product, a producer doubled down on paraquat under a "freedom to sell" campaign. According to the reporting, a manufacturer of paraquat used techniques designed to underestimate the chemical's toxic effects, hid the results of its own research from regulatory authorities, and sought to systematically discredit the work of an academic researcher who demonstrated the link between paraquat and Parkinson's. A company even sought to prevent her from serving on an Environmental Protection Agency (EPA) advisory panel because it would be a "real disaster" for many of its projects.[45] According to the journalist Carey Gillam, who obtained the company's secret files and revealed their contents in a series of reports, "There is abundant evidence from the company's own internal documents demonstrating that the company prioritized its business interests over the health and safety of the public."

If the company's actions—concealing research, attacking scientists, promoting unsafe products—sound familiar, they should. Many have been adopted by the tobacco industry,[60] lead paint manufacturers,[61] opioid producers,[47,62] and, most recently, social media companies.[47] There is even a new word for the practice: *agnotology*.[63]

Science is the production of knowledge. Agnotology is the deliberate production of ignorance, often for commercial gain.

To this day the company still maintains, "There is no causative link, at all, between paraquat exposure and Parkinson's disease."[64] In fact, the company's principal science advisor says, "No scientist or doctor has ever concluded in a peer-reviewed scientific analysis that paraquat causes Parkinson's"[64] (see **Skeptics' Corner**). The manufacturer makes these statements after having withheld information from the world that could allow scientists and the public to reach that very conclusion.[45]

SKEPTICS' CORNER: **PROOF**

In the early twentieth century, rates of lung cancer, which was previously rare, were soaring in England, and no one knew why. Asphalt from new roads, delayed effects from toxic gases from World War I, and the recent influenza pandemic were all proposed as explanations.[65]

Sir Bradford Hill, a British epidemiologist (a scientist who studies disease patterns in humans), and his physician colleague Dr. Richard Doll thought the culprit was a relatively new habit: smoking. So they surveyed British doctors in the 1950s on their smoking habits and then waited for them to die. They found that doctors who smoked were far more likely to die from lung cancer than those who did not.[66] But this finding did not necessarily "prove" that smoking caused lung cancer. Maybe smokers were more likely to drink coffee, for example, and it was the coffee that was causing the cancer.

In medicine, the best evidence comes from randomized controlled trials. But Hill knew that such trials would not be feasible, practical, or ethical. He could not randomly assign people to smoke or not smoke and then follow them for years to see who developed cancer. Similarly, scientists today cannot randomize farmers, consumers, or children to pesticide exposure or placebo for years and then see who develops Parkinson's disease decades later.

Hill wanted to know when we can "pass from [an] observed *association* to a verdict of *causation*."[67] So, in 1965, he put forth nine aspects of an association that should be considered "before deciding that the most likely interpretation of it is causation."[67] These included the strength of the association, the consistency of the findings, the presence of a dose-response relationship, the biological plausibility, and experimental studies. Across all these dimensions, pesticides like paraquat satisfy most, if not all, of Hill's criteria.

On a practical level, "A demand for scientific proof is always a formula for inaction and delay and usually the first reaction of the guilty. . . . In fact scientific proof has never been, is not, and should not be the basis for political and legal action." The author of these words? A scientist at British American Tobacco.[68]

In 2021, the EPA reapproved the continued use of paraquat, even though its own website (**Figure 5**) states, "One sip can kill."[47] With support from the Michael J. Fox Foundation, farmworker groups, environmentalists, and health organizations represented by Earthjustice (a nonprofit focused on environmental litigation) sued the EPA over its reauthorization.[69] As a result, the US Department of Justice instructed the EPA to review its decision,

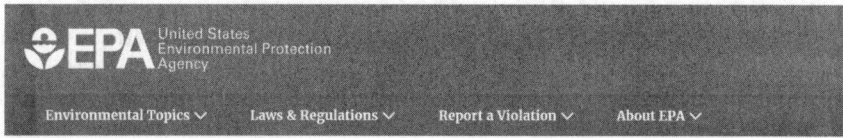

EPA United States Environmental Protection Agency

Environmental Topics ∨   Laws & Regulations ∨   Report a Violation ∨   About EPA ∨

Paraquat Dichloride: One Sip Can Kill ☠

Figure 5. The US Environmental Protection Agency's webpage about paraquat. Image modified for clarity.

again to no avail. In 2024, the EPA reauthorized the continued use of paraquat.[47]

ON THE VINE

Pesticide use remains an international problem. The French consumer association Que Choisir was curious about whether pesticides get into wine. In 2013, they tested ninety-two bottles of French wine from various regions of France "ranging from a $2.20 bottle of generic red to a $20.25 bottle of Châteauneuf-du-Pape."[70] Que Choisir detected traces of pesticide in every bottle.[71]

According to the *Wine Spectator*, the study "caused a furor in France."[72] Among the chemicals found were pesticides that had supposedly been banned.[72] Another study of more than three hundred French wines found remnants of pesticides in 90% of the bottles tested.[73]

None of this should be surprising as vineyards are large consumers of pesticides. While they cover just 3% of agricultural land in France, vineyards account for 20% of pesticides used in the country.[73] The good news is that organic wineries are growing, but they face strong resistance.

In April 2014, Emmanuel Giboulot, a grower of organic wines, was, according to the *New York Times*, "charged with breaking the law for refusing to use" a pesticide that is a known nerve toxin.[74] The French were worried about an insect spreading a plant disease.[75] The French agricultural ministry prosecuted Giboulot under Article 251-20 of the rural code for "failing to apply an insecticide [a chemical that kills insects] treatment to his vineyard."[75]

The class of pesticides that Giboulot did not use is associated with an increased risk of Parkinson's, Alzheimer's, and death.[76–78] He was convicted and fined €1,000.[79] The grape disease that was the target of the French government's action never materialized. The pesticide was not needed. Giboulot "became a hero for organic food and wine supporters around the world," and an appellate court eventually reversed course and ruled in his favor.[79]

Not all wine growers are so fortunate. Because French vineyards are among the most intense users of pesticides, the risk of Parkinson's may be higher among wine growers.[80] Indeed, researchers found that those working with pesticides in the South of France were twice as likely to have Parkinson's as those who didn't.[81]

A more recent study sought to determine whether the increased risk of Parkinson's extended beyond winemakers to those living near vineyards. French researchers looked at nearly 70,000 individuals who were newly diagnosed. They found that these individuals were much more likely to live in rural areas. Next, they discovered that the French districts or "cantons with high density of vineyards, showed the most consistent and robust association with [Parkinson's disease]." Moreover, the association was found for farmers and nonfarmers, women and men. The researchers note that pesticides used on farms can spread into the air, water (including well water), and homes of those who live nearby. In short, the harmful effects of pesticides are not restricted just to those who work with the chemicals.[80]

You do not need to live in France to be at risk. Similar studies have found higher rates of Parkinson's among those living near areas of high pesticide use from Israel to California.[49,82] A California study found that living within five hundred meters (1,650 feet) of where paraquat and another dangerous pesticide was used "greatly increased the risk of developing [Parkinson's disease]." Moreover, the risk may be especially high among individuals who were children, teenagers, or young adults when they were exposed.[49]

CRY BABY

Despite the best efforts of some pesticide producers to conceal risks, a few farmers are getting the message. After twenty-five years of growing millions of onions in upstate New York, Matt Mortellaro, a second-generation farmer, called it quits. The main reason—pesticides. Every onion season since he was in his twenties, Matt had loaded a sprayer with nerve toxicants designed to kill tiny insects that wreak havoc on onion fields. He sprayed his onion crops every seven to ten days, about twenty times during a growing season. To do so, he diluted pesticide concentrate, which could cost up to $2,000 per gallon.

For many years, the pesticide of choice for onion farmers was chlorpyrifos, a chemical that has been used worldwide since 1965.[83] In addition to farms, it is found on utility poles, wood fences, and golf courses.[84] The chemical, which works by slowing the breakdown of a neurotransmitter (a chemical that allows nerve cells to communicate with one another), has cost twenty-six million American children an estimated seventeen million IQ points.[85] Like paraquat, chlorpyrifos can produce the pathology of Parkinson's in laboratory animals and is associated with an increased risk of Parkinson's in humans.[86,87] Because of pesticides like chlorpyrifos, farmers are at a higher risk for Parkinson's[88] and cancer.[89] For Mortellaro, that is too much. He says, "Not handling pesticides is the most significant reason why I left farming."

Today, three years after selling his Cry Baby onion business, Matt misses farming. He and his wife, Stephanie, have just purchased a small farm where they can grow fruits and vegetables and raise some livestock. But this time, the farm will be different. It will be organic.

But even organic produce is not completely safe from pesticides. A 2024 analysis by *Consumer Reports* found that organic fruits and vegetables had lower levels of pesticides than conventionally grown foods. However, some organic foods, including imported green beans, carried a moderate or worse pesticide risk. Scientists at the magazine also found that "pesticide residue posed a significant risk in roughly 20% of the 59 common foods examined in its research." Among the high-risk foods were conventionally grown kale, blueberries, potatoes, and bell peppers.[90]

Pesticides have become endemic in the food supply. They are found on fruits and vegetables and even in a popular cereal fed to toddlers.[91–93] They are also found in us. In a small 2023 study, 90% of American adults had a pesticide used in oat-based foods present in their urine.[94]

NEW KINDS OF SICKNESS

In 1962, Rachel Carson warned about the indiscriminate use of pesticides in her era-defining book *Silent Spring*. She expressed grave concern about the impact of pesticides like DDT, a widely used chemical during World War II, not only on the environment (a "silent spring") but also on our health. She wrote, "The farmers spoke of much illness among their families. In the town the doctors had become more and more puzzled by new kinds of sickness appearing among their patients."[95] These new kinds of sicknesses could include Parkinson's and related conditions.

Dementia with Lewy bodies is the second most common cause of dementia after Alzheimer's disease.[96] It affects an estimated one million Americans,[97] and it disabled the late Robin Williams, who grew up in a farmhouse complete with an orchard located right next to a golf course.[98,99] However, as prevalent as it has become, dementia with Lewy bodies may be another new disease.

Thirty years after Dr. Zimmerman saw high rates of ALS on Guam, Dr. Kenji Kosaka, a Japanese psychiatrist with a penchant for the microscope, saw something new in 1976. He had just finished examining the brain of a sixty-five-year-old woman who had a combination of early-onset Alzheimer's disease and features of Parkinson's. Her symptoms began at age fifty-six with forgetfulness and involuntary movement of her neck. Over years, she developed severe dementia and eventually could not walk. After her death, when Dr. Kosaka looked at her brain, he saw Lewy bodies throughout. They were not just isolated to the parts typically affected by Parkinson's. Kosaka had never seen a brain look like that before and said, "As far as we know, no similar case has been reported."[100]

Eight years later, Kosaka and colleagues reported additional, similarly affected individuals in Japan, Germany, and Austria. Kosaka wondered whether this dementing illness with features of Parkinson's was actually "a new disease."[101]

What caused the possibly "new" disease that Kosaka first described fifty years ago? No one knows for sure, but thirty years before Kosaka's seminal report, following World War II, Japan began using fat-loving organochlorine pesticides, such as DDT and chlordane, on its rice paddies.[102] Paddy fields cover more than half the farming land in Japan.[103] During World War II, DDT was sprayed to kill mosquitoes, preventing the spread of malaria and saving millions of lives. Afterward, its use soared, and its applications multiplied.[104]

Japan used 30,000 tons of DDT and even larger amounts of related chemicals from the mid-1940s until the country banned their use in 1971.[105] Rice production is a major source of pesticide pollution with up to 50% running off from fields into lakes, rivers, wetlands, and groundwater.[103] DDT and similar chemicals can also be found in rice itself[106] and in increasing concentrations as they make their way up the food chain to humans.[107] Because they dissolve in fat like BMAA, they can be found in breast milk and in the fatty tissue of humans.[105] Indeed, the concentrations of DDT in samples of fat tissue of Japanese men (aged forty to ninety-three), which were absent in the 1930s, rose quickly beginning in the late 1940s and peaked in the early 1960s. Following restrictions on its use, the concentration of DDT fell in both food products and in the fat of the Japanese population.[105]

Pesticides similar to DDT can damage the dopamine-producing nerve cells that are lost in Parkinson's.[108] A recent study found that Greek patients with Parkinson's had higher levels of a DDT breakdown product than did individuals without the disease.[109] Whether DDT or related chemicals may have contributed to the early reports of dementia with Lewy bodies is uncertain. But the relationship between ingested pesticides and subsequent development of dementia with Lewy bodies requires much further study.

Parkinson's disease and dementia with Lewy bodies share striking similarities. Unlike strokes, seizures, and migraines, these diseases have emerged only in the industrial age. At the time Parkinson and Kosaka described them, they struck the surgeon and the psychiatrist as something novel. Neither had been classified in the medical literature, the two were almost certainly rare when described, and both are increasingly common. And pesticides may be part of the reason why.

MYSTERY IN HEBRON

On March 18, 2024, Sarah Teale, an Emmy-nominated documentary producer, emailed Ray, one of the authors of this book. She wanted to speak about the EPA's recent decision to reapprove paraquat. She was also concerned about what was happening in a rural, upstate New York town called Hebron, where eleven farmers, including her husband, had been diagnosed with Parkinson's.

One month later, I visited Hebron to give a talk about the disease. Before I could get out of my car, George Flint, a fireman, city councilman, and life-long resident of the community, greeted me. I asked him about his interest in Parkinson's, and he said words that I had never heard before: "Everyone here is concerned about Parkinson's disease."

He then proceeded to tell me about Hebron, its residents, their work, and the plague of Parkinson's that had hit this 1,800-person farming town. No one had any idea why so many in this community near the border between New York and Vermont (**Figure 6**) had developed the disease. Most of the individuals did not have a family history of Parkinson's, yet it was affecting many Hebron families. And the numbers only seemed to be increasing.

Some were concerned about the proximity of a nearby orchard that was suspected of spraying large amounts of pesticides. Some, like Sarah's husband, had used paraquat on their farms. Others thought that the uptick in Parkinson's could be related to a nearby chemical company. Another possibility was the water, as almost everyone in the community relied on private

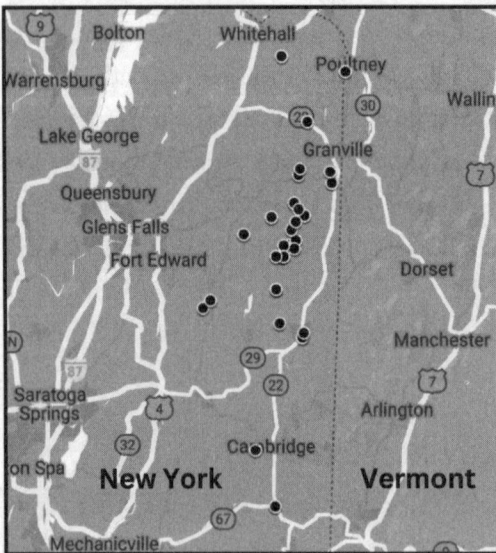

Figure 6. Location of individuals with Parkinson's disease in Hebron, New York, and the surrounding community. Image courtesy of Sarah Teale.

wells, which are prone to contamination from pesticide runoff from nearby farms or from chemical contaminants upstream.

On a cold, gray Sunday afternoon in April before spring arrived in upstate New York, about sixty people crammed into the Hebron firehouse (**Figure 7**) to find answers to their concerns. Many had Parkinson's, some were caregivers, and others had lost family members to the disease. Like the residents of any small town, most knew one another. However, everyone, including Ray, was uncertain of what to expect. After a brief overview of Parkinson's disease, dozens of questions were asked by farmers, longtime residents, migrants from cities, and even a former employee of the state department of health. They wanted to know what the cause of Parkinson's was for them, their loved ones, and their neighbors. They agreed testing the water seemed like a good idea and that additional investigation was warranted.

A couple months later, Sarah emailed again to indicate that after some additional digging, they had found that multiple pesticides linked to Parkinson's had been used by farmers in the community. She also wrote to say that after some additional discussions, the number with Parkinson's in the community had now increased to thirty-six.

The culprit for the large number of affected individuals in this community remains uncertain. These clusters of Parkinson's are likely found

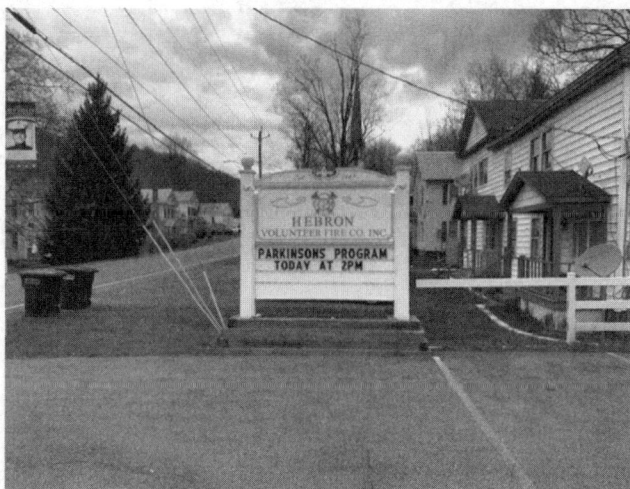

Figure 7. Photograph outside the firehouse in Hebron, New York. Photo taken by authors.

throughout the country and around the world, but only a handful have been investigated.[110] Chance may be an explanation for some, genetics for a few, but most likely have an environmental cause.[110]

Like the Chamorro people, residents of Hebron now find themselves overwhelmed with not only a debilitating illness but also relentless questions about how and why they are in this situation. They want answers and relief.

In the interim, given the link between pesticides and Parkinson's, we can all take actions to reduce our exposure. These include banning the most dangerous pesticides, reducing our use of others, and informing and protecting those who work with them. The sooner we take these steps, the faster we will create a world where consumers, veterans, farmers, scientists, rural residents, and all of us are spared the wrath of Parkinson's.

2

TOXIC WATER

The benefit of the doubt should go to
the people, not the chemical.

—Master Sergeant Jerry Ensminger, US Marine Corps (Ret.)

On May 12, 2006, Phoenix Suns power forward Brian Grant (**Figure 1**) played two minutes in a National Basketball Association (NBA) playoff game against the Los Angeles Clippers. He did not have a point, a rebound, or an assist. However, in the last game of his NBA career, the thirty-four-year-old power forward made history. He had played an entire basketball season with Parkinson's disease. He just didn't know it.

While he was not diagnosed with the condition for another two years, Brian had first noticed the symptoms of the disease a season earlier while with the Los Angeles Lakers. There the 6'9", 250-pound player was puzzled that he could no longer jump off his left leg like he once could. Sometimes the leg gave out. The next season his left hand started shaking. After his career ended, profound depression and periods of anxiety, all common early features of Parkinson's, followed. He says, "It was like falling off a cliff."[1]

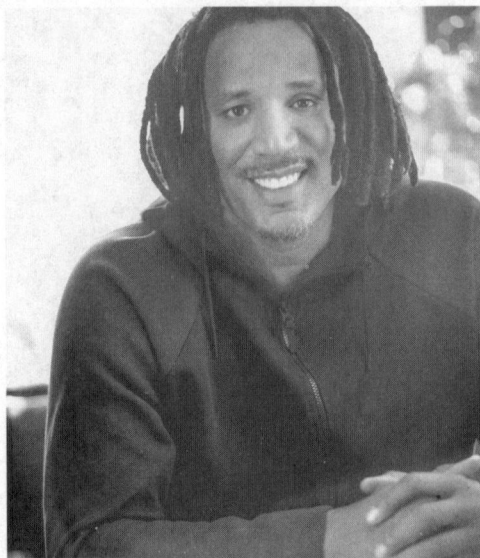

Figure 1. Photograph of Brian Grant. Courtesy of Brian Grant.

At his peak, Brian was one of the top power forwards in the league. He was a relentless rebounder and tenacious defender for his beloved Portland Trail Blazers. At the pinnacle of his twelve-season career, he held one of the game's greatest scorers to just eight points in an NBA playoff game.

However, the NBA was a world away from his roots. As he wrote in his auto-biography, *Rebound*, Brian grew up as a "Black kid from a little farming town on the banks of the Ohio River who expected to be in a field picking tobacco and potatoes his whole life."[1] Indeed, beginning in the sixth grade, Brian spent his summers toiling on a tobacco field under the eye of his grandfather. In high school, he was a lightly regarded athlete before he was given a chance to become a star basketball player at Xavier University in Cincinnati, Ohio.

But before the NBA or the Xavier Musketeers or even the tobacco fields, Brian lived at a Marine Corps base called Camp Lejeune. He was a three-year-old boy, and his father, a Marine, was stationed there. His family lived in a trailer park on a dirt road in Jacksonville, North Carolina. His dad would take his young son around the 246-square-mile training facility and show him the fighter planes. Brian liked those but not his neighbor's pet boa constrictor. Other than the snake, though, the three-year-old enjoyed life at Camp Lejeune. He liked his preschool and the freedom to explore the vast base. Unbeknownst to Brian, his father, and his family, that freedom would come with a price. The water that Brian used for bathing, swimming, and drinking was likely contaminated with toxic chemicals.

Military officers need spotless uniforms. Unfortunately, the chemicals from a local dry cleaner and from underground storage tanks contaminated the base's water supply.[2] Among the contaminants were two closely related chemicals called trichloroethylene (TCE) and perchloroethylene (PCE). The contamination was extensive (at least seventy times levels thought to be safe) and prolonged (at least from 1953 to 1987).[2] According to the National Academy of Sciences, it was the "largest human exposure to TCE from drinking water in this nation's history."[3]

TCE and PCE are remarkably simple molecules (**Figure 2**).[4] Both have just six atoms: two carbons, one hydrogen, and three chlorines for *tri*chloroethylene, and two carbons and four chlorines for *per*chloroethylene (the prefix *per-* means "four"). Chemists first created TCE in the lab in 1864, and commercial production began in the 1920s. One of its earliest uses was in dry cleaning. In addition to not shrinking clothes like water, TCE is also not flammable like earlier dry-cleaning agents, such as kerosene. In the 1950s, the clear, colorless, and volatile (readily evaporating) TCE was replaced by PCE in dry cleaning. Today, most dry cleaners in the United States still use PCE (often called "perc").[5]

Beyond dry cleaning, TCE has had a myriad of uses, including decaffeinating coffee and degreasing metal. If you are a longtime drinker of decaffeinated coffee, you may have consumed some TCE along with your brew, until the US Food and Drug Administration banned such use in 1977.[6] At its

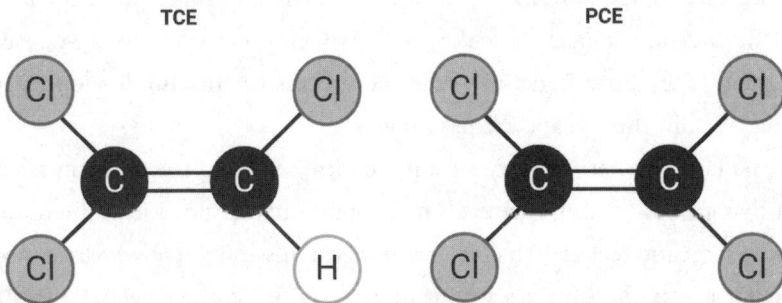

Figure 2. Chemical structures of trichloroethylene (TCE) and perchloroethylene (PCE). Created by the authors.

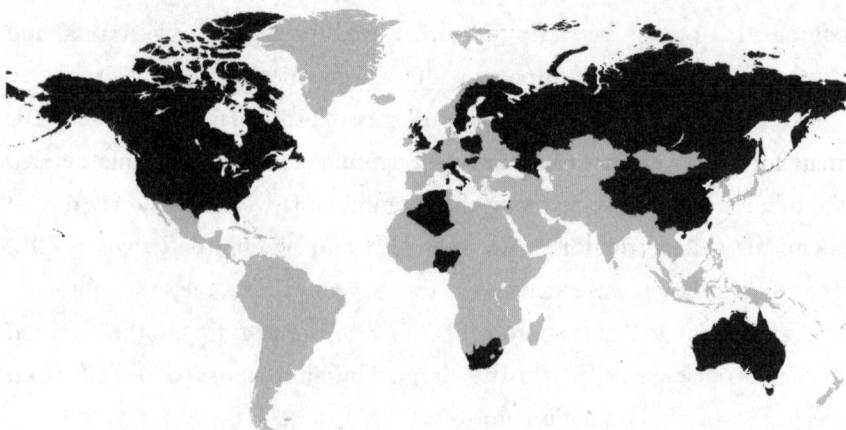

Figure 3. Countries with published studies of sites of groundwater TCE contamination.[7]

peak, the United States used six hundred million pounds annually of TCE, more than two pounds per American. Not all of it was disposed of properly. Some of it leaked from sewer lines, some escaped from fifty-five-gallon drums, some was dumped into rivers and streams, and some was just poured into the ground. As a result, up to 30% of the groundwater in the United States has been contaminated with TCE. And like pesticides, TCE contamination is a global problem (**Figure 3**).[4]

TCE's adverse health record is long. As detailed in the book and movie *A Civil Action*, TCE polluted the water in Woburn, Massachusetts, outside Boston, in the 1970s.[8] A decade earlier, the same occurred in Toms River, New Jersey, as described in the Pulitzer Prize–winning book *Toms River*.[9] In both cases, large numbers of children in the communities developed and died from cancer, especially leukemia.[10] At Camp Lejeune, the six-year-old daughter, Janey Ensminger, of a Marine drill instructor also developed leukemia. Within three years, she passed way.

Years later, her father, Jerry Ensminger, learned from the news on television that cancer-causing chemicals had contaminated the base.[11] The retired master sergeant realized that it was not just his daughter who had been affected: it was the Marines whom he had trained to be "always faithful," their families, and all who supported them. After a twenty-four-year career as a Marine, he dedicated the next twenty-seven years (and counting) to bringing justice to the one million Marines, dependents, and civilians who lived and worked at the base between 1953 and 1987.

In 2001, a US House of Representatives oversight subcommittee found that "for thirty years, Marines and their dependents serving at Camp Lejeune were exposed to toxic chemicals in the drinking water. It took the [US Marine Corps] more than four years to shut down drinking water wells they knew to be contaminated with toxic chemicals and another 24 years and an act of Congress to force them to inform veterans about this contamination and its potential health problems. For two decades the U.S. Marine Corps prevented full disclosure regarding the true extent of contamination at Camp Lejeune."[12]

TCE causes a host of health problems affecting nearly every organ system.[13] Cancer is the biggest concern, as TCE causes cancer and PCE likely does.[14,15] In addition, TCE can cross the placenta and may lead to low-birth-weight babies, congenital heart disease, disorders of the nervous system, and miscarriages.[7] According to one news report, "Hundreds of mothers [at Camp Lejeune] suffered miscarriages or gave birth to stillborn babies or infants with birth defects."[16] A local cemetery just off the base called "Baby Heaven" is filled with scores of children, infants, and babies, some born without a brain.[11]

In 2012, Drs. Sam Goldman, now a professor of medicine at the University of California, San Francisco, and Caroline Tanner, helped add Parkinson's to this grim list.[17] They interviewed ninety-nine pairs of twins, one with Parkinson's and one without, from a World War II twin registry. They asked the twins if they had exposure to chemicals like TCE or PCE at work or in their hobbies. About 10% of the twins had been exposed, often from work as an electrician, dry cleaner, or artist.

Twins who had been exposed to TCE had a six-fold increased risk of Parkinson's compared to their twin who did not have such exposure. For PCE, the risk was likely similar. In both cases, the Parkinson's was diagnosed ten to forty years after the exposure began, suggesting that exposure triggered a process that decades later ultimately led to the disease.[17] This lag corresponds to the time between Brian's childhood exposure and his own diagnosis.

Brian's family was not spared. His younger brother was born at Camp Lejeune and nearly died, suffering disabling allergies possibly due to the toxic effects of TCE and the other chemicals in the water. After they left the base two years later, his brother's health dramatically improved. Unfortunately, the same was not true for other family members. In March 2020, Brian's father, who had become his best friend, died at age sixty-five of esophageal cancer. That condition is also linked to TCE.[7]

Two years after his diagnosis, in 2010, Brian formed the Brian Grant Foundation to provide resources to help people "who wanted to use exercise and nutrition to manage and slow their symptoms and get on with the business of living."[18] Brian, the proud father of five college graduates, is fighting to help end Parkinson's.[19] As he wrote in his autobiography, "Basketball gave me a life; Parkinson's taught me how to live it."[1]

A COVER-UP

From 1984 to 1988, a young Navy officer, Amy Lindberg, was stationed at Camp Lejeune on the Atlantic coast of North Carolina. On hot, humid days, Amy swam, ran, trained, and outworked her peers. She also drank lots of water. Amy did not know, of course, that the water was contaminated with TCE, PCE, and other chemicals.

At Camp Lejeune, Amy served as the hospital's food service director. The new 205-bed hospital, just opened in 1982, was replete with five operating theaters, five labor rooms, and three delivery rooms.[20] Amy and her team were eager to provide healthy meals for the physicians, nurses, and staff who worked there and the patients they cared for. They set the menus, ordered the food, cleaned it, cooked it, and served it in the hospital's cafeteria and in patients' rooms. All of it was contaminated with TCE.

Amy says, "I was oblivious to it." She did not know that the food and water they were preparing and serving every day had cancer-causing chemicals in it. In considering the implications, including serving patients recovering from cancer surgery with TCE-contaminated water, Amy pauses. "I can't even wrap my head around it, the more I think about it."

Thirty years after serving at Camp Lejeune, Amy, then a fifty-seven-year-old woman who had risen rapidly through the ranks and managed large health programs, could no longer find the right words to say or stay on task. She developed anxiety, depression, and a "brain fog." She saw a neuropsychologist who asked her about her loss of smell, decreased right arm swing, and dragging of her right leg. She also had a mild rest tremor in her right hand and long-standing constipation. She was referred to a neurologist who diagnosed her with Parkinson's.

Drs. Goldman and Tanner wanted to see if veterans like Amy, who served at Camp Lejeune during the period of maximum contamination (1975–1985), had higher rates of Parkinson's. To do so they compared the proportion of service members who developed the disease after serving at Camp Lejeune to those who served at the less contaminated Camp Pendleton, just north of San Diego. The Marines who served at the polluted base were young (average age twenty), healthy (almost by definition), and there for a short time (just over two years on average). Yet thirty-four years later, Camp Lejeune veterans had a 70% increased risk of developing Parkinson's compared to those who served at Camp Pendleton.[21]

The thirty-four-year lag between exposure and diagnosis was similar to what both Brian and Amy experienced and to what Goldman and Tanner had found in their twin study. As with smoking and lung cancer, individuals do not get exposed to a toxic chemical one day and develop the disease the next. It takes time. This gap makes such studies hard to conduct, risks difficult to identify, and findings especially concerning when they are observed.

The story, unfortunately, is not complete. Those who served at Camp Lejeune not only had a higher risk of having Parkinson's but also were more likely to have early features of the disease, such as tremor and anxiety, that put them at high risk for a future diagnosis. In addition, the average age of the cohort examined was just sixty. As the incidence of Parkinson's triples every decade, many more service members are likely to be diagnosed.[21]

Today, Amy, her husband, Brad, and their adult children live in Wilmington, North Carolina, an hour's drive south of the Marine base. Amy and Brad, a retired military officer himself, have a new hobby: beekeeping. They have about a dozen beehives in their backyard and enjoy contributing to a healthy environment. Amy is also an active member of a group of more than one hundred Marines who served at Camp Lejeune and now have Parkinson's.

Amy, who is remarkably fit, remains an avid runner who enjoys pickleball, boxing, and working out constantly. She is still disabled by the disease's nonmotor features, including digestive and urinary issues, pain, and mood changes. At this stage of her disease, her medications compensate for her lost motor skills. However, she has chronic worry over the "inevitability" that the medications will become less effective and that her graceful, coordinated movements will become jerky and unpredictable. She fears that she will become physically and mentally disabled. Looking back, Amy is "astounded . . . that these chemicals are still being used today . . . when they have been proven to be neurotoxic."

The Camp Lejeune story has been a tragedy for a generation of Marines, their families, civilians, the Marine Corps, the military, and the country. A cemetery is filled with deceased children, parents are scarred, Marines feel betrayed, hundreds are dead, and thousands are disabled. And many more are still unaware of their exposure to this day.

From this tragedy, we know that TCE and PCE are unsafe, that their connection to Parkinson's is real, and that we must find and notify those who have been exposed. If we inform those who may have been exposed, they can have questions answered, better understand their current health, pursue cancer screening, and possibly avoid the suffering borne by those who served our country. We should learn these lessons, but as we shall see, in many cases, we fail to confront the truth. The result is unnecessary and avoidable suffering—from miscarriages, cancer, and Parkinson's.

Unfortunately, Camp Lejeune is just the most widely known TCE-polluted site. Scores of military bases, including many in the Air Force where Jana and Sara served, have been contaminated with this ubiquitous chemical.[22] But members of the military are far from the only ones at risk. TCE and PCE have contaminated half of the most toxic sites in the country. The contamination is widespread, is usually invisible, and affects the tap water of fourteen million US veterans and civilians, including numerous communities in the Hudson River Valley in New York state.[23]

THE PHYSICIAN AND THE SUPERFUND SITES

In the 1970s, the residents of Love Canal, which was designed to be a model city near Niagara Falls, confronted one of the greatest environmental disasters in human history. The ground underneath their homes, playgrounds, and schools had been contaminated with numerous cancer-causing chemicals, including TCE. A chemical company had used an abandoned canal to dispose of over 21,000 tons of hazardous chemicals.[24] The company later sold the land—with a disclaimer related to the contamination—to the local school board for $1 in one of the worst purchases ever made.

As chemicals surfaced in the backyards and basements of homes, trees turned black, and stories of miscarriages and cancer multiplied.[25,26] Residents led by Lois Gibbs formed the Love Canal Homeowners Association and pressured the state and federal government into unprecedented action. In 1978, New York governor Hugh Carey ordered the evacuation of pregnant women and young children from the contaminated suburb, and President Jimmy Carter later ordered further evacuations. The state subsequently purchased over two hundred homes, and the federal government provided aid to clean up the pollution. In the aftermath of Love Canal, the federal government created a "Superfund" program to clean up the country's most toxic sites and to hold responsible parties accountable for the costs.[27]

Today, there are about 1,300 Superfund sites in the United States.[28] Over seventy million Americans and over 20% of all children live within three miles of one. More than 5% of the country's population and 7% of children under age five live within one mile of a Superfund site.[29] Jesh Mittal was one of those children.

Dr. Jesh Mittal is a fifty-year-old endocrinologist who was raised in upstate New York. His first home in East Fishkill, a town of 30,000, had its own well for water. Unfortunately, it was located less than a mile from a Superfund site where TCE, PCE, or both had contaminated sixty residential wells.[30] The contamination was not identified until 2000, long after Jesh and his family had moved out.

Today, one in eight Americans, forty million people, receive their water from wells.[31] Private wells tap into underlying groundwater fifteen to fifty feet or more below the surface. Such water is prone to contamination from pesticides from nearby farms or industrial chemicals from military bases or local businesses. And drinking well water may be associated with Parkinson's.[32–34]

These wells, which are usually located on an individual's private property, are not regulated by the Safe Drinking Water Act, which was created in 1974 to ensure that public ("city") drinking water is safe.[33,35] As a result, private wells are tested infrequently, often only when a property changes hands. And when testing is done, it is usually for bacteria and other infectious agents, not for pesticides or industrial chemicals like TCE and PCE.

As part of its investigation into the East Fishkill site, the Environmental Protection Agency (EPA) and the New York State Department of Environmental Conservation "discovered a 1,200-gallon metal septic tank containing materials exhibiting extremely high concentrations of PCE." The tank was found at a commercial facility that had cleaned microchip holders from the late 1960s until the mid-1970s.[30] During this same time, TCE and PCE were widely used to clean silicon chips, and fifteen Superfund sites are located along a seven-mile stretch of US Route 101 in California's Silicon Valley.[36]

Before he started high school, Jesh's family moved. Unfortunately, their second home, which also had a private well, was located near another TCE-contaminated Superfund site.[7] The likely source was a former metal-fabrication plant, which had used TCE to degrease metal. Even though the Mittal family did not live right near the factory, they may have been affected by an underground "plume." The EPA found that TCE had contaminated the groundwater and resulted in an underground collection of polluted water, or plume, that extended for 1.5 miles from the plant.[37] Contaminated plumes are found throughout the country from Phoenix, Arizona, to Antrim County, Michigan, and this plume had polluted the private wells of homes like the Mittals'.[38] In 2017, both sites near where Jesh lived were listed among the "20 most toxic places in Upstate New York."[39]

However, Jesh's potential exposure did not end at home. The future physician attended high school adjacent to a large computing firm where his father, a metallurgical engineer, worked. The soil and groundwater at a manufacturing site right next to the school were contaminated with TCE and PCE. Long before his freshman year, the well at the high school was found to have "slight contamination" with TCE even *after* a filtration system was installed.[7] Wherever Jesh went, he encountered TCE.

In 2010, after a nurse noticed that his handwriting was becoming smaller, Jesh was diagnosed with writer's cramp. Two years later he developed constipation, a "twitch" in his right hand, and stiffness in his right arm. He was subsequently diagnosed with Parkinson's at age thirty-eight. He had no family history of the disease and carried no genetic markers. Two years earlier, his mother had been diagnosed with breast cancer, and three years after his Parkinson's diagnosis, his father was found to have prostate cancer. Both cancers are linked to TCE.[40]

Jesh's symptoms progressed over time, and uncontrollable movements of his head, neck, and trunk led him to undergo deep brain stimulation, which helped. Unfortunately, Jesh, like Jana, is no longer able to practice medicine.

WELL WATER

Fifty miles up the Hudson River from East Fishkill is the town of Saugerties, New York. There, Adeline Cassin and her two sisters grew up on seven acres near the foot of the Catskill Mountains. Adeline enjoyed the idyllic community as a child and always wanted to be outside on the jungle gym or just playing around. What she loved most, though, was the stream in their backyard. Every summer she would spend countless hours wading there and chasing fish. Her love of nature never left her, and as an adult Adeline joined the board of the nonprofit Amazon Watch to help protect the Amazon rainforest and the rights of its Indigenous guardians.

Like many in their neighborhood, the home where she grew up was supplied by a well located on their property that was infrequently tested. Although crop dusters sprayed pesticides on the cornfields near Adeline's home, pesticides may not have been the only issue for her, her family, and her community. From 1961 to 2001, a company manufactured electronic components in this small town. Like many manufacturing plants, it used degreasing agents including TCE and PCE to clean its parts. Unfortunately, in 1986, high concentrations of these chemicals were found in the groundwater. The chemicals were also found in several nearby residential wells.[41] Adeline does not know if her family's well was tested or contaminated. Regardless, she is concerned.

Next to and across the road from their home lived three families. All were affected by cancer. In two, female residents had cancer of the uterus. In the third, the daughter had uterine cancer, and the mother and father died thirteen months apart from ovarian and brain cancer, respectively. Neighbors became concerned about their drinking water. Adeline's father started buying bottled water.

Amid the stories of cancer in her community, Adeline was a star student and a great athlete and, like Jana Reed and Sara Whittingham, wanted to serve her country. She was admitted to West Point, but she opted for the University of Notre Dame and the Reserve Officers' Training Corps. After graduation, she became an officer in the US Army Signal Corps, focused on satellite communications and information systems.

She then pursued a career in global media and tech where she quickly rose through the ranks at Discovery Channel, Paramount, and CNN International, working around the world. Adeline loved her profession. "I was one of those people who wanted to work until I was ninety." However, that all changed when, at the height of her career, she was diagnosed with Parkinson's.

Because of her young age and her grandfather's history of young-onset Parkinson's, her physician recommended genetic testing. Adeline agreed and found that she did not carry any of the genetic mutations linked to the disease (see **Skeptics' Corner**).

SKEPTICS' CORNER: **GENETICS**

Following important contributions from Dr. Rosalind Franklin, Drs. James Watson and Francis Crick in 1953 identified the molecular structure of DNA, which contains the genetic code for humans.[42] With their publication in *Nature*, a new era of genetics was launched that continues to the present day.

Today, genes determine an estimated 20% to 30% of a person's health.[43,44] The genetic causes of many diseases, including Parkinson's, have been identified. In 1997, researchers discovered the first genetic cause—a mutation, or change, in the alpha-synuclein gene.[45] Today, changes in seven genes, including *LRRK2* (the most common genetic cause), have been determined to be "causal contributors."[46]

In all, ninety different genetic risk variants for Parkinson's have been found.[47]

These genetic advances have increased our understanding of Parkinson's.[47] The genetic forms have shown, for example, that the energy-producing parts of cells—the mitochondria—are damaged.[48,49] Genetic variations also contribute to differences in how individuals break down (or metabolize) medicines and other chemicals, including pesticides.[50] These variations may help explain who among the exposed does and does not develop Parkinson's.[50] Finally, the genetic causes have also opened the door to gene-based therapies and personalized medicine.

All of these are important. However, despite these immense advances, the overall heritability of Parkinson's is low, the genetic causes are rare, and their ability to cause disease is limited.[51] A study by the Parkinson's Foundation, called PD GENEration, is trying to determine exactly how common these genetic variants are in North Americans with the disease. As of June 2023, over 10,000 individuals across eighty-five centers have enrolled in this landmark study. Of these, only 13% carry a reportable genetic variant for Parkinson's;[46] 87% do not. This is consistent with what we have known for one hundred years—that 85% of people with Parkinson's do not have a family history of the disease.[52]

While additional genetic causes will be found in the future, they will likely be rare. Since Watson and Crick's paper, over 37,000 studies have examined the genetics of Parkinson's. It is unlikely that they have missed the major ones. Moreover, a 1999 study in twins, led by Dr. Caroline Tanner, concluded "that genetic factors do not play a major role in causing typical [Parkinson's disease]."[53] It is time that we heed the words of Dr. Tanner, change the paradigm, and search in greater earnest for Parkinson's environmental causes.

Adeline's symptoms were progressing and beginning to interfere with her work. She felt like a "big claw had suddenly reached out and snatched away" her life as she knew it. Adeline is struggling with her Parkinson's. She has not been able to tolerate levodopa, and other medications have been less effective.

Unlike Sara, she cannot complete an Ironman. In fact, she can barely walk. When Ray visited her at her home in Miami, she had trouble walking down a couple of stairs, even with assistance. It took her countless steps and three minutes just to get into a car. The former Army officer, who graduated at the top of her class, has lost thirty pounds and now weighs ninety-four pounds.

Parkinson's has robbed Adeline of a promising career and a happy life. "I don't know if there would ever be a way to prove it, but I wonder about our groundwater contributing to the Parkinson's." She is grateful that her two sisters have not developed the disease. Her mom, a retired nurse, is really concerned about her and calls her daily. Her father, an engineer, still lives in the same home where she grew up. "I am sure [my Parkinson's] is distressing for him," she says. "I worry about him most."

Researchers do not know why some individuals exposed to TCE (or any chemical) develop a disease while others do not. The timing, extent, and route of exposure, interaction with other factors (e.g., genetic and environmental), and modifiers like other diseases and stress may all play a role.[54] There may be protective factors (e.g., exercise) that are valuable as well.

Today, Adeline is "grieving, frustrated, and furious, all at once." Yet, she says, "I am intent on igniting the hope within myself and the Parkinson's community that together we will triumph in this battle of a lifetime."

WHY IT HAPPENS

The human studies linking TCE exposure to Parkinson's are supported by laboratory research. Dr. Tim Greenamyre, who showed that the pesticide rotenone causes Parkinson's in rats and then later developed Parkinson's himself, has been leading this research with his former postdoc, Dr. Briana De Miranda, now a toxicologist at the University of Alabama at Birmingham. Like many pesticides, TCE impairs the function of mitochondria, which supply the immense energy needs of nerve cells by turning sugar (glucose) into energy. TCE and PCE, along with many pesticides linked to Parkinson's, readily dissolve in fat. While this proves useful in degreasing, this property also allows TCE ready entrance into the brain, cells, and mitochondria.[55]

De Miranda and Greenamyre showed that rats fed TCE for six weeks lose dopamine-producing nerve cells in the brain region affected by Parkinson's.[56]

In addition to damaging the cells that are lost in Parkinson's, TCE also replicates the activity of the most common genetic cause of the disease. Mutations in a gene called *LRRK2* account for about 2% to 3% of individuals with Parkinson's.[57] Genes provide instructions for the production of proteins, which carry out the various functions of a cell. Experiments performed by Greenamyre and De Miranda show that both the *LRRK2* gene mutation and TCE increase the activity of the LRRK2 protein.[58] In other words, a likely environmental cause of Parkinson's may mimic the actions of a genetic one.

For one hundred years, TCE (and likely PCE) has been causing cancer and quite likely Parkinson's disease. In 2013, the European Union severely restricted most of its uses.[59] Minnesota and New York followed with bans in their states, and California has banned the use of PCE in dry cleaning.[5,59,60] In 2023, the EPA concluded that both chemicals "pose an unreasonable risk to human health" and proposed bans.[61,62] The bans were finalized in 2024 and are the result of over forty years of advocacy from a mother (Ms. Anne Anderson) who lost her son Jimmy to leukemia in Woburn, Massachusetts.[63] Lawsuits from the manufacturers of the chemicals are expected.

While use of TCE peaked in the United States in the 1970s, today an astounding 250 million pounds are still used annually.[64] Global use, especially in China, which accounts for about half the world's market, continues to rise.[7] A ban would help counter the rise of Parkinson's; however, it would not address the thousands of contaminated sites around the world, many of which remain hidden even to those near them.

For too long, we have assumed that the water we drink is safe. This is not a safe assumption. We know that "forever chemicals" in water can cause cancer, so we test for them. We know that lead in water can impair intellectual development, so we eliminate it. We now have good evidence that TCE and PCE can contribute to Parkinson's, so we should test for and eliminate them. Unfortunately, these chemicals may have poisoned not only the water we drink but also the air we breathe.

3

AN INVISIBLE CAUSE
INSIDE OUR HOMES

[The] most likely [cause of my Parkinson's disease] I
think is, that I was exposed to some kind of chemical.

—Michael J. Fox[1]

FORTY YEARS AGO, ENGINEERS WERE BUILDING A NUCLEAR POWER
plant along the Schuylkill River in Pottstown, Pennsylvania, about thirty
miles outside Philadelphia. As part of the plant's safety measures, a monitor was installed to make sure workers at the plant were not being exposed
to unsafe levels of radiation, including from a radioactive gas called radon.
Radon is a decay product of uranium, which is used in nuclear facilities. It
is also found in nature, usually in low levels, from the normal decay of the
metal uranium in soil and rocks. Too much radon, though, can be deadly.

One day in December 1984, Stanley Watras, a construction engineer at the plant, walked through the monitoring doors and set off the
radiation-exposure alarms. Concerned, the plant's health physicist immediately phoned the Pennsylvania Department of Environmental Resources.
However, the incomplete plant could not be blamed for the alarm. It had

not yet commenced operations and was still free of radioactive material. Moreover, Watras had set off the alarms while walking *into*, rather than out of, the plant. Something was amiss.[2,3]

After much confusion, physicists at the plant decided to assess the levels of radon in Watras's home in Boyertown, seven miles away from the plant. Watras, his wife, and his two young children had just moved into the one-story ranch earlier that year. After testing the indoor air, the scientists identified an entirely new way to be exposed to cancer-causing chemicals. They found radon gas in his home.[2,3]

The radon levels in Watras's home were six hundred times what the US Environmental Protection Agency (EPA) currently deems to be safe; that level of exposure is equivalent to smoking 135 packs of cigarettes a day.[2-4] The gas in Watras's home had coupled with dust particles and gathered on his clothing. His clothing was radioactive—so much so that it set off the detectors at work.

Seeking a source for this radon, geologists located an underground rock formation that had high levels of uranium—something that's actually common across the United States. Radon is a clear, colorless gas that moves through the ground, and via holes or cracks in foundations, radon can enter homes, schools, and buildings.[5,6] The gas causes 21,000 cases of lung cancer per year in the United States alone, the vast majority of which are preventable through simple testing (e.g., a do-it-yourself kit costs less than $100) and remediation that costs about $1,000 to $2,000 per home.[7,8]

At the recommendation of the secretary of the Pennsylvania Department of Environmental Resources, Watras and his family were evacuated from their home. Over the next two years, over 18,000 homes in the area were assessed for radon, and nearly 60% had unsafe levels.[2] A few schools and other public buildings were also affected.[2]

The Watras home was remediated via a simple pump that moves radon gas from below a building's foundation into the outside atmosphere. Once outside the home, the radon quickly dissipates and no longer poses a health hazard. After the pump was installed, the air inside the Watras home was found to be safe.[3] The family moved back in, and as of 2015, they were still living there happily.[3]

Today, the EPA estimates that one in fifteen homes in the United States contain unsafe levels of radon.[9] While no state currently requires testing, many require disclosure of radon testing results to prospective homebuyers. Some local governments, such as Montgomery County, southwest of Baltimore, Maryland, require testing before a home is sold.[6] The Montgomery County requirement was implemented in 2015, and in the year after the law went into effect, the average value of a home in the county was $18,000 higher, suggesting that testing and disclosure need not reduce a property's value.[10]

Radon, of course, is not just a US problem. In China, 19% of kindergartens tested in Beijing had levels that exceeded the standard for new construction.[11] In Brazil, the indoor air levels of radon have been found at ten times the threshold set by the World Health Organization.[12] Few individuals around the world are aware of radon's danger, even though it is the second leading cause of lung cancer.[13] Many of these radon-associated cancers are avoidable through simple testing, remediation, and protective barriers that prevent radon's entry into a home or building.

Unfortunately, radon is not the only invisible indoor air pollutant. Although radon does not cause Parkinson's, the villains of Chapter 2, trichloroethylene (TCE) and perchloroethylene (PCE), can also evaporate from contaminated soil and water and invade the indoor air of homes, schools, and offices. They can also cause exposure at work.

Despite the risks, these exposures and their link to Parkinson's have been little studied (see **Skeptics' Corner**). But the absence of evidence is not necessarily evidence of absence.[14] It just means we need to look hard, sometimes very hard, to find the truth.

SKEPTICS' CORNER: **ABSENCE OF EVIDENCE**

Our understanding of the genetics of Parkinson's disease has soared since the identification of the first genetic cause in 1997. The same cannot be said of the environmental causes. Even though environmental factors are the principal causes of Parkinson's, six times as

many papers have been published on the genetics of the disease
(**Figure 1**).[15]

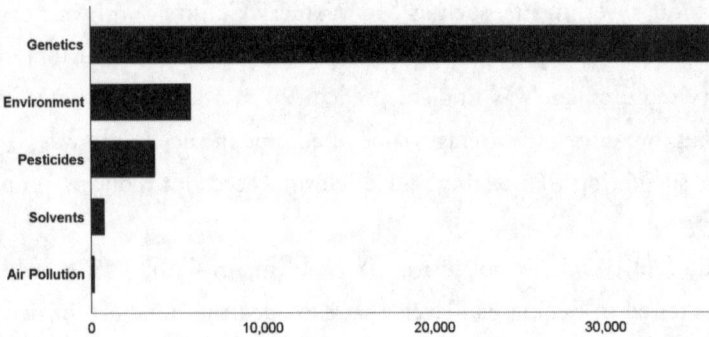

Figure 1. Publications on Parkinson's disease and various topics,
1953–2024.[16]

For TCE and Parkinson's disease, the situation is even worse.
According to the US National Library of Medicine's PubMed database, a grand total of forty-two papers have been published on the
topic. Four times as many papers are published on the genetics of
Parkinson's disease *per month* as have been published on TCE and
Parkinson's in over fifty years. (The situation for PCE and Parkinson's is even worse, with just six total papers published.) This is a failure of funders, scientists, and science.

The result is that many researchers in the field are deeply skep-
tical of both the environmental contributions to Parkinson's in general and the effect of TCE in particular. A reviewer of one of Ray's
recent grants asked, if TCE is such an important factor in Parkinson's, why hasn't anyone heard about it? Indeed, neither Ray nor
Michael, despite their extensive training, knew about the chemical
and its link to Parkinson's until Dr. Caroline Tanner introduced Ray
to the chemical and the Camp Lejeune story during his sabbatical
around 2017.

This knowledge gap is addressable. But doing so will require
both an increase in funding and a change—or, at a minimum, an

expansion—of priorities.[17] Science has done an incredible job of advancing our understanding of the genetics of Parkinson's. It is time it does the same for its likely environmental causes, especially TCE and PCE.

DRY CLEANING STRIKES AGAIN

With the large number of white-collar workers in Rochester, New York, dry cleaning was in high demand there in the 1980s and 1990s. For over forty years, a large downtown dry cleaner sought to meet this burgeoning demand. The problem was how to get rid of all of the chemicals that it was using. Rather than discard the chemicals off-site, the dry cleaner apparently opted to create an open pit in the basement of its downtown processing site where it would pour the used solvents into a "dry well." A dry well is a simple hole dug into the ground for the purpose of disposing of unwanted liquids. However, chemicals, like TCE and PCE, did not all stay in this well. Instead, they contaminated the soil and then made their way down to the groundwater, from which they could evaporate, like radon, and enter nearby buildings.

The dry cleaner was right in the midst of downtown Rochester.[18] Across the street was a large plaza, home to the country's first indoor mall. In a city where seasonal snowfall can begin on Halloween and continue until Mother's Day, an indoor shopping mall was a great idea. In addition to a wide array of stores, the mall area included an eighteen-story building with a hotel, restaurants, and high-end offices for accountants, consultants, and attorneys. A three-story underground garage was also constructed (**Figure 2**).

Among the many who worked in the building was ambitious twenty-six-year-old attorney Dan Kinel. Born and raised in Rochester, Dan had taken a job in New York City after graduating from law school but was excited to return to his hometown to practice law, close to family and friends. He joined one of the city's top firms and focused his practice on corporate finance and securities law. The expectations were high, and he worked long hours, sometimes seven days per week, on stock offerings, mergers

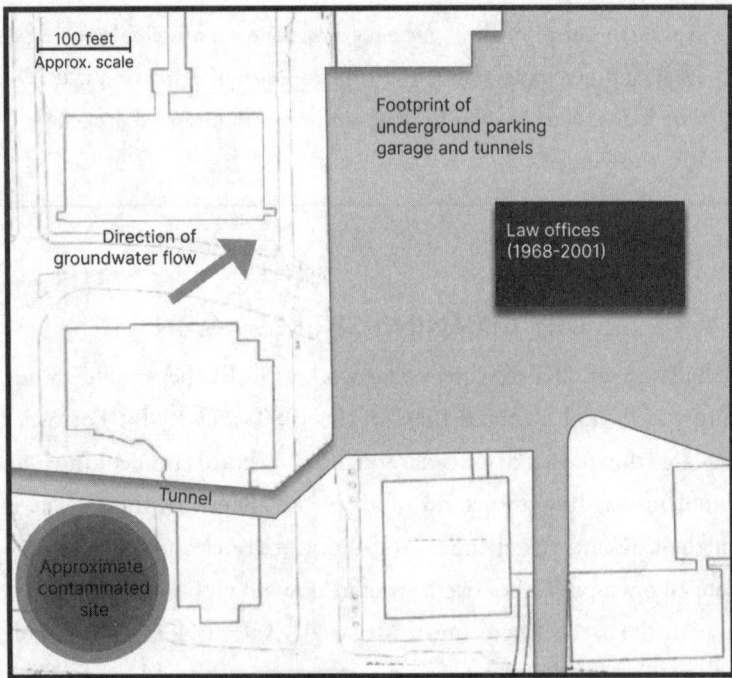

Figure 2. Map of contaminated dry-cleaning site and office building.[18]

and acquisitions, and financings of all kinds. He was often the first in the office, located on the building's seventh floor, and usually one of the last to leave. He parked in the underground garage's lowest level, which, like many garages, had poor ventilation. Dan's hard work paid off. After just seven years, he was made a partner in the firm.

Unbeknownst to Dan and his colleagues, the chemicals from the dry cleaner had likely seeped toward them. In 1992, a medical device company was looking to build a new downtown headquarters in Rochester at the same location where the dry cleaner had long operated. As part of the planning process, the company requested an environmental inspection, which revealed that the soil and likely the underlying groundwater had been contaminated with extremely high levels of TCE, PCE, and other dry-cleaning chemicals.[18]

The City of Rochester embarked on a lengthy, multi-million-dollar cleanup that included excavation of thousands of tons of polluted soil and hundreds of gallons of TCE and PCE. Unfortunately, toxic chemicals don't obey property boundaries, and the contamination almost certainly did not stop at the border of the new corporate headquarters. It likely extended under the ground, and the chemicals may have entered the indoor air of the building where Dan worked, along with the garage where many others parked their cars to work, shop, or visit.

TCE and PCE can evaporate from contaminated soil and water and enter people's homes, schools, and workplaces through cracks in the floor and foundation, gaps for utility lines, or other openings. The migration of gaseous chemicals from underground sources into buildings, known as vapor intrusion (**Figure 3**), happened to the Watras home in Pennsylvania in the 1980s.[19]

Once they enter the groundwater, these chemicals can also form underground rivers, or "plumes," concentrated areas of liquid contaminants that can migrate with the groundwater sometimes a mile or more from the original source. After traveling underground, these volatile chemicals can then make their way to the surface, enter buildings, and be "breathed in" by their

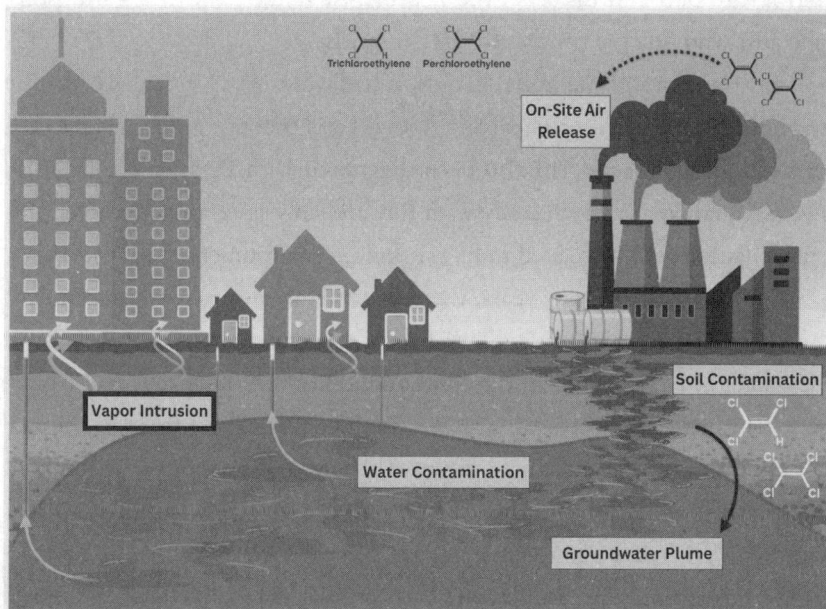

Figure 3. Model of vapor intrusion due to soil or water contamination from TCE and PCE.[18,20]

occupants.[19,21] In most cases, residents or workers are unaware that they may be inhaling dangerous chemicals daily for months or years.

Dan worked in the tower with the indoor shopping mall for six years before moving to a new space in 2001. Many of his colleagues worked there for decades. In 2013, Dan started experiencing a frozen left shoulder and then back problems. He went to a physical therapist, and while completing the prescribed exercises, he noticed that the left side of his body did not respond the same way as his right. Shortly thereafter, he developed a small tremor in his left pinky finger.

His concerned primary care physician advised him to see a neurologist as soon as possible. At his neurologist visit, after a quick exam, Dan, forty-three, was found to have the symptoms of Parkinson's. However, he, like the Air Force physicians Jana Reed and Sara Whittingham, thought he was "much too young" to have the disease. The general neurologist left the examination room to consult a colleague while Dan and his wife sat shell-shocked. They thought of how the disease would affect them and their two young sons, who were then only ten and eight. After what seemed like an eternity to Dan and his wife, the neurologist returned with a Parkinson's specialist who quickly confirmed the diagnosis.

After the shock of the initial diagnosis had worn off, Dan realized that he was not the only person in his law firm who was becoming sick. He recalled former colleagues who had also been diagnosed with Parkinson's. In 2019, he embarked on a research study with Ray and colleagues to determine if his health issues could be related to his workplace environment.[18]

Over the course of four years, the research team assessed seventy-nine of the eighty-two law partners at Dan's firm who worked for at least one year in the office tower next door to the contamination.[18] Of the seventy-nine partners, four had Parkinson's, and fifteen had a cancer related to TCE (**Figure 4**). Eighteen of the seventy-nine partners had died. Even more disturbing, of the fifteen for whom health records existed, eleven (73%) had died with at least one TCE-related condition.

The proportion with Parkinson's was higher than expected based on age and sex, and the percentage with a TCE-related cancer was three times higher than in a comparison group of attorneys who were not partners in

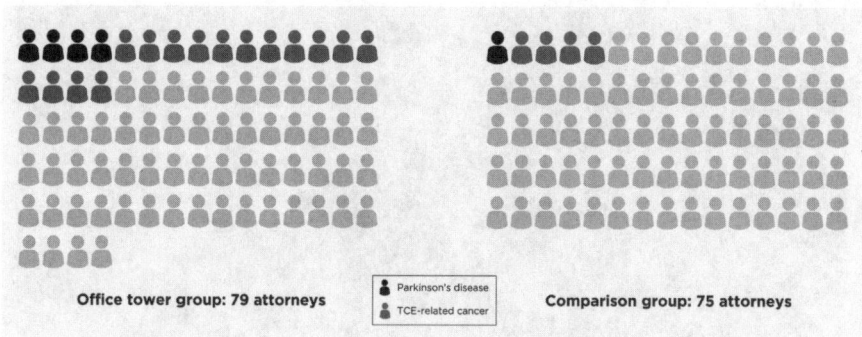

Figure 4. Medical conditions in office tower group versus a comparison group of attorneys.

the firm.[18] While not definitive, the results were concerning for the role TCE and PCE may have been playing in the health of Dan and his peers. According to Dan, "It was a running joke among my former colleagues that something in the former building was making people sick. Unfortunately, it was likely not a joke. I now know that my Parkinson's disease was probably entirely preventable. It makes me angry that we can prevent people from becoming sick, disabled, and dying, and we don't do anything about it."

Last year, Dan had deep brain stimulation surgery to help reduce the fluctuations in his symptoms. Due to the relentless progression, Dan has also retired from his work as an attorney. He remains dedicated to finding and eliminating the root causes of Parkinson's.

Following the study, Dan has helped his colleagues identify and map out other sites in Rochester contaminated by TCE, PCE, or both. It turns out that in Monroe County, where Rochester is located, there are over one hundred sites contaminated with at least one of the dry-cleaning and degreasing chemicals (Figure 5). Some of these sites are former dry-cleaning stores, others are small manufacturing facilities, and a few are large industrial sites.

Dan says, "My hope is that this research is building a foundation that allows us to keep future generations from suffering from terrible diseases like Parkinson's and cancer. I have had Parkinson's disease for eleven years, and it is too late for me. I don't expect a cure for my disease. But it is not too late for my children and grandchildren. Parkinson's disease and many forms of cancer are likely entirely preventable. We have to reduce and limit

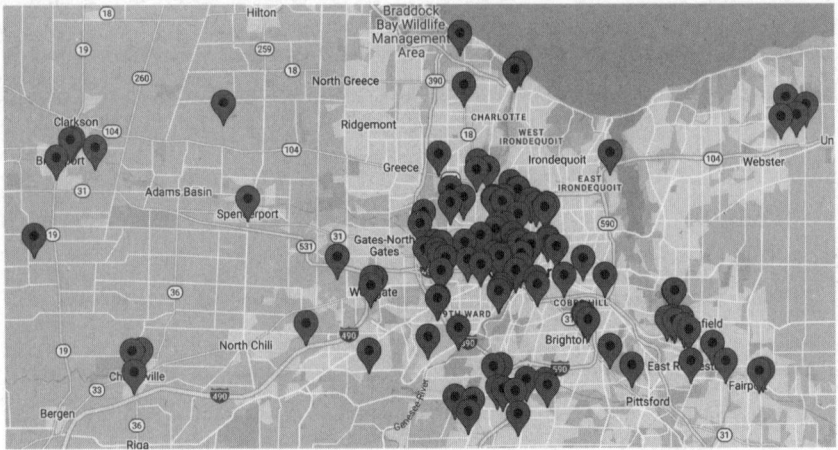

Figure 5. Map of sites contaminated with TCE, PCE, or both in Monroe County, New York, based on analysis of data from the New York Department of Environmental Conservation.[22]

the exposure of people to dangerous chemicals like TCE and PCE. If we do so, we can create a world without Parkinson's disease. We just have to have the will."

THE SMELL OF PERCHLOROETHYLENE

After World War II, Samuel Toth wanted to expand his father's dry-cleaning business from Syracuse, New York. So he opened Toth's 3 Hour Laundry about ninety miles west in downtown Rochester. The laundry was located across a small city park, just blocks away from the large dry cleaner site that may have caused Dan's Parkinson's disease. There, Toth created a drive-through service, not for hamburgers and fries but for clothes. Busy commuters dropped off their dirty laundry as they drove into the bustling city that was home to the headquarters of corporate behemoths, including Eastman Kodak, Bausch & Lomb, and Xerox. On their way home, these working individuals could pick up their crisp, clean clothes.

Sammy, as he was known to his friends and colleagues, was an honest businessman with high integrity. The large family had always been very involved in the community, and Sammy officiated hockey games for the local professional team and was even inducted into the Rochester War

Memorial Hockey Hall of Fame. He had no idea that the chemicals he was using at work were toxic.

Like many cleaners in the United States, the laundry business was a family affair. Sammy and his wife had six children, all of whom were involved in the business. Growing up, the two eldest children, Dave and Patti, would accompany their mother to the dry cleaners. They were there when their mom was pregnant, when she nursed, and when they came home from college to earn some spending money. As children, they would "crawl all over the floor" and hide in the large bins of dirty clothes. As they grew up, they would help make hangers and fold laundry. As teenagers, they would help manage the drive-through window. According to Patti, "We loved it there."

PCE was the cleaning agent of choice at Toth's 3 Hour Laundry. Dave recalls, "I loved the smell of perchloroethylene." The sweet-smelling chemical was used not only in dry cleaning but also to clean machine grease at home. An extra bottle of the liquid was kept at the Toth house to clean spots off clothing.

After twelve years serving the community, the Toth family business left Rochester. They expanded to cleaning sports teams' uniforms, and eventually the family left dry cleaning altogether. The Toth family now sells scoreboards, video displays, and sound systems to professional and amateur sports teams in western New York.

Even though the business changed, the likely effects of PCE were lasting for the two oldest Toth children. In 2011, Dave was diagnosed with Parkinson's. Two years later, Patti followed with the same diagnosis. While determining the exact cause of their Parkinson's is not currently possible, their early and likely extensive exposure to PCE as children and teenagers is deeply problematic. One small Danish study suggested that compared to other workers, women who worked in laundry and dry cleaning had a *fifteen times* higher risk of Parkinson's.[23] No other occupation examined had such a high risk.

Today, Dave lives in Victor, New York, where he enjoys mentoring young men in their spiritual journeys. He still works part-time for a technology company that measures the nutritional contents of many food products, babysits his grandchildren, and, like the anesthesiologist Sara, bikes a lot. "I love riding a bike because all my symptoms go away when I do." He is trying to find the right combination of medications to keep his symptoms at bay and is considering deep brain stimulation surgery.

Patti, who had deep brain stimulation a year ago, lives in Dillon, Colorado, and recently wrote a book titled *Chronic Hope* to help individuals who are hurt, convalescing, or simply in need of encouragement. She is also an ambassador for the Davis Phinney Foundation and enjoys skiing, biking, hiking, and spending time with her family. Both Dave and Patti remember their childhood fondly, but they are saddened that their health was likely harmed by a dangerous chemical used in the family business.

Their father, who spent the most time of anyone in the family working with PCE, was never diagnosed with Parkinson's. However, before he died in 2021, his family noticed that he had tremors that were increasingly affecting his whole body. In the last years of his life, he had trouble finding the right word or replying quickly in conversations. Eventually, the previously gregarious Sammy Toth could not say more than a word or two.

AT THE CORNER OF HEALTH AND HAPPINESS

After several years of investigating TCE's role in Parkinson's, Ray began thinking that the chemical might be everywhere. He thought of the least likely place to be contaminated: Newport Beach, California. So Ray, who went to high school in the beautiful coastal town, googled "trichloroethylene + Newport Beach." What he found shocked him. Not only was there a contaminated site in the wealthy city, but it was just a quarter mile away from his alma mater.

With its year-round sunny skies, strong universities, and entrepreneurial spirit, Southern California has long been a major hub of the aerospace industry. During World War II, the region employed two million aerospace workers and produced 300,000 airplanes. In the 1980s, one-third of the nation's aerospace engineers were located in the region.

In 1957, a large aerospace unit opened in Newport Beach to conduct "research, engineering and manufacture of . . . missile guidance components, rocket motors, and computer hardware."[24] Not surprisingly, the work generated a lot of grease, which was easily and conveniently cleaned with chemicals like TCE and PCE. Following the end of the Cold War in the early 1990s, the aerospace industry shrank, and the plant, located three miles from the Pacific Ocean, closed its doors.[25-28]

When the facility was demolished, TCE and PCE were found in the soil and groundwater, and cleanup efforts began in 1996. The land was subsequently rezoned from industrial to residential use. However, the remediation was not completed, and the pollution did not just disappear. In the early 2000s, TCE and PCE were still found in the soil vapor and shallow groundwater. This did not raise health concerns, at least at that time, perhaps because the water was not being used for drinking. By 2017, the Santa Ana Water Board, however, had become concerned that the TCE and PCE vapors could migrate and enter the air of homes, churches, and other buildings.

Scores of monitoring wells were placed throughout the region (**Figure 6**). In multiple wells, the soil gas levels were elevated, in some cases one hundred times above screening levels. Among the locations near these wells were homes close to the corner of La Salud (Spanish for "health") and La Felicidad ("happiness").

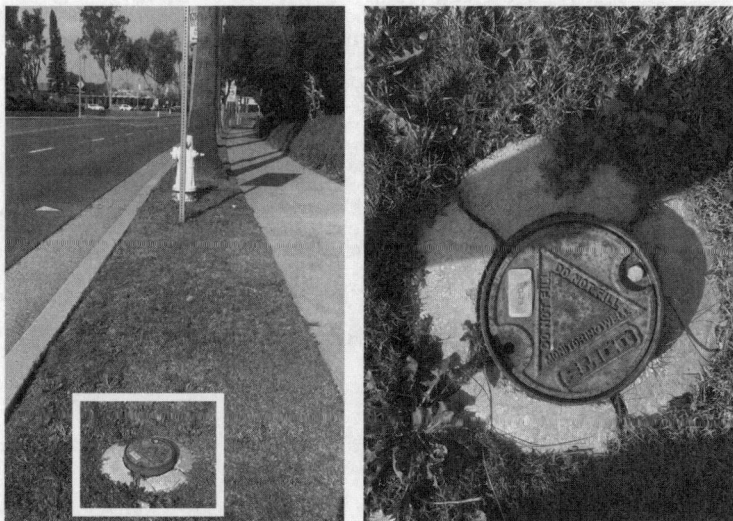

Figure 6. A monitoring well for TCE and PCE near Ray's high school in Newport Beach, California.

Beginning in 2018, the indoor air of homes in Newport Beach was tested, and TCE and PCE were found above screening levels for about a third of the approximately 390 homes sampled.[26] Elevated concentrations were found in bedrooms, living rooms, and kids' playrooms. In twenty-nine of these homes, vapor intrusion was thought to occur "based on property-specific evaluations."[26] The remedy offered to remove these cancer-causing chemicals in the indoor air of people's homes has included both air purifiers and remediation systems.

Despite the extensive contamination, many in the community remain unaware of the risks. Catherine Keligan, a lifelong resident of Newport Beach, learned of the pollution by listening to a podcast featuring Ray as a guest. When her hometown was mentioned, her ears perked up. While she never lived in the area that was formerly occupied by the aerospace company, her friends did. She spent many afternoons and nights there. She also recalled the whispers of cancer in the community that affected numerous parents of her classmates. "It was known that people in that neighborhood got cancer. Everyone thought it was due to a landfill," but the nearest one Ray could locate was miles away.[29]

Today, she sees solutions, such as testing and remediation, as accessible. She says that most residents can readily afford $1,000 or $2,000 to remediate their home, but no one is telling them about breast cancer or Parkinson's. Her fiancé, Harrison Avisto, echoes Catherine's impressions. He recently asked a friend who grew up in the affected neighborhood whether he had heard about the contamination. He said, "Ohhhhhhh, yeahhhhhhhh. Tons of people talked about it, and the soil was tested super often. There were higher levels of chemicals in certain areas, [and] there were tons of cancer cases in the neighborhood." Harrison says, "If this is happening in one of the most beautiful, affluent areas, what does it mean for other areas?"

CONCRETE JUNGLE

TCE and PCE do not have to migrate from contaminated soil or groundwater to enter homes. Sometimes they can come from downstairs.

In the early 1990s, the New York State Department of Health evaluated the concentration of PCE in the indoor air of apartments over ground-level dry cleaners in Albany and New York City. In thirty-nine (98%) of forty buildings tested, the level of PCE in the indoor air was found to be unsafe.[30] In some cases, the concentration of PCE was more than *1,000* times the safety threshold.[30] In a 1992 letter to the EPA, the New York State Department of Health wrote, "[Our] data suggest that even state of the art equipment may not adequately protect the many people living in apartments adjacent to dry cleaners."[30]

Many New Yorkers live near one of the more than 1,000 dry cleaners in the state.[31] In the 1990s, about five hundred dry cleaners were located in residential buildings in New York City alone.[30] A study performed during this time found that twenty-four (83%) of twenty-nine apartments tested had elevated levels of PCE in the indoor air (**Figure 7**). The researchers thought that the exposure posed "a danger to the health of the residents."[30] Because PCE's (and TCE's) contribution to Parkinson's may not appear for decades, that risk may only become apparent in the future. Unfortunately, residents are unaware of that risk. The researchers wrote, "As far as we know, however, no responsible government agency has systematically sought to identify people exposed to high [PCE] levels in apartments above dry cleaners, to inform them of the potential hazards of [PCE], or to determine their exposure and to evaluate their health."[30]

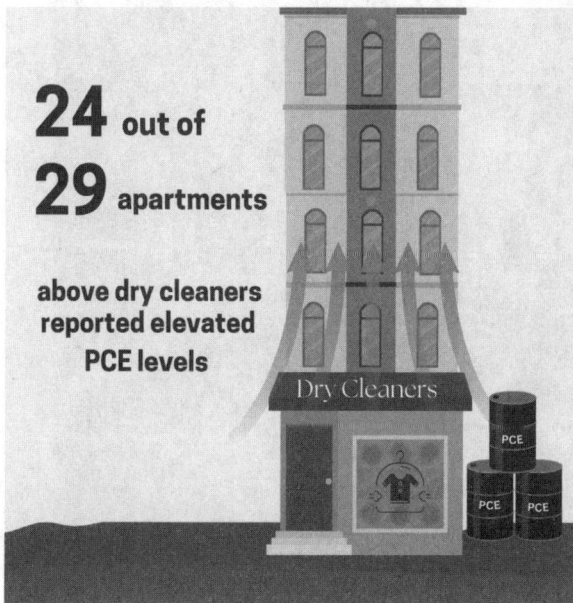

24 out of
29 apartments

above dry cleaners reported elevated PCE levels

Figure 7. Apartments above dry cleaners had elevated levels of PCE in the indoor air.[30]

Unfortunately, the exposure did not end in the 1990s. Between 2001 and 2003, researchers assessed sixty-five apartments across twenty-four buildings where PCE was used on site. A quarter of the apartments sampled had unsafe levels of PCE in their indoor air. "Moreover, the mean [average] indoor air [PCE] levels in minority neighborhoods . . . were four times higher than in nonminority households . . . and were > 10 times higher in low-income neighborhoods . . . than in higher income neighborhoods."[32] In 2020, New York became the second state (after Minnesota) to ban TCE and prohibited dry cleaners from using PCE in residential buildings.[31,33]

Unfortunately, these bans do not affect the thousands of already contaminated sites in New York, the tens of thousands nationally, and the hundreds of thousands globally. These contaminations persist, despite the now well-documented risks. In 2021, toxic fumes were found at a popular shuffleboard club in New York City.[34] Concentrations under the building were more than *10,000 times* those allowed by the state.[34] According to a New York Public Radio website, the *Gothamist*, "Thousands of people have

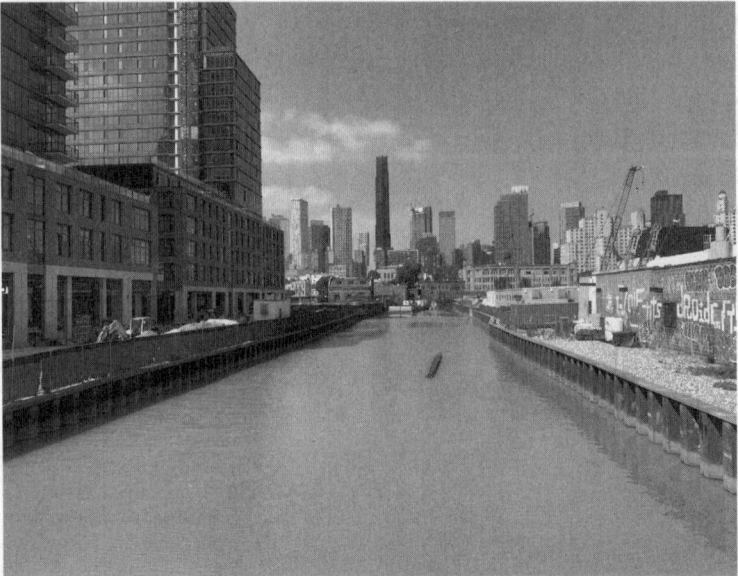

Figure 8. Picture of the Gowanus Canal in Brooklyn, late 2020.[34]

likely been exposed to trichloroethylene" at the popular club, which was located at a former contaminated "brownfield" site.[34]

The contamination, known as "black mayonnaise" by local residents, in the area includes the Gowanus Canal, which runs through Brooklyn (**Figure 8**).[34] Over one hundred blocks in the city are now under investigation. In 2024, buildings in the area were reported to have TCE in the indoor air that was 450 times the level deemed to be safe. In another area that was home to twenty-two businesses, the TCE concentration was more than 250 times higher than the safety threshold.

As with many of these contaminated sites, most people were unaware of the dangers. A local real estate agent said, "I am shocked by how little the [contaminated] site comes up in Gowanus. I'm usually the one who brings it up, when people start talking about gardening—this is the soil you can't plant anything in if you want to eat it."[35] One advocate said, "There's no signage anywhere—no warnings" of the contamination.[36]

In 2010, the Gowanus area was declared a Superfund site, among the most toxic in the country.[35] These roughly 1,300 Superfund sites litter the United States. Twenty million people live within a mile—the distance many underground plumes of TCE or PCE often travel—of a Superfund site.[37-39] As we have seen, these sites are just the tip of an enormous iceberg of polluted locations nationally and globally.[40]

The United States does not have the monopoly on dry-cleaning-related air contaminants. Apartments in Mülheim in western Germany have had high levels of PCE and TCE in their indoor air, and residents have measurable levels of TCE in their blood.[40,41] Grocery stores may also be at risk. TCE and PCE are both excellent degreasers because they can dissolve in fat. Unfortunately, this property is not specific to grease. In German grocery stores located near dry cleaners, PCE has been found in the butter and in the cheese.[40]

SAFE AT WORK?

Not surprisingly, degreasing is important in the automobile industry. A physician at Chrysler Corporation was worried about the health effects of the miraculous degreaser TCE.[42] Dr. Carey McCord from Cincinnati, Ohio, recognized the value of the compound for the automobile industry but was worried about its "toxic nature." He applied TCE to the skin of rabbits. They died in weeks, if not days. He had rabbits inhale TCE. They died in days, if not hours.

He concluded, "Any manufacturer contemplating the use of trichloroethylene may find in it many desirable qualities. Too, in the absence of closed systems of operation, he may find in this solvent the source of disaster for exposed workmen." The results of his experiments were published in the *Journal of the American Medical Association* in *1932.*[42]

That prescient warning has largely gone unheeded. The first known case report linking TCE to Parkinson's did not occur until 1969. A fifty-nine-year-old man in Germany had worked with TCE for over thirty years and later developed symptoms of the disease. Following his death, an autopsy revealed that his brain had lost dopamine-producing nerve cells in the substantia nigra, the part of the brain affected by Parkinson's.[43] Thirty years later, a French woman worked for months as a house cleaner in a poorly ventilated room with TCE, followed by six years in an even smaller room in the plastics industry with TCE and other volatile compounds. Three years later, she was diagnosed with Parkinson's at age thirty-seven.[44]

In 2008, investigators at the University of Kentucky were enrolling an individual with Parkinson's in a clinical trial when the prospective participant mentioned that his factory coworkers in Berea, Kentucky, were also affected. Led by Dr. Don Gash, researchers embarked on an unprecedented effort to evaluate at least thirty individuals who worked at the small plant, which produced metal gauges and other instruments.[45,46]

For twenty-five years, the forty-nine-year-old research participant had worked with TCE to degrease metal parts. He and a colleague would dump metal parts into a large open vat of TCE in an effort to clean them. They wore no protective gear—no gloves, no masks, no apron. They then passed the cleaned parts by hand to a fifty-six-year-old woman who would dry them. All three developed Parkinson's.[45]

The researchers evaluated other individuals who worked on the same factory floor. They found, "Coworkers more distant from the trichloroethylene source, receiving chronic respiratory exposure, displayed many features of parkinsonism, including significant motor slowing."[45]

As with certain pesticides, numerous studies by investigators around the world have demonstrated that laboratory animals, when fed TCE, develop the symptoms and pathology of Parkinson's.[47,48] Given that most human exposure to TCE is from inhalation, Dr. Briana De Miranda at the University of Alabama at Birmingham wanted to know what would happen if mice and rats inhaled the chemical.[48]

She found that compared to laboratory animals breathing in filtered room air, those breathing in TCE for eight weeks lost 50% of their dopamine-producing nerve cells. In addition, they walked slower. The inhaled dose was also lower than the dose fed in previous laboratory studies. To De Miranda and her colleagues, the results suggested "that TCE inhalation caused potent dopaminergic neurotoxicity at much lower doses than previously examined, providing a mechanistic link between TCE exposure and [Parkinson's disease] risk."[48]

These exposures through work are common. In the 1970s, an estimated ten million Americans worked with TCE or similar chemicals. In the United Kingdom, one in twelve workers may have been exposed to TCE through

Example occupations where trichloroethylene exposure may occur

Aircraft maintenance workers	Painters
Automotive factory workers	Pesticide manufacturers
Communications equipment repairers	Pharmaceutical manufacturing workers
Computer specialists	Printers
Corrosive control technicians	Radar technicians
Distillery workers	Refrigerant manufacturers
Dry cleaners	Resin workers
Electronics manufacturers	Rubber cementers
Embalmers	Sewerage workers
Food manufacturers	Shoe makers
Insecticide manufacturers	Silk screeners
Jet engine mechanics	Systems technicians
Leather manufacturers	Taxidermists
Machinery installation workers	Textile and fabric cleaners
Mechanics	Textile manufacturers
Metal treatment workers	Tobacco denicotinizers
Missile technicians	Varnish workers
Nautical equipment workers	Waste treatment workers
Oil processors	Weapons specialists

Table 1. Example occupations where exposure to TCE may occur. Modified from the source.[47]

their jobs.[49-51] The list of occupations with potential exposure to TCE is long (**Table 1**) and includes everyone from painters and printers to mechanics and embalmers. One rocket scientist said that he was "swimming" in it.[47]

A LIKELY SOURCE

Among those who were likely exposed to TCE are Jana Reed and Sara Whittingham. In his effort to find a likely cause for their Parkinson's, Ray emailed them asking where they served while in the Air Force. What he found surprised them all.

Year	Role	Base	TCE Contamination?
1991–1995	Cadet	US Air Force Academy	
1996, 1998	Active duty	Brooks Air Force Base	✓
1997	Active duty	Travis Air Force Base	✓
1998	Active duty	Wright-Patterson Air Force Base	✓
2002–2006	Emergency physician	Andrews Air Force Base	
2006–2007	Emergency physician	Bitburg Air Force Base	✓
2007–2011	Emergency physician	Ramstein Air Force Base	
2009–2010	Emergency physician	Forward Operating Base Lightning, Afghanistan	
2011–2012	Emergency physician, reservist	Wright-Patterson Air Force Base	✓
2012–2016	Flight surgeon, reservist	Wright-Patterson Air Force Base	✓
2016–Present	Flight surgeon, Air National Guard	Moffett Air National Guard Base	✓

Table 2. List of bases where Dr. Jana Reed served.

Year	Role	Base	TCE Contamination?
1992-1996	Cadet	US Air Force Academy	
1996-1998	Aircraft maintenance officer	Kelly Air Force Base	✓
2002-2003	Intern	Lackland Air Force Base	
2003	Aerospace Medicine School	Brooks Air Force Base	✓
2003-2004	Flight surgeon	Kunsan Air Force Base	
2004	Medical member	Osan Air Force Base	✓
2004-2005	Flight surgeon	Ramstein Air Force Base	
2004-2006	Flight surgeon	Travis Air Force Base	✓
2009-2011	Anesthesiologist	Nellis Air Force Base	✓
2010-2011	Anesthesiologist	Bagram Air Force Base	
2011-2019	Flight surgeon, reservist	Hills Air Force Base	✓

Table 3. List of bases where Dr. Sara Whittingham served.

Since enrolling at the US Air Force Academy in the early 1990s, Jana has served at eight different Air Force bases. Five have been contaminated with TCE (**Table 2**).[52-59] For Sara, the story was no better. She has served at ten Air Force bases, and six were polluted with TCE (**Table 3**).[52,53,60-64]

Before applying to medical school, Sara served as an aircraft maintenance officer at Kelly Air Force Base in San Antonio, Texas. There she oversaw the cleaning and degreasing of jet engines that were flown from all over the world to the base for periodic maintenance. Her small office was located above where much of the degreasing was done. The base and the surrounding civilian community were contaminated with TCE, and cries of cancer and birth defects came from those living near the base.[60] The experience, twenty years before she developed symptoms of Parkinson's, was not Sara's favorite and led her to pursue a career in medicine.

In the past two chapters, we have seen how two simple chemicals, which are ingested and inhaled, have likely contributed to Parkinson's at military bases and in countless communities, office towers, dry cleaners, city apartments, worksites, and even hospitals. In a small twin study, the chemicals are associated with a 500% increased risk of the disease.[65] In a large observational study, the increased risk was 70%.[66] TCE mimics the biological effects of the most common genetic cause of the disease.[20] The chemicals damage the energy-producing parts of cells that we know are impaired in Parkinson's.[45] In animal studies, TCE leads to loss of dopamine-producing neurons and parkinsonian features.[47] The chemicals are ubiquitous, yet in the vast majority of cases, the individuals never knew of their exposure.[49,66]

In the United States, TCE and PCE may be the most important causes of Parkinson's disease. Certain pesticides are likely the dominant factors in rural areas. But in more populous suburban and urban areas, TCE and PCE likely reign.

Additional investigations into TCE and PCE and Parkinson's are long overdue.[18] In the interim, we can take several actions to lower our risk. First, we can ban TCE and PCE, as the United States has recently done. However, as of January 2025, that ban has been "frozen" or delayed.[67] The use of TCE in the United States and globally must end. Companies already advertise safer alternatives, and many countries use them.[68–71] No one needs to get Parkinson's so that our clothes don't shrink.

Second, individuals who work with the chemicals or spend time near contaminated sites have the right to know the risks. Only with such knowledge can individuals take actions to protect the health of their colleagues, their families, and themselves. Third, testing of water (especially wells) and indoor air for these chemicals should become commonplace. Such testing for lead and radon has had enormous health benefits and protected millions from their deleterious effects. The same should happen for TCE and PCE.

Fourth, the risks should be mitigated. Protective equipment for workers, carbon filters for water, and home mitigation systems are all far more affordable than Parkinson's disease and cancer.[72,73]

Finally, contaminated sites need to be cleaned up. Of all the recommendations, this is the only one that requires substantial resources. However, there are parties responsible for this pollution. They—not members of the military, workers, residents, and children—should pay the price.

4

THE BRAIN'S FRONT DOOR

For as long as humans have burned things, . . .
air pollution has been a killer.

—Tim Smedly, author of *Clearing the Air*

In Mexico City, children used to color the sky brown. Birds fell dead mid-flight. In 1992, the country's capital had the world's worst air pollution.[1]

The population of the largest city in North America is young. As was Dr. Lilian Calderón-Garcidueñas, who started at Mexico City's National University Medical School at age fifteen. She was worried about the effects of air pollution on the country's youth. Of its twenty million inhabitants, eight million are children.[2] So, she did something unprecedented. Under the microscope, she looked at the brains of 203 individuals in Mexico City who had died prematurely, usually from car accidents or gun violence. The average age of the cohort was twenty-five years. The oldest was forty, and the youngest was an eleven-month-old baby.[3-5]

Of course, none of these young individuals had been diagnosed with Parkinson's disease. They were too young (see **Skeptics' Corner**). However, in

their brains, Calderón-Garciduañas found Parkinson's pathology. In nearly
one-quarter of the individuals under twenty-five, she found the misfolded
alpha-synuclein protein that marks the disease. She found it in the brain's
smell center, the substantia nigra, and other areas known to be affected by
Parkinson's.[4] She also found the pathology of Alzheimer's in 99% of the brains
she examined. The harmful effects of air pollution on the brain begin early.[5]

SKEPTICS' CORNER: **LONGEVITY**

Perhaps the greatest accomplishment of the twentieth century was
a thirty-year increase in life expectancy in almost every part of the
world.[6] And in most cases, a long life is a prerequisite for Parkinson's. The disease is very rare before age forty, after which the number of new cases, or incidence, begins to triple with every passing
decade (see **Figure 1**).[7]

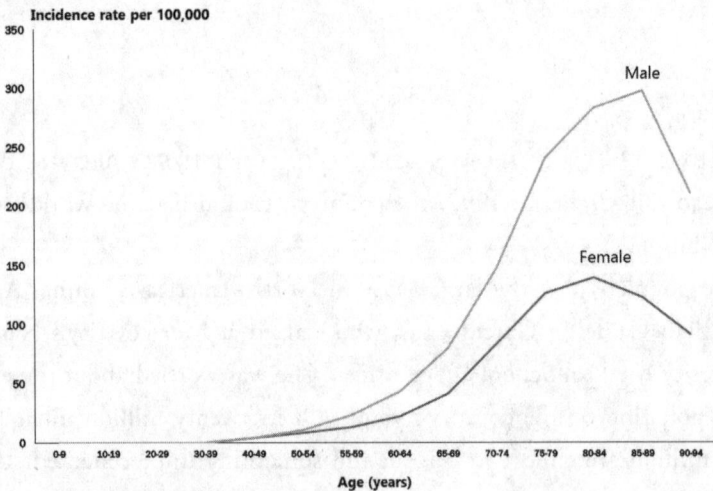

Figure 1. The number of new cases of Parkinson's disease by age in the
United Kingdom.

Without longevity, the disease would rarely become apparent. Dr.
Calderón-Garciduañas's research shows us that the initial pathology of
the disease is present long before symptoms appear. It takes years or

decades for the misfolded alpha-synuclein to spread and for symptoms to emerge. For example, Brian Grant was likely exposed to trichloroethylene at Camp Lejeune when he was just three years old. He did not develop symptoms of the disease until thirty years later.

However, longevity alone is insufficient to explain the rise of Parkinson's. Parkinson's is one of the world's fastest-growing brain diseases even after adjusting for age.[8] By contrast, the global burden of Alzheimer's has more than doubled in the past generation but, after controlling for aging populations, its prevalence has changed little.[8] In addition, there is hardly any evidence that aging alone causes Parkinson's. Animals in the laboratory do not spontaneously develop the disease unless their genes are manipulated or they are exposed to toxic chemicals.

Parkinson's is also not the only disease that is rare before age forty and triples every decade thereafter. Lung cancer is the same (**Figure 2**).[7] Aging does not cause lung cancer. Smoking does. In fact, lung cancer was "a once-in-a-lifetime oddity" before the advent of cigarettes.[9] Even today, over 80% of lung cancer is due to smoking.[10] For most: no smoking, no lung cancer.

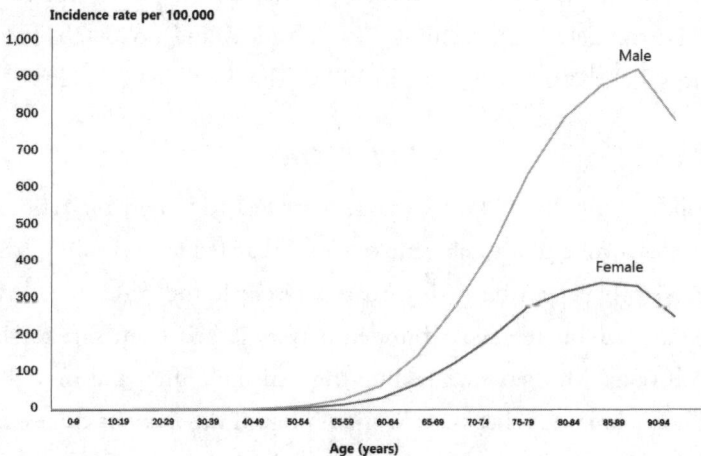

Figure 2. The number of new cases of lung cancer by age in the United Kingdom.

The same is likely true for most Parkinson's: no chemical exposure, no Parkinson's.

The origin of the pathology that Calderón-Garcidueñas, now a physician, toxicologist, and professor at the University of Montana, observed may be the brain's smell center, called the olfactory bulb. In toddlers, she has identified signatures of Parkinson's in this network of nerve cells located just above the nose and behind our eyes. When she looked at the brains of fifty-seven individuals who died before age twenty, two-thirds had diseased nerve cells with the abnormal alpha-synuclein protein.[3] Some of the nerve cells had already died. Her findings are consistent with other studies that have found Parkinson's pathology in the smell centers of over 90% of individuals with the disease.[11]

Consistent with this damage to the smell center, teens and young adults from Mexico City score low on tests of smell.[3] Loss of smell precedes Parkinson's symptoms in up to 90% of young individuals with the disease.[12,13] Based on her results, Calderón-Garcidueñas advocates for actions to protect children, teens, and young adults. She wrote, "Pollution control should be prioritized. . . . Preventive medicine ought to be our goal and we must consider the ramifications of lifelong air pollutant exposures on children and we must do what we can to protect them."[3]

Air pollution has many sources, and for Mexico City, it was the automobile.[1,14] Fortunately, with technological advances and policy changes, the city's air is 75% better than it was in 1992.[1] The skies are again blue.

AN LA STORY

On Monday, July 26, 1943, two years after Pearl Harbor, the residents of Los Angeles awoke to a thick, smoky cloud that reduced visibility to three city blocks. Their eyes burned, throats scratched, and noses recoiled. On the streets, bedlam reigned. "Blinded drivers jerked from side to side to avoid collisions. Mothers snatched up frightened children and moved them into ornate lobbies for shelter."[15] Workers "found the noxious fumes almost unbearable," and judges sought to close their courtrooms.[15] However, the culprit behind this chaos was not the Japanese army but Californians' newest love—the automobile.[16]

Los Angeles was not always dominated by the car.[17] In fact, electric streetcars once connected the sunny city through 1,500 miles of track.[16] However, an alleged conspiracy involving car, tire, and oil companies undermined the electric vehicles and fueled the rise of the automobile.[16,18] In 1915, only 55,000 cars drove the streets; a generation later, there were 1 million.[19]

Gas-fueled cars pollute the air by releasing noxious gases and "particulate matter," which includes soil and dust, soot and smoke. Some particles are big enough to see in the clouds of smog that engulf Los Angeles. These larger particles irritate our eyes and throats but are usually filtered out by nose hairs or coughed out by our lungs.

However, the most dangerous particles are the ones we cannot see. The smallest particulate matter, some thirty times smaller than the width of a hair (**Figure 3**), can bypass our normal filtration systems and be inhaled directly into our lungs. Air pollution is tied to asthma, heart attacks, lung cancer, strokes, and male infertility.[20–22] Dirty air is not only disabling; it's deadly. Air pollution costs each of us, on average, nearly three years of life.[23]

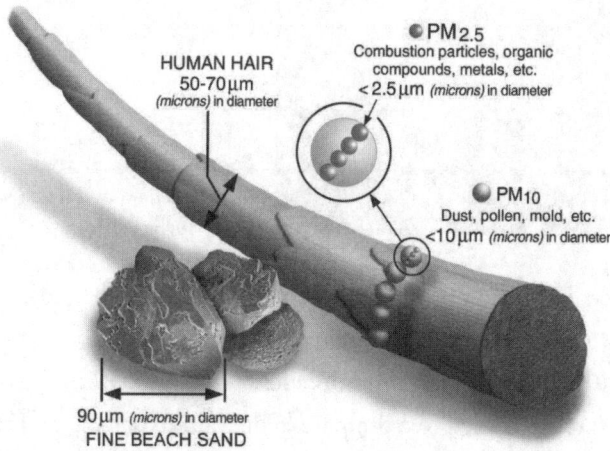

Figure 3. Relative size comparison of particulate matter (PM), fine beach sand, and human hair.[24]

And this loss does not even account for its harmful effects on the brain. The nerves responsible for smell hang down into our upper nasal passages.[25] These nerves, which exit the skull through small holes, provide a path for tiny air particles to enter the brain. Once these particles arrive at the brain's smell center, they can then spread to regions that are responsible for memory or movement.

These small air particles carry dangerous hitchhikers. The unwanted travelers include metals, such as lead from leaded gasoline, platinum from catalytic converters, and iron from brakes. The brains of individuals exposed to air pollution have these metals at levels one hundred times what is considered normal.[26] These metals can damage nerve cells and lead to misfolding of proteins.

The air pollution (**Figure 4**) in Los Angeles would not be addressed until 1967, when Ronald Reagan, California's governor at the time, helped create the California Air Resources Board to set limits on car pollution.[27] California's pioneering efforts eventually led President Richard Nixon, a Southern California native, to sign the Clean Air Act of 1970, which restricted air emissions from factories, steel mills, and cars for the entire country.

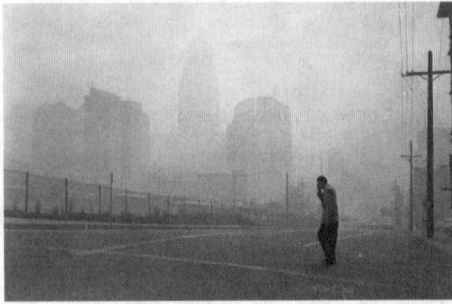

Figure 4. Air quality in Los Angeles in 1955. Photo by *Los Angeles Times* via Getty Images.[28]

With new legislation and reduced emissions, air quality in Los Angeles began improving in the 1980s. The number of smoggy days in Los Angeles decreased 40% over the next three decades.[29] The peak of the Covid-19 pandemic in March 2020 led to a dramatic reduction in driving and the "cleanest air ever recorded."[29] Unfortunately, the fresh air did not last. Six months later, fueled by warm weather and wildfires, Los Angeles experienced its worst smog in nearly thirty years.[30]

THE PARKINSON'S LINK

Today, Los Angeles remains among the country's most polluted cities, and the incidence of Parkinson's in the county is among the highest in the country.[31] Researchers at the University of California, Los Angeles, have demonstrated that traffic-related air pollution in California is associated with an increased risk of Parkinson's.[25,32,33] Similar studies have linked air pollution from cars to Parkinson's across the world from Denmark to Taiwan.[32-35]

In 2023, Drs. Brittany Krzyzanowski, a geographer, and Brad Racette, a neurologist, from the Barrow Neurological Institute in Phoenix conducted a landmark study. They wanted to know if prior exposure to high levels of particulate matter was associated with Parkinson's for the whole country. So they looked at sophisticated maps of air pollution in the United States and linked the data to diagnoses of the disease. They found "a nationwide association" between particulate matter and Parkinson's risk. Those living in areas with typical air pollution levels had a 56% greater risk of developing Parkinson's than individuals breathing in the cleanest air. As **Figure 5** suggests, they found that the risk of Parkinson's was greatest in Southern California and in the Mississippi-Ohio River Valley, where air pollution is among the country's worst. By contrast, those living in the Rocky Mountains enjoy clean air and lower rates of Parkinson's.[36, 37]

Air pollution did not begin with the automobile and did not start in North America. The first area of the world to develop high levels of particulate matter is also the place where Parkinson's was first described.

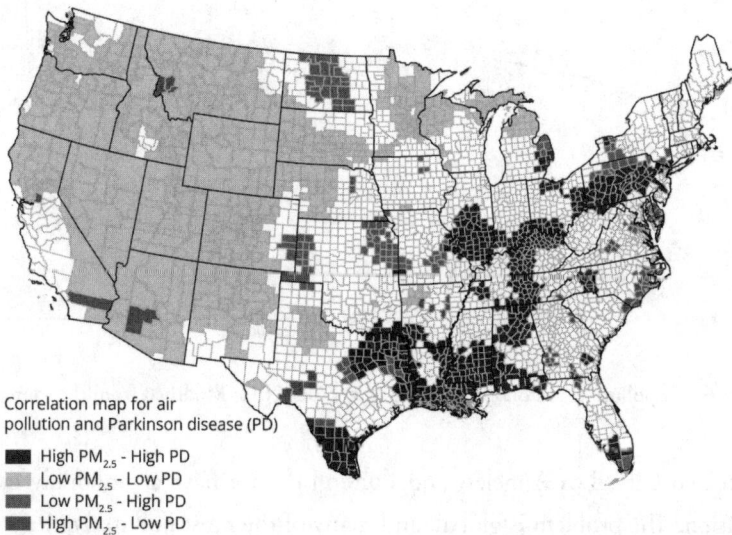

Correlation map for air
pollution and Parkinson disease (PD)

■ High PM$_{2.5}$ - High PD
■ Low PM$_{2.5}$ - Low PD
■ Low PM$_{2.5}$ - High PD
■ High PM$_{2.5}$ - Low PD

Figure 5. Levels of air pollution ("fine particulate matter") in the United States by county, 2000–2016.[36]

PEA SOUP

Air pollution, principally from coal-burning factories, has plagued London since at least the 1600s. In the nineteenth century, London was periodically "plunged into darkness."

There, in the midst of an impenetrable London "fog," Dr. James Parkinson originally described six individuals in his essay.[38] These individuals had an "[involuntary] tremulous motion, with lessened muscular power . . . a propensity to bend the trunk forwards, and to pass from a walking to a running pace."[38] The level of air pollution in 1800 London was actually twice as bad as during the "pea soupers," the euphemism for London's dense air pollution, of the 1950s (**Figure 6**). The air pollution in London two hundred years ago was on par with that in Delhi, India, today. Consistent with the rise in air pollution in London in the nineteenth century, Parkinson's was becoming modestly more common in both the clinic and the morgues.[39–41]

Average concentration of particulate matter in London versus Delhi, 1700-2016

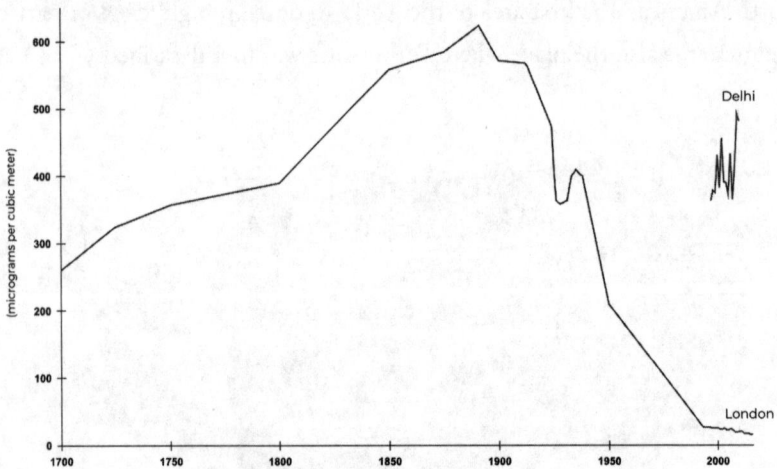

Figure 6. Air pollution in London versus Delhi, 1700–2016. Modified from the source.[42]

Mexico City, Los Angeles, and London do not have a monopoly on air pollution. The problem is global, and many of the most polluted cities in the world are located in Asia (**Figure 7**), where rates of Parkinson's are increasing most rapidly.[43,44]

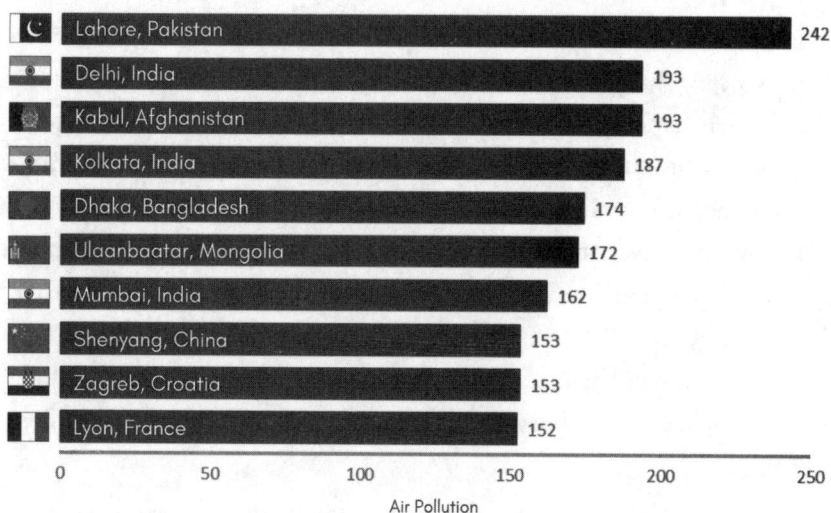

Lahore, Pakistan		242
Delhi, India		193
Kabul, Afghanistan		193
Kolkata, India		187
Dhaka, Bangladesh		174
Ulaanbaatar, Mongolia		172
Mumbai, India		162
Shenyang, China		153
Zagreb, Croatia		153
Lyon, France		152

0   50   100   150   200   250

Air Pollution

Figure 7. The ten most polluted cities in the world by Air Quality Index. Modified from the source.[4]

Cars and coal are far from the only sources of outdoor air pollution. The list is long and includes emissions from power plants, household fuel, shipping, aviation, agriculture, landfills, and mining.[45] The latter may have had the unlikeliest of victims.

THE POPE AND THE QUARRY

When he became pope in 1978 at age fifty-eight, Pope John Paul II was the epitome of health. He hiked, jogged, lifted weights, skied, and swam so much that a newspaper article called him the "keep-fit pope."

But possibly as early as 1991, doctors diagnosed the pontiff with Parkinson's (or a closely related disease).[46] Initially, the pontiff, who was a champion of democracy, was undaunted. In response to his aides encouraging the globe-trotting pope, who visited 129 countries during his papacy, to slow down, he said, "Si crollo, crollo" ("If I collapse, I collapse").[47] And collapse he did. In 1993 he fell and dislocated his shoulder; the next year, he fell and broke his leg.[48]

It was not until 2001 that one of his physicians publicly disclosed his Parkinson's diagnosis.[49] By then, Parkinson's experts were commenting on his drooling, stooped posture, and soft voice.[50] His once warm smile disappeared, and his "face refused to express what was in the heart."[51] By then, "a visibly shaky John Paul II [was] unable to finish [a] speech in Armenia."[52] After thanking an Armenian patriarch for a kind welcome, the pope "slumped in his chair, he drooled, his breathing became audible, and his hands shook uncontrollably. For 22 awkward seconds, the pope seemed to be struggling to recover and read on." Eventually, an Armenian priest stepped up to the microphone and delivered the rest of the speech. Two years later, the pope was, according to British journalist and author of *The Pope in Winter*, John Cornwell, having difficulty identifying close colleagues, including the archbishop of Canterbury, saying after a visit, "[Tell] me, who were those people?"[53]

By 2005, the formerly gregarious pope could no longer speak. Because of his increasing difficulties swallowing, doctors placed a breathing tube into his trachea. On Easter Sunday of that year, he appeared at his apartment window and, according to the Vatican, "in silence, with his right hand, blessed the city and the world."[54] That would be his last public appearance. Days later, the pope developed a bladder infection and died. According to one commentator, Parkinson's had, over fourteen years, "robbed John Paul of all the things that seemed to typify his office and his life."[51]

The roots of that theft may have been planted sixty-five years earlier. In 1940, during World War II, Nazi Germany occupied Poland, and to avoid deportation and concentration camps, all men between fourteen and sixty were required to have a manual labor job.[55] The future pope, then called Karol Wojtyla, was twenty and began working at the Zakrzówek quarry, just outside Kraków in the south of Poland.[56,57] There he broke apart limestone and hauled wheelbarrows full of crushed stone from deep inside the quarry. The temperatures inside the quarry were regularly well below zero. Later, Wojtyla, who had yet to begin studying in a seminary, used explosives to help blast away at the large stone walls.[55] The resulting rocks were used by a chemical company to create soda ash and produce everything from baking soda to glass.

In addition to limestone, the quarry had high concentrations of a metal called manganese, which, when mined, is released into the air.[58] Inhaling manganese can result in Parkinson's disease or a condition very similar to it.[59,60] The neurological toxicity of manganese was first described in 1837 among five individuals who crushed manganese ore in France.[59,61] Since then, numerous descriptions of a similar disorder have been reported among miners, smelters, and welders, all of whom have likely breathed in the toxic metal.[59,62] Chronic exposure to heavy metals, especially manganese, is associated with Parkinson's.[63] One study found that the risk of Parkinson's among miners quadrupled.[64]

Determining and proving the exact cause of Pope John Paul II's parkinsonism would be difficult, if not impossible, but we have clues. The deeper Wojtyla and his fellow laborers mined, the more likely they were to encounter manganese-polluted air. At depths greater than twenty meters, the concentration of manganese in the mine in which he worked increased by tenfold or more.[58] Ventilation was likely limited and air quality likely poor. Generations later, Pope John Paul II would display many of the symptoms caused by manganese exposure, including a stooped posture, impaired balance, falls, a softened voice, diminished facial expression, and drooling.[59]

Today, the Zakrzówek quarry has an entirely new life.[65] In the 1990s, a limestone quarry operator pierced the water table, leading to flooding of the mine. Once a forced labor camp, the quarry is now a park, complete with five enclosed swimming pools, including one for children. Admission to the reservoir is free, and on warm summer afternoons, tourists from all over the world wait for hours to enjoy the idyllic setting and lovely views.[66,67]

Visitors can even go scuba diving and explore the remains of the mine.[65] There they can search for a memorial plaque in Polish that reads, "In this quarry worked physically one of the greatest Poles, late Karol Wojtyla Pope John Paul II—Beneath your care, we give ourselves, the divers."[55]

TOO GREEN?

Like most exercises, golf can be beneficial for individuals with Parkinson's. One small study even found that golf improved performance on a walking test more than tai chi and was more likely to be continued by those with the disease.[68] A 2021 review concluded that "regularly playing golf can lower the risk of falls in . . . older adults with Parkinson's disease and demonstrates the potential to improve quality of life."[69]

However, we've recently had to ask a more ominous question: Could living near a golf course increase the risk of Parkinson's? In 2013, two neurologists thought that question was worthy of investigation after they found that nineteen of twenty-six patients in their cohort with Parkinson's lived within two miles of a golf course. And sixteen of the nineteen lived downwind.[70]

Beginning at age ten, Karl Robb, a tech entrepreneur, lived in suburban Charlotte, North Carolina, right next to the thirteenth hole of a golf course. If it rained, golfers would cross his family's white picket fence and take shelter under their covered porch. As a teenager, Karl was looking for a summer job and joined the golf course's "sod squad." Every morning, he would help redo the greens and repair divots on the course. He liked the camaraderie of the team and the opportunity to play tennis after work.

At age seventeen, Karl's left foot started to twitch. Then he noticed that he dragged his left foot and that the wear on his tennis shoes was uneven. His voice became softer, and family members would tell him to sit straight.

Karl was concerned, and in the era before the internet, he started visiting the library. He read medical books and became convinced that he had a brain tumor. He saw nine different doctors over six years before being diagnosed with Parkinson's at age twenty-three.

Karl, a graduate of the University of North Carolina, was working in Washington, DC, when he became an early adopter of online dating in the early 1990s. He began corresponding with a web developer at AOL. Their conversations were going well, and eventually Karl disclosed his condition. She was not fazed by the disclosure because Karl made her laugh. His future wife, Angela, later said, "I love the man, not the diagnosis."

Karl says, "Parkinson's disease has given me a purpose. It's brought me a wife and a business partner." Angela and Karl have worked together on numerous entrepreneurial endeavors, including the development of a stylus to use on touch screen computers. The US Postal Service became their biggest customer.

Both Karl and Angela are fierce advocates for the Parkinson's community. For twenty consecutive years, Karl visited Capitol Hill on behalf of those affected by the disease, and for six years, he served on the board of the

Parkinson's Action Network. Angela has given voice to caregivers across the country, and in 2015 the White House recognized her as a "Champion for Change" for Parkinson's disease.

Today, the couple lives in Fairfax, Virginia. They recently spent a month in Europe. Karl has increasing difficulty managing involuntary movements that are a side effect of his levodopa medication but thinks that he "may write another book or two." Asked about his likely pesticide exposure from living and working near a golf course, he says, "I am not embittered, but there needs to be a better understanding of the consequences of exposure to these chemicals while playing or working. It is very scary stuff."

In the 1990s, the New York state attorney general produced a report titled "Toxic Fairways."[71] The report examined the use of pesticides on golf courses on Long Island and found that, in a single year, fifty-two golf courses used 200,000 pounds of dry pesticide products and 9,000 gallons of liquid pesticide formulations. This amounted to two tons of pesticides per course per year, costing some courses more than $50,000 annually.[71] One weed killer used on courses was also one of the two main ingredients in Agent Orange.[72] These pesticides, used on some of the country's top golf courses, can contaminate underground water supplies, and some can be inhaled.[71]

"Greenspace" workers (e.g., gardeners, landscapers, golf course employees) have an increased risk of Parkinson's.[73] For fifty years, Joe Smith worked on golf courses spraying pesticides. He holds a degree in horticulture and has worked on some of the country's top golf courses. In all of them, he used pesticides. He says, "There was a lot of pressure to make golf courses look a certain way." He would sometimes push back on the amount of pesticides used, but he may not have pushed back hard enough.

At age sixty-five, Joe's right and then left hand started to shake. He saw a neurologist, who ordered a sophisticated imaging test that yielded results consistent with his Parkinson's diagnosis. The drug levodopa has worked wonderfully to reduce his symptoms, though he does have a few regrets. "I still think that I would . . . have done the job, but I would have worn personal protective equipment like a spray suit more often." Now he does "not want to get near a drop of pesticide. I know that is why I have Parkinson's."

PUTTING IT ALL TOGETHER

In 2003, a brilliant German pathologist, Heiko Braak, first postulated that Parkinson's, a brain disorder, does not begin in the brain.[74] Instead, based on a review of brains with the disease, he observed that the disease's pathology was first present in the brain's smell center (olfactory bulb) or in the nerve cells that innervate the gut (the vagus nerve). He thought that Parkinson's may be due to "neuroinvasion," perhaps by an infectious agent that enters through the gut and then spreads upward through the nervous system to the brain like "a falling row of dominos."[74]

Sixteen years later, Per Borghammer, a Danish scientist and physician, and his colleague, Nathalie Van Den Burge, built upon this model and proposed that Parkinson's disease and the closely related dementia with Lewy bodies begin in either the nose or the gut.[75] Dementia with Lewy bodies has features of Parkinson's, like tremor and slowed movements, but also impairs thinking and produces hallucinations early in its course.[76] The disease, which may be present in a million Americans, also affected the late, great actor and comedian Robin Williams.[77]

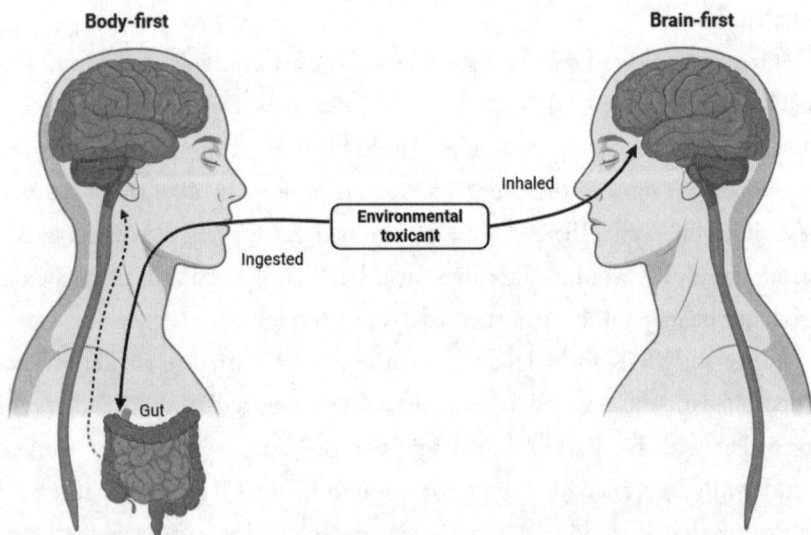

Figure 8. Body-first and brain-first model of Parkinson's disease and other Lewy body disorders.[75]

Borghammer and others[78] have argued that dementia with Lewy bodies and advanced Parkinson's disease (with dementia) are "one and the same."[79] When Borghammer and colleagues compare the symptoms of both diseases, the imaging (his specialty), and the pathology, they find the diseases to be "indistinguishable."[79]

The major difference may be where they begin. Most Parkinson's may begin in the nose, and most dementia with Lewy bodies may start in the gut. The former gives rise to a "brain-first" model of the disease; the latter to a "body-first" model (**Figure 8**).[75]

This model fits well with the likely inhaled or ingested environmental causes of the diseases.[80] For example, chemicals or particles that are breathed in could lead mainly to Parkinson's disease, starting in the nose. On the other hand, chemicals in food or water that are swallowed could result primarily in dementia with Lewy bodies that begins in the gut.

Inhaled pollutants, as we have seen from Dr. Calderón-Garcidueñas's studies in Mexico City, can lead to misfolding of alpha-synuclein beginning in the brain's smell center. This pathology can then spread backward from the brain's smell center with just one stop (in the amygdala, which processes emotions) before reaching the substantia nigra. The misfolded protein can continue to spread like Braak's falling dominoes to nerve centers that control sleep and automatic functions like digestion. As the pathology spreads throughout the brain, different symptoms emerge, beginning with early loss of smell (perhaps) and then slowness of movement and tremor (usually on one side). These symptoms are followed by sleep disturbances (like acting out one's dreams) and constipation, and, much later, dementia.[80]

By contrast, ingested chemicals from contaminated well water or food could lead to the pathology beginning in the gut, as suggested by Braak. The misfolded protein could then spread upward to the lower parts of the brain and eventually to the movement center (substantia nigra) and the higher areas of the brain that control thinking. Again, the symptoms of the disease roughly match the spread of pathology.

When beginning in the gut, constipation is an early feature, followed by sleep disturbances. Because the gut receives nerves from both sides of the body, individuals may have a more symmetric tremor or slowness in

movements and are more likely to develop problems thinking and hallucinations.[80] According to Dr. Honglei Chen, a physician and epidemiologist at Michigan State University, and Dr. Beate Ritz, an epidemiologist
at the University of California, Los Angeles, the nose and the gut "are the
two anatomic sites . . . [that] directly interact with the environment, where
inflammation commonly occurs, and where paths to the brain are well
established."[81]

In both cases the spreading of the misfolded protein can take place over
years, decades, or even generations. Symptoms are only produced when a
sufficiently large number of nerve cells have died off, and this takes time.

The "windows of vulnerability" to these toxic chemicals may be greatest
earlier in life.[82] The relevant exposure may be in a mother's womb or as a child
(like the basketball player Brian Grant), a teenager (Karl Robb), a young adult
(the Navy captain Amy Lindberg), or an adult (the attorney Dan Kinel).

More generally, the risk of Parkinson's may reflect three sets of factors
(**Figure 9**).[80] The first is exposure: the dose, duration, timing, and route.
Inhaled toxicants may be especially concerning for Parkinson's disease.[83]
Next, as we will discuss in subsequent chapters, interactions with genes or
other environmental factors (e.g., head trauma) may help determine who
among the exposed develops the disease. Chance may play a role as well.

Finally, there are likely numerous factors that modify the likelihood of
developing Parkinson's. As we age, some biological functions, including our

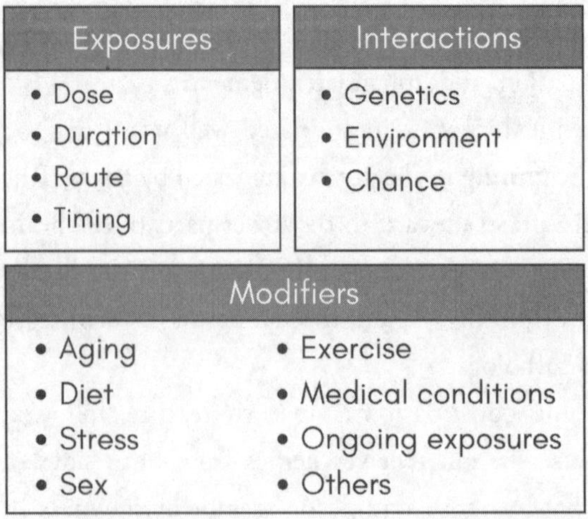

Exposures	Interactions
• Dose	• Genetics
• Duration	• Environment
• Route	• Chance
• Timing	

Modifiers	
• Aging	• Exercise
• Diet	• Medical conditions
• Stress	• Ongoing exposures
• Sex	• Others

Figure 9. Factors determining who develops Parkinson's disease.[80]

ability to remove misfolded proteins, decline.[84] Diet, exercise, sex, sleep, other medical conditions (e.g., diabetes), new illnesses, stress, and continued or new exposures to toxicants could all influence the onset and progression of the disease.

Like chemicals in our food and water, air pollution is addressable. In fact, air quality in the industrialized West is 50% to 90% better than it was just decades ago.[85] This relationship may be helping slow the rise of Alzheimer's and could do the same for Parkinson's.[85-87] We need to continue to extend and expand these efforts so all children breathe clean air and see blue skies.

Our risk of Parkinson's and our health in general reflect our past environments. These environments are due to decisions we make as individuals, communities, and, most importantly, societies. We now know what the likely causes of Parkinson's are. If we want to bring about the end of Parkinson's for us, for our children, and for all time, we can. We just need to eliminate its causes.

PART 2

LEARN

5

LEARN WHY

The Start, the Spread, and the Progression

Illnesses do not come upon us out of the
blue. They are developed from small daily
sins against nature. When enough sins have
accumulated, illnesses will suddenly appear.

—Hippocrates

PARKINSON'S DISEASE HAS MULTIPLE CAUSES. IN THE PREVIOUS chapters, we have detailed how chemicals in our food, water, and air are causing the disease. However, not every farmer who works with paraquat, not every Marine who drinks contaminated water, not every person who works in a dry cleaner, and not every child from Mexico City will develop Parkinson's disease. In fact, only a minority will.

Only about 10% of smokers will develop lung cancer.[1,2] This should not be interpreted as meaning that smoking does not cause lung cancer or that paraquat does not cause Parkinson's. They do. It means there must be more to the story. And there is. We must learn why.

This chapter examines why Parkinson's starts, why it spreads, and why it progresses. The answers to these questions hold the key to preventing, slowing, treating, and curing Parkinson's.

THE START

A Greek Story

Alexander the Great liked to drink wine, lots of it. Wine was a customary part of Macedonian military life. Alexander's doctor, Philip, sought to alleviate the effects of his drinking by supplementing his diet with radishes. We know today that radishes are filled with antioxidants, vitamin C, and fiber. Now, antioxidants may support gut health, but they wouldn't be enough to counteract excessive alcohol use.

During Alexander's final drinking party, "he drank unmixed wine from his cup, and then shouted with pain as if struck through the liver with an arrow. After a few minutes, he could bear it no longer, and left for his bedroom. Subsequently, he remained bed bound, with the occasional desire to vomit, growing weaker and weaker."[3] Some historians believe that Alexander died of something that is largely preventable and curable today: stomach ulcers.

Alexander the Great built one of the largest empires in history. Hippocrates, who also lived during this time, declared that every illness must have an underlying cause. The source of Alexander's fatal ailment was never officially discovered, and he died when he was only thirty-two. If Alexander's doctors had known the reason for his disease and successfully eliminated the cause, what would Alexander have accomplished? What would the world look like today?

In the late 1960s, bleeding ulcers were one of the leading causes of death globally.[4,5] Many claimed to know the cause. Experts were convinced that stress, spicy foods, and excess stomach acid were the trifecta of sins. For years, doctors recommended stress reduction and job changes, bland foods, and invasive surgeries. Yet people continued to suffer, bleed, and die.

A radical new idea of why people developed gastric ulcers was minted by two Australian scientists, Barry Marshall and Robin Warren. Their answer was that stomach ulcers (also called peptic ulcer disease) were caused by an infection. They said that a curve-shaped bacterium caused the disease and that all our advice about reducing stress and spicy foods was a waste of time.

Rather than welcome the new ideas, many of their colleagues labeled Marshall and Warren quacks. The orthodoxy was that bacteria could not survive in a bath of acid located inside the human stomach. Warren recalled, "Every time I spoke to a clinician they would say, 'Robin, if these bacteria are causing it as you say, why hasn't it been described before?'" After studying about one hundred patients and growing a bacterium called *Helicobacter pylori* in the lab, Marshall was ready to share his results, but his colleagues still were not receptive. But Marshall and Warren persisted.[6]

The resistance was brutal and unrelenting. Expert journal reviewers did not consider their findings important or even interesting enough to publish.[6] Finally, Marshall took matters into his own hands—or, more precisely, into his own stomach. He drank a solution of the *H. pylori* bacteria, and he developed inflammation of the stomach. He then underwent a biopsy to prove the cause. He then treated himself with antibiotics and demonstrated the cure. Marshall painfully and personally proved both the cause and the cure for peptic ulcer disease. Yet it *still* took years for the medical community to accept the work.[7-11]

Today, due to the persistence of these two Australian physician scientists, stomach ulcers are cured every day. The solution is a simple cocktail of antibiotics along with a pill designed to suppress stomach acid. Deaths and hospitalizations due to peptic ulcer disease have plummeted.[6]

The "why it started" in the peptic ulcer story was the discovery of a simple corkscrew-shaped bacteria. This led scientists and doctors down the road to the disease's true cause. Once we learned why, the path became obvious. A treatment was already available and on the shelf. It was waiting to be pressed into action.

An insane number of scientists from every corner of the earth have tried to learn and to track down "why Parkinson's starts." Frustratingly, we remain mostly in the dark. For Parkinson's disease, our efforts to learn why are hampered by limited funding, inadequate tools to study exposures, and, in the case of the makers of paraquat, concealment of evidence.

Genetics and Beyond

Dan Kinel was a young, forty-three-year-old lawyer in Rochester, New York, when he was diagnosed with Parkinson's. Why did Dan get Parkinson's, while other partners in his law firm got cancer? Why were some partners spared and others affected?

In Dan's case, we suspect that the man-made chemical trichloroethylene (TCE), which originated from the contaminated dry cleaner next to his law office, was the culprit. If true, the TCE would have attacked critical parts of Dan's brain cells called the mitochondria. Mitochondria are the powerhouses of human cells and are critical for the production of the brain's energy. If chemicals damage the brain's powerhouses, terrible diseases like Parkinson's can result. Without learning about "why it starts," how can we expect to find out why some suffer and others don't? How can we slow disease progression or find a cure?

Though genetic causes of Parkinson's represent a minority of all cases, in 2024 Thomas Gasser, Andrew Singleton, and Ellen Sidransky were awarded the Breakthrough Prize in Life Sciences for their groundbreaking work on the genetics of Parkinson's disease.

When Thomas Gasser was growing up in Stuttgart, Germany, his father was a member of a team of engineers who advanced archaic telephone rotary dialing into the touch-tone dialer. Thomas, like his dad, wanted to be part of a discovery that benefited society.

As a student, Thomas debated pursuing biochemistry or medicine. When he finally settled on the latter, he was determined that he must be a "switch-hitter," practicing both medicine and science. While training as a neurologist in Munich, Thomas was accidentally introduced to Parkinson's disease. Fate tied the funding for Thomas's position to a company interested in developing medications that worked on dopamine receptors, an area in which he had no experience. Though the work was interesting, it would not be his touch-tone phone.

Thomas wondered whether a chunk of Parkinson's disease could be related to abnormalities in DNA. If his hypothesis proved true, uncovering Parkinson's genes (pieces of DNA) could lay the groundwork for addressing an emerging societal need. The time was right for Gasser, as new genomics techniques were emerging to hunt the DNA aberrations underpinning neurological diseases. Maybe if there was a Parkinson's gene, it could be used to learn why Parkinson's starts?

Gasser journeyed to Harvard to launch his postdoctoral studies under a mid-career professor named Xandra Breakfield. Xandra had cloned the first gene for a disease (called dystonia) that had similar features to Parkinson's. In Gasser's mind, if there was a gene for dystonia, there must be one for Parkinson's.

While Thomas was climbing the ladder to unlock the genetics of Parkinson's disease, Andy Singleton was living on a small island. Guernsey is the second-largest and southernmost of the Channel Islands between Britain and France, with a population of only about 60,000 people. Andy loved the island of Guernsey, but school and work were not stimulating. Singleton was so bored in high school that he flunked out. He was also bored of his office job and wondered what life beyond Guernsey and in a university setting would be like.

Andy's mom died from breast cancer when he was twelve. He was raised by his dad, a carpenter. His grandmother was a good influence and a compelling woman. She convinced Andy that he was smart enough to make the leap from high school dropout to college graduate. There was a school that took a chance on him. Today, Singleton is one of its most famous graduates.

Singleton was instantly noticed for his excellent work in the laboratory. He was invited to northeastern England to Newcastle University to study the chemicals, tissue, and genetics of a disease called Alzheimer's. Andy loved this work and was so prolific that he was invited to complete a doctorate. Andy learned how to separate DNA fragments by using simple gel solutions, and he quickly absorbed an emerging field of radioactive sequencing. Andy could painstakingly determine the sequence of nucleotides in DNA and search for abnormalities, which were possibly tied to neurological diseases. The work was slow, and he frequently failed. However, as Andy read off each DNA sequence, the inner feeling of excitement was exhilarating. Though the technique would later be automated, the experience and wisdom provided critical building blocks for his scientific future. Singleton, like his father, was becoming a carpenter, building the genetics of neurodegenerative diseases. His work with Thomas Gasser culminated with the discovery of the most common Parkinson's gene, *LRRK2*.[12–14]

The third hero in this genomics story is Ellen Sidransky. Ellen was born in New Orleans but grew up in Pittsburgh. She loved archeology, history, and science. During her undergraduate studies at Brandeis University in Boston, Massachusetts, she fell in love with the new and emerging field of medical genetics. Later, as a senior medical student at Tulane University, she visited the National Institutes of Health (NIH) for a rotation. Instantly, she was in complete wonderment of the technology, the machines, the people, and, of course, the science. NIH at the time was changing the genetic landscape of science and medicine.

Ellen pivoted course when she completed her residency in pediatrics and moved to Israel. She would practice as a general pediatrician for four years. Ellen could not, however, shake her love of genetics. She not only returned to NIH but would spend the next thirty-five years studying the gene responsible for a rare disorder called Gaucher's disease. In Gaucher's, an enzyme is either scarce or missing, leading to a buildup of fat in the liver, spleen, bone marrow, and, in some cases, the brain. It wasn't immediately obvious to Ellen or to anyone that the gene for Gaucher's, *GBA*, would turn out to be an important risk factor for Parkinson's disease.

Ellen started with three brain samples wrapped together in aluminum foil and sent through the mail by a pathology resident who was training at Harvard Massachusetts General Hospital and who had read her recent paper. When she checked the sequence of *GBA*, she was astonished to discover that all three samples carried *GBA1* mutations. Ellen was able to confirm both Gaucher's and Parkinson's in the same tissue samples. This was groundbreaking. Gaucher's also turned out to be highly associated with another disease called dementia with Lewy bodies, which is a close cousin of Parkinson's.[15–17]

Thomas, Andy, and Ellen all believe that Parkinson's research should start with a simple premise: "We don't yet understand 'why it starts.'" Thomas says, with no pun intended, that "our current understanding is shaky at best."

Though the genomics story is now a quarter century old, it remains incomplete and cannot be the whole story. An astounding 87% of Americans with Parkinson's disease do not carry mutations in either of the two most common

Parkinson's-related genes (*LRRK2* or *GBA*),[18] and not everyone carrying a Parkinson's gene mutation actually gets Parkinson's. It turns out that genetic causes of Parkinson's, like the environmental ones, are generally insufficient to cause the disease in most people. For example, only 30% of individuals who carry a mutation in *LRRK2* will develop the disease; the majority will not.[19-21] For *GBA* mutation carriers, the lifetime risk of Parkinson's is even lower, at less than at 10%.[22-24] What flips the switch on or off for Parkinson's? We need to learn why it starts. Scientists believe that those with Parkinson's genetic mutations may actually be more susceptible to pesticides and to chemical exposures. And indeed, that appears to be the case.[22,25-27]

Genes have played an important role in uncovering critical clues in our understanding of the causes of Parkinson's disease. Genomics has enlightened the importance of functions within the tiny confines of brain cells. The genes have pointed us toward an important part of the Parkinson's story, the mitochondria, or the energy producers for each cell. Many of the likely environmental causes of Parkinson's, including paraquat, rotenone, and TCE, all damage the mitochondria. Interestingly, the genes (and some of the chemicals) have also directed us toward the lysosomes, which help to digest waste and debris in each cell.[28] For the 87% without a Parkinson's-related genetic mutation, what is the cause, and what is the role of the environment?

Some of the explanation may be that genetic differences may not cause the disease or be a risk factor. Instead, they may lead to differences in how individuals break down chemicals. We know that genetic differences affect the way patients break down (or metabolize) medicines. The same may apply to the breakdown of pesticides.[29,30] For example, variations in some genes are linked to a twofold increased risk of Parkinson's following exposure to a certain class of pesticides.[31] Finally, understanding interactions among environmental factors (e.g., head trauma and pesticides or different pesticides with one another) may be important to discovering why Parkinson's starts.

THE SPREAD

A Mad Cow

In the mid-1980s, farmers in the United Kingdom noticed that their usually calm cows were becoming irritable. They were uncharacteristically clumsy, and some animals even had difficulty standing. The cows developed a never-before-seen disease. Those who lived through the era will recount the pervasive fear of eating meat and developing what became known as mad cow disease. Scientists coined the name bovine spongiform encephalopathy based on the combination of the symptoms and how the disease gave the brain a sponge-like appearance under the microscope.[32-34]

The cause of mad cow turned out to be an infectious protein, first described in 1982 by Stanley Prusiner at the University of California, San Francisco.[35-42] Prusiner, like Barry Marshall and Robin Warren in the peptic ulcer story, was described by his colleagues as completely crazy, because his hypothesis challenged fundamental ideas about both how diseases are transmitted and how proteins function. The human version of the disease had been named after the two German neurologists who first described it in the 1920s, Hans Gerhard Creutzfeldt and Alfons Maria Jakob. Prusiner, who described the infectious protein, would go from mad scientist to Nobel laureate for his groundbreaking discovery.

Today, we accept that proteins can behave like infectious agents (e.g., viruses) and can spread widely throughout the brain and nervous system. The term *prion-like* has emerged and reflects the idea that, in Parkinson's disease, proteins can spread from brain region to brain region, but this does not mean that Parkinson's is an infection. How do they spread? We think that the secret is in how the protein folds. Certain shapes impart to the protein the superpower to move from brain cell to brain cell.

Fifteen years after Prusiner's discovery of a misfolded protein spreading through the brains of cows, the German pathologist Heiko Braak thought that the pathology of Parkinson's might also spread from nerve cell to nerve cell "like a row of falling dominos."[43] Braak was proposing that Parkinson's could start in the gut and spread to the brain. Later, in 2008, Dr. Jeffrey Kordower, a neuroscientist now at Arizona State University, saw something that supported this notion and stunned the field. Kordower looked under a microscope at brain tissue collected from people who had undergone dopamine cell transplants for their Parkinson's disease. The cells inserted were all healthy dopamine-producing "mini-factories." When Kordower examined the tissue, the healthy cells had become sick with classic changes of

Parkinson's disease.[44-46] The pathology of Parkinson's was able to spread from sick regions of the brain to healthy ones. We must learn why.

Based on this research, a new Parkinson's diagnostic test can be used to find elements of this misfolded protein in the spinal fluid. The test has set off a race for other biological markers of the disease with the ultimate prize hopefully being the development of a simple blood test.[47-49] Such tests will help diagnose the disease and ideally help measure its progression and the effects of new treatments. Simple blood tests can both measure levels of cholesterol and evaluate the response to cholesterol-reducing medications. The result has helped prevent heart attacks. Maybe the same can be done using blood in Parkinson's disease.

A New Theory

Per Borghammer grew up in Aarhus, the second-largest city in Denmark, which has been home to his family and ancestors for over 1,000 years. His father taught physics and math, and his mother delivered the mail. He grew up with a burning desire to determine the origins of the universe. Instead of becoming an astronomer, he would try to learn the "why" of something equally mysterious, Parkinson's.

Borghammer's fate was sealed twenty years prior, when Danish politicians fell in love with a field called nuclear medicine. Today, there are more positron-emission tomography (PET) scanners in Denmark per capita than in any other country. A PET scanner can be used to measure chemicals in the brain and in the body. Additionally, more than half of all Danish nuclear medicine doctors have two degrees, an MD and a research degree, the PhD. In Denmark, studying nuclear medicine is a natural fit for those wanting to become doctors and scientists.

Nuclear medicine is a lesser-known specialty where radioactive tracers can be used to identify and diagnose disease. The procedure begins with injecting a tagged molecule into a person's vein and sending it on a journey to a specific brain region. A special camera creates a pictorial diary like the procedure NASA uses to document space travel. In a marvel of modern technology, scientists have fused the PET scan, which measures radioactivity, with traditional imaging from brain computed tomography (CT) or

magnetic resonance imaging (MRI) scans. The result has been an unprecedented view of Parkinson's. Borghammer has found patterns that identify
different ways the disease spreads and symptoms develop.

As discussed, Borghammer has postulated that there are two forms of
Parkinson's and related diseases—one that begins in the gut ("body-first")
and one that starts in the nose ("brain-first"). Chemicals that are eaten or
ingested could lead to a body-first form that begins in the gut, while those
that are sniffed or inhaled could result in a brain-first form of Parkinson's that starts in the nose.[50] With his sophisticated imaging techniques,
Borghammer and his colleagues are now mapping out the spread of Parkinson's from these starting points.[51]

Many scientists believe that to learn "why Parkinson's spreads," we will
need to uncover a big bang and to trace the origins of all the brain proteins
involved in the genesis of the disease. In Parkinson's disease, in addition to
developing new MRI and PET technologies, we are hot on the trail of blood
tests, which can detect small amounts of one of the abnormal proteins in
the Lewy body, alpha-synuclein. Borghammer believes that improved brain
imaging and blood tests will be a winning combination. Such tests could be
used to study individuals at genetic or especially at environmental risk for
the disease.

THE PROGRESSION

Better Models for Parkinson's

Parkinson's in mice is far from the human form of the disease. One of the
cruel jokes in the field is that a different research group publishes a "cure"
for Parkinson's every month. These cures are, of course, not in humans but
in mice. Unfortunately, these therapies all fail to translate from the mouse
to the human. We will need to develop better animal models for Parkinson's
and, when possible, to develop models not requiring the use of animals.

Ron Mandel, a professor of neuroscience at the University of Florida, and
Jeff Kordower have both struggled with the limitations of animal models.
Their advice is "to go bigger." We need models that are closer to humans.
We know the human brain uses a ton of energy to run, and we should, if

we have to use animal models, mirror the human condition as closely as possible.

Primates (monkeys), pigs, and sheep are large animals with neurocircuitry and immune systems highly similar to humans'. This similar neurocircuitry is important to movement, to reward, and to Parkinson's disease. The most unique aspect of the human substantia nigra is neuromelanin. Neuromelanin is similar to a pigment found in the skin called melanin. Melanin is also found in hair and in the eyes, but in the brain it is important for movement, mood, and sleep. However, no other species has true neuromelanin. Scientists can now insert genes to create mice with humanlike neuromelanin, and hopefully one day soon they will translate this to larger animal models.[52]

Also unique to primates relative to rodents is the circuitry that underlies their memory and thinking. Cognitive decline and dementia are common and devastating symptoms in Parkinson's, and currently there are few treatments. Testing novel therapies in nonhuman primates may lead to treatments that are desperately needed. We should also focus as we move forward on choosing animal models with immune systems and inflammatory responses similar to humans'. Animal models are critical for developing and understanding the progression of Parkinson's, and scientists who employ them should be sure to protect, care for, and minimize harm to them.

Another challenge is that there are only seven NIH-funded primate research centers in the United States. Unless a Parkinson's researcher holds an NIH grant for a specific project, they are prohibited from using primates in one of these designated centers, even if they arrive at the table with institutional or private money to reimburse the costs. Kordower puts it succinctly when he says, "The cost of monkeys and providing us with primates is far less than the cost of another failed clinical trial." And failure has been the norm for Parkinson's clinical trials this century.

One recent shift in the landscape for animal models has been the recognition that the presence of Lewy bodies is not the only important finding in the disease. A well-kept secret is that most Parkinson's brains, when examined at autopsy by a pathologist, contain more than one disease (copathologies), including both Lewy bodies and two proteins (tau and amyloid) implicated in Alzheimer's disease. Kordower and his colleague John Morrison, who is at the Icahn School of Medicine at Mount Sinai in New York, have been working on a fix that would allow scientists to study brains with multiple diseases at once. They are hard at work creating Parkinson's models that have the pathologies of both diseases, and these may better reflect the human form of Parkinson's.[53,54] Such models will attract more research funding and drive better treatments.

Mini-Brains in a Dish

The search for "why" Parkinson's disease progresses will also require that we build a better and more "human and humane system" to study the disease. Many experts believe using stem cells to build mini-brains in a dish will catapult our efforts and eventually help reduce the need for experiments on laboratory animals.

A stem cell has a unique ability to turn into different types of cells. Stem cells can either make more stem cells or can develop into specific cells of many kinds of tissues. Stem cells are important for growth, healing, and repair. The development of new brain cells with massive connectivity that can replicate the architecture of a mature dopamine-producing brain cell in a dish could be transformative. Stem cells can be used to drive research and learn how Parkinson's disease progresses.

Organoids—three dimensional structures that can be made from stem cells—are mini-brains in a dish. They are nifty in that they can mimic the architecture and function of real human organs, including brains. Can we make an organoid to mimic a Parkinson's brain? Can we sprinkle in some dopamine-producing neurons and include the brain circuits responsible for movement, mood, and thinking? This is important because we desperately need models of Parkinson's that include more than just motor dysfunction. This technology is rapidly evolving and will be very powerful.

How the Brain Defends Itself

Matthew Lavoie, the son of a chemist, grew up in the tiny Revolutionary War town of Yorktown Heights, New York. There he watched his dad unlock the mysteries of anticancer drugs. Matthew was drawn to science and particularly to the idea that if he earned a PhD, he could become an expert in one specific area of scholarship. He was interested in catching frogs and turtles and in understanding the "why" of biology.

After two decades of research into both Parkinson's and Alzheimer's, he now directs a neurodegenerative research center at the University of Florida. Matt believes that it is time to rethink why Parkinson's disease is a progressive syndrome at all. Shouldn't the cells in our bodies be equipped to slow the progression of Parkinson's? Once Parkinson's disease starts, why don't our immune system and our built-in cell-based protective mechanisms stop the progression?

Matt thinks we should shift some of our effort toward understanding what allows a brain cell to survive. What are the weaknesses in our brain cells and our brain circuitry? Matt reminds us that the strength of our cells and the connections between them matter. We must delve deeper into what makes these connections important to aging and how Parkinson's overcomes our own defenses as it progresses.

Though many scientists investigating Parkinson's have overlooked the normal function of cells in pursuit of a treatment, Matt thinks this is a mistake. We are lost in a very dark forest, and we need to understand the terrain to find our way out. Every cell in the human body is at risk or vulnerable to something. Scientists call this property of cells *selective vulnerability*. Why, if the Parkinson's-related protein alpha-synuclein is found normally all over the brain, does it get entangled into a progressive degenerative process and in just certain parts of the brain? Just as some individuals may be more susceptible to chemicals or to pesticides, some may be more susceptible to faster progression. We need to invest in sorting this out.

Buz Jinnah, a neurologist-scientist from Emory University, suggests that how "Zen" your brain cells are may be critical. The big scientific word to describe this is *homeostasis*. If your cells lose their homeostasis, Buz and other experts believe, this will be a crucial factor determining not just whether one day your brain will succumb to Parkinson's. It may also determine the type of Parkinson's you will get and the rate of progression. Could modifiable lifestyle changes or choices impact disease progression? Could sleep flush out brain toxicants, and could exercise strengthen brain connections? We need to invest in understanding what we can do to keep the Zen of our brain cells.

Dopamine neurons are hungry brain cells. They communicate by firing constantly to keep up with the billions of connections all over the brain. Dopamine-producing brain cells, especially those located in the substantia nigra and in other areas affected by Parkinson's, are constantly releasing chemicals and creating communication with close and faraway groups of cells. Firing of these brain cells is critical to functions such as movement, reward, and cognition. All require substantial energy. These cells must be constantly fed. Understanding what makes these hungry cells happy or unhappy will likely provide clues as to why Parkinson's progresses. Whether exercise, aging, stress, infections, or medications (like GLP1 weight-loss drugs) could be used to keep cells happy could all impact progression.

Better Tools Can Help Us Unlock Why Parkinson's Progresses

While other boys were talking about the Dallas Cowboys, nine-year-old Ed Boyden was deeply philosophizing about the meaning of life. In a northern suburb of Dallas called Plano, he opined on the meaning of life, the purpose of religion, and ultimately the value of science. Ed was chosen as one of the elite 150 kids in the state of Texas to attend the Texas Academy of Mathematics and Science. This opportunity meant he would have to leave home at the age of fourteen instead of eighteen, and ultimately he skipped four grades (eighth, tenth, eleventh, twelfth). When he arrived, he was armed with some "big questions." How can we better understand the human condition? How do we explain the true nature of our existence? Can we change our DNA? Ed fell in love with chemistry and started working in a laboratory, where he spent his days mixing and matching chemicals to recreate DNA. At age sixteen, he transferred to the Massachusetts Institute of Technology, where his passion and creativity for science would build into an unstoppable, high-intensity momentum. He was a natural, clear, and critical thinker, and he understood the power of the hypothesis. At a young age, Ed learned he could both shape and break an argument, and he became a champion of challenging dogma.

Although no one would label Ed primarily a Parkinson's researcher, many of his methods and techniques have been applied by leading scientists in the field.

To Ed it comes down to one key question: "What is the approach that will offer you the best chance for impact?" Nurturing novelty involves operating from the bottom up to develop and deliver crucial engineering "know-how," which is necessary to create the impact. We frequently forget the importance of the engineering and of developing the tools necessary to drive the science. If we can't adequately visualize it, how can we treat or cure it? Ed points to the field of physics, where the microchip was a necessary innovation to convert many theories into impact.

To Ed it is imperative that we fully visualize the structure underpinning a disease, in order to reach the "aha" moment of understanding its function. We must invest in the tools necessary for visualization and for imaging Parkinson's, especially the tiny things that escape our human field of view. Enhanced MRI, improved microscopes, and refined techniques, such as novel calcium-based imaging, will allow us to peek inside the actual activity of brain cells. To nurture the novelty, Ed reminds us that we must understand the orchestra of cells and how they fire together, or not. We must appreciate the dynamics of the pipes connecting them. For example, scientists have been hard at work optimizing a green-glowing protein (called GCaMP6) to visualize living cells in action. Another example is the development-visualization technique called voltage imaging, which can measure brain-cell firing through changes in electrical activity. Ed is convinced that development of such bottom-up engineering advances can and will move the needle in Parkinson's, especially when paired with the top-down big picture of the suffering human.

The brain has over 1,000 different types of cells, so mapping, dynamically controlling, and developing a new brain technology for Parkinson's disease will require the use of artificial intelligence. He is applying a technique called *expansion microscopy*, which has nanoscale precision. Ed can snap pictures at around seventy-nanometers resolution, which is 1,000 to 1,400 times smaller than the width of a human hair and 35 times the diameter of a single strand of human DNA. This tool will allow mapping of proteins in the gaps between brain cells, facilitate identification of new proteins at cell junctions, and enable analysis of gene-expression profiles at the level of a single brain cell.[55-58] Recently, Ed and colleagues can image things as small as five nanometers, which is only twice the width of human DNA.

To learn why Parkinson's starts, spreads, and progresses, we need to understand its structure, observe the dynamics of the process as it unfolds in real time, learn to control the process, and apply machine learning to answer critical questions. Ed, along with many researchers in the field, is increasingly concerned that we are blinded by brain plaques and deposits and may be overlooking upstream changes that are critically important in Parkinson's.

What are we missing because we have yet to develop the tools to find it? The answer to the start, spread, and progression questions in Parkinson's will be highly dependent on what is in our toolbox.

Swim Upstream for the Answers

The 1937 Nobel laureate Albert Szent-Györgyi declared, "It is important to swim upstream in science." Szent-Györgyi was most famous for elucidating the role of vitamin C in the prevention of the disease scurvy.[59] He felt that "discovery consists of seeing what everybody has seen, and thinking what nobody has thought." He emphasized the importance of swimming against the "prevailing currents of thought in scientific research." In Parkinson's disease, we have been stuck sifting through all the sediment that has accumulated downstream, including the pile of alpha-synuclein and Lewy bodies. We need to look upstream for the three "why" questions (start, spread, and progression) of Parkinson's.

There have been some attempts to look upstream, including examining the dysfunction in the energy-producing parts of cells called the mitochondria. The mitochondria have been linked to early changes in Parkinson's disease, including those in energy production. There have also been attempts to characterize abnormalities in oxidative stress resulting from an imbalance in the brain's production of chemical troublemakers. These troublemakers are produced when cells use oxygen to make energy. We must better understand how to help the brain detoxify them.

Further, in Parkinson's we do not know if chronic inflammation is an early event that may trigger neurodegeneration. We know that the brain's immune system has an army of scavenger cells (called *microglia*) that become activated in the disease and release pro-inflammatory factors. We know fluctuations in calcium levels can damage or even kill a cell or cells. We know in Parkinson's disease that we can't efficiently get rid of the waste in the brain. Where and when do these changes start? How do they contribute to spread and progression?

These areas represent potential avenues for early intervention in Parkinson's and, if understood, could one day be harnessed to halt or slow the progression of the disease well before the toxic accumulation of clumps of alpha-synuclein. Donald Rumsfeld, the former US secretary of defense, in a 2002 briefing famously said, "Reports that say that something hasn't happened are always interesting to me because as we know, there are known knowns; there are things we know we know. We also know there are known unknowns; that is to say we know there are some things we do not know. But there are also unknown unknowns—the ones we don't know we don't know." Albert Szent-Györgyi, if he were alive, would surely encourage Parkinson's researchers to swim upstream to answer the three "why" questions of Parkinson's disease by going after what "we don't know we don't know."

The Impact of Learning Why

We must learn "why" to reach new treatments and cures for Parkinson's disease. You cannot cure a medical disease without knowing and understanding its cause. Polio was the most feared disease in the world. If you survived, leg braces, crutches, or a wheelchair were the norm, and some people required an iron lung for breathing. Without identification of the cause, there was no hope for a cure. The same will be true for Parkinson's disease.

In 1908, the Viennese immunologist Karl Landsteiner identified the poliovirus as the cause of the disease. Within two years of that discovery, antibodies were uncovered in the blood of people infected. Later, in 1949, the poliovirus was cultivated in human tissue by John Enders, Thomas Weller, and Frederick Robbins at Boston Children's Hospital. In 1954, together they received the Nobel Prize for their efforts that helped answer the "why" questions of polio: why it starts, why it spreads, and why it progresses.

These answers helped Jonas Salk and Albert Sabin create vaccines to prevent polio. To help produce a world nearly free of polio, Salk and Sabin needed the why. For us to prevent, slow, and one day cure Parkinson's, we will also need to invest in answering the three "why" questions and to keep in mind that "illnesses do not come upon us out of the blue. They are developed from small daily sins against nature. When enough sins have accumulated, illnesses will suddenly appear."

6

THE PARKINSON'S 25

An ounce of prevention is worth a pound of cure.

—Benjamin Franklin

IF PARKINSON'S IS DUE TO CHEMICALS IN OUR FOOD, WATER, AND air, it must be preventable. And it is.

Here we detail twenty-five actions individuals can take that could reduce their risk of Parkinson's. These recommendations may be especially important for those at genetic risk, those with a family history of the disease, those who have been exposed to toxic chemicals, and even those who already are affected. By the time someone is diagnosed with Parkinson's, about 60% of the nerve cells that produce dopamine in the substantia nigra have died.[1] We need to protect the remaining 40%.

It is also never too late to get started. We take a lesson from smoking. For smokers, cessation helps all regardless of age, and the benefits accrue fast.[2,3] Twenty minutes after the last cigarette smoked, an individual's heart rate returns to normal. A day later, the risk of heart attack lowers. By nine months, coughing is reduced, and a decade later, the risk of lung cancer is halved.[2] The same could be true for environmental toxicants and Parkinson's.

Let's stop waiting passively for Parkinson's to surface. Let's apply what we have learned and begin preventing the disease now.

FOOD

1. Wash Your Produce, Even if It's Organic

Pesticides have made their way into our food supply. In 2024, *Consumer Reports* found that remnants of pesticides posed a significant health risk in 20% of common foods that it examined, including blueberries, bell peppers, and potatoes.[4] Purchasing organic produce, dairy products, and meat can all help reduce exposure. However, even organic produce can have unsafe pesticide residues.[4] So what to do?

Regardless of whether you buy organic or conventional fruits and vegetables, wash them. Use water and possibly a vegetable wash, because, like dirt, many pesticides do not dissolve in water. These washes are available in many grocery stores. The one Ray uses costs $4 and lasts months. Vinegar and salt solutions are good options too.[5] To determine what levels of pesticides are safe, the US Department of Agriculture measures them after food has been washed with water for fifteen to twenty seconds.[4] If that is their practice, yours should be even longer.

Another way to reduce your overall exposure to pesticides without buying entirely organic produce is to consult the reports of the Environmental Working Group, which lists foods with a lot of exposure (the "Dirty Dozen") and those with much less (the "Clean Fifteen"). These can be viewed at www.ewg.org/foodnews. Another good way to learn what pesticides are being used is to go to a farmer's market or join a community-supported agricultural farm where you can speak to the farmers who grow the crops.

2. Change Your Diet

Individuals who eat a Mediterranean diet—high in fruits and vegetables and low in animal products—may lower their risk of Parkinson's.[6,7] Such a diet may also be beneficial for those who already have the disease.[8] The reasons for the benefit are not certain and may be multiple. These include reduced exposure to dangerous pesticides and other toxic compounds in meat and dairy and increased exposure to healthy compounds (e.g., antioxidants) in whole plant foods.

In addition to pesticides, other chemicals, including PCBs (polychlorinated biphenyls), widely used in the electronics industry, can concentrate in animal fat.[9] PCBs are structurally similar to DDT and related pesticides linked to Parkinson's. Like BMAA and the flying foxes in Guam, PCBs can accumulate in animals as they make their way up the food chain. Whales can concentrate PCBs in blubber much like cows do for pesticides in their milk. And high consumption of whales is associated with an increased risk of Parkinson's.[10] Another reason to go easy on animals.

3. Make Sure Your Grocery Store Is Safe

Perchloroethylene (PCE), the dry-cleaning chemical, can readily spread beyond the walls of a dry cleaner. In Germany, PCE, which dissolves in fat, has been found in dairy products in supermarkets near dry cleaners at two to twenty times the levels found in shops farther away.[11,12] Germany now prohibits supermarkets from being located close to dry cleaners.

Next time, before you shop at your local market, look around to see what is located nearby.

4. Enjoy Wine Without Pesticides

Like produce, organic wines are not immune to pesticide contamination, but they have lower levels and thus reduced health risks. In addition, organic vineyards are likely safer for those who work there and for those who live nearby. Currently, organic wines represent only a small slice (3%) of global sales, but their share is rising.[13] Organic choices in what we eat and drink could improve the health of consumers, farmers, and communities.

5. Avoid, or At Least Manage, Diabetes

Numerous studies have shown that diabetes is associated with a higher future risk of Parkinson's and may lead to a faster rate of progression.[14–18] While it is unlikely a root cause of the disease, diabetes is probably an important accelerator of progression, and its burden is increasing globally.[19] So avoid diabetes by eating a healthy diet and staying active, and if you already have it, control your blood sugar levels.

6. Have a Cup of Caffeinated Coffee

Research has repeatedly demonstrated that caffeine consumption is associated with a decreased risk of Parkinson's.[20,21] Caffeine may protect the dopamine-producing nerve cells from the damage that results from exposure to environmental toxicants.[22]

The benefits appear to be present regardless of your beverage of choice (e.g., coffee or tea) but are not present with decaffeinated beverages.[20,21] Of course, caffeine has its own health risks, such as anxiety and headache. But you now have another reason to enjoy your morning cup of coffee.

7. Farm Safely

Farming is the world's most common job. Approximately 1.8 billion people, more than 20% of the world's population, are engaged in agriculture.[23] Unfortunately, most use pesticides and in increasing amounts.[23,24] Pesticides have improved crop yields and reduced disease, and they can be beneficial. However, widespread, indiscriminate, unprotected use is not.

Farmers who work with certain pesticides have a higher risk of Parkinson's.[25–27] Farmers can lower their risk by decreasing the amount of pesticides used, reducing their frequency of administration, and using lower-risk pesticides. Not every pesticide is linked to Parkinson's.[27] Most likely aren't. Avoiding the ones with the greatest risk, such as paraquat (sprayed on fields of corn, cotton, and grapes), chlorpyrifos (used on apple orchards), and a class of pesticides called organochlorines (DDT is the poster child), is a good place to start. Personal protective equipment (PPE) including gloves, masks, and goggles can also help reduce exposure to many of these dangerous chemicals and lower the risk of Parkinson's.[26,28]

Farmers can also unknowingly bring pesticides into the home on their shoes and clothing. Keeping shoes and work clothes out of the house can protect a farmer's family.

WATER

8. Check Your Well

Up to forty million Americans get their drinking water from a private well. Unlike municipal or "city" water, these wells are not regulated by the Safe Drinking Water Act. As we have seen, these wells, which are infrequently tested, are prone to contamination from pesticides and industrial chemicals.

If you have a private well, test it regularly (e.g., annually) and ensure that you test it for pesticides and chemicals like trichloroethylene (TCE) in addition to the usual bacteria. Testing for these chemicals is often not done and may need to be specifically requested. The Environmental Protection Agency (EPA) provides a list of laboratories that are certified to test water, and mail-in options are available.[29]

Outside the United States, one in four people do not have access to safe water.[30] As pesticide use increases globally and the threat of contaminated wells rises, the need to ensure clean water for everyone will only heighten.

9. Use a Water Filter

Just as air filters can reduce exposure to particulate matter in your home, a water filter can do the same for pesticides and TCE. A simple carbon filter, widely available in supermarkets, can reduce exposure to pesticides, TCE, and other chemicals.[31,32]

These carbon filters can be installed for the whole house at the "point of entry" or at the point of use, such as faucets or even water pitchers.[33]

INDOOR AIR

10. Consider Air Purifiers

Air purifiers are an easy and effective way for people to control their environment and lower their risk of disease from indoor air pollution. They may also benefit individuals who already have Parkinson's, as high levels of air pollution have been associated with an increased risk of hospitalization.[34] It is important to note that air purifiers do range in cost (from as low as $10 to as high as $1,000), require periodic cleaning and filter changes, and may need to be installed in multiple places depending on the size of the home, school, or workplace. Also be sure to use air purifiers with carbon filters designed to remove "volatile organic chemicals," like TCE.[35]

11. Don't Poison Yourself

Sometimes the remedy is worse than the disease. Insects, including fleas, ants, and moths, can be unwanted guests. Unfortunately, some commonly used pesticides can increase the risk of Parkinson's.

A synthetic class of pesticides called pyrethroids are widely used to kill insects.[36] Among these is the pesticide permethrin.[37] Research has tied permethrin exposure to loss of dopamine-producing nerve cells in laboratory animals, and early-life exposure may set the stage for the later development of Parkinson's.[38,39] The pesticide is found in flea collars, ant sprays, mothballs, and outdoor apparel. Some of the products containing this and related pesticides are household names that are commonly sold in stores and are likely in millions of homes and garages, including possibly yours.

The solution may be to avoid exposure when at all possible and to minimize any necessary exposure by wearing a mask, increasing ventilation, avoiding spraying near children, and considering safer alternatives.[40,41]

12. Choose Your Home Carefully

Over seventy million Americans (22% of the US population) live within three miles of a Superfund site.[42] Twenty million live within a mile. Most of these Superfund sites are unmarked, unfenced, and largely invisible to residents around them. The EPA has a database where you can search for these sites,[43] but less contaminated sites may be harder to find. Some states have their own databases, and internet searches can uncover many.

If you live near a TCE- or PCE-contaminated site, all is not lost. In fact, preventing the effects of TCE and PCE pollution in your home, school, or office is readily achievable. Testing (usually through an environmental testing company) of one's indoor air can determine if TCE or PCE is present.[44] If either is, a mitigation system that pumps air from below your foundation to above your roof can be installed and looks just like ones used for radon (**Figure 1**).[45]

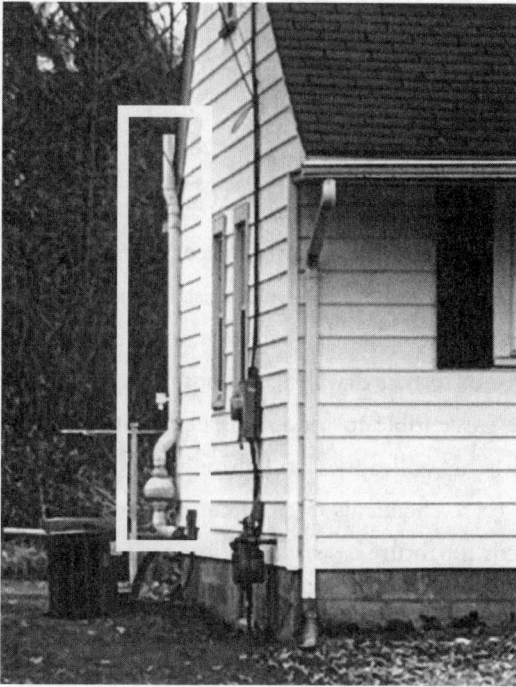

Figure 1. Picture of a mitigation system for trichloroethylene and perchloroethylene.[45]

13. Dry Clean Cautiously

Newly dry-cleaned clothes release dangerous chemicals ("off gas") like TCE and PCE. If you put your dry cleaning in your car, you may be breathing in PCE on your way home.[46] Once you take the clothes into your closet, the chemicals can spread throughout the air inside your home.

To limit exposure, first, find a dry cleaner that does not use PCE. If you cannot, consider minimizing your dry cleaning, and when you do have to dry clean, "air" out your clothes before taking them inside the home. Take off the plastic bag and let the clothes breathe, so you don't have to breathe the chemicals in yourself.

14. Check the Ground Floor

Before moving into a high rise of apartments or condominiums, you may want to check out what is on the ground floor. Because if there is a dry cleaner, the air inside may not be safe.

If a dry cleaner is located in your current or future residence, ask them if dry cleaning is done on site (sometimes it is just a storefront with dry cleaning done off-site) and whether they use PCE (commonly known as "perc" in the industry). If they do, you should test your indoor air.

15. See What Is Near Your Child's Day Care Center

Dry cleaners can also contaminate soil and groundwater, and these volatile chemicals can enter nearby homes, schools, workplaces, and child-care centers. In Washington state, Elmer Diaz, a toxicologist from the state's Department of Health, has identified eighty day-care centers that are within three hundred feet of a current or former dry cleaner. Those that are nearby (often in strip malls) can be susceptible to indoor air pollution from the dry-cleaning chemicals. With his colleagues and through education, he works to mitigate the risk of these chemicals to children. Early exposure to chemicals could plant the seeds for future cases of Parkinson's, so look for a child-care center that is not near a dry cleaner.

OUTDOOR AIR POLLUTION

16. Roll Up Your Windows in Traffic

Traffic-related air pollution, like that found on congested highways, is associated with an increased risk of Parkinson's and Alzheimer's. Next time you find yourself stuck in traffic or traveling through a tunnel full of cars, roll up your windows, and circulate the air within your car (**Figure 2**) to avoid bringing toxic fumes inside.

17. Garden with Care

Plants, like chrysanthemums, do not like to be eaten by insects, so many of them produce their own pesticides. Humans have used dried chrysanthemums to kill insects for over 2,000 years.[47] The flowers produce an oil

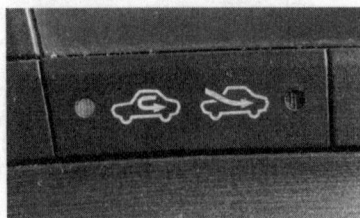

Figure 2. Car button to press to recirculate the air when driving in polluted areas.

called pyrethrum that contains six naturally occurring insecticides called pyrethrins, which can be inhaled or eaten.[48] In addition to damaging the nervous systems of insects, pyrethrins can damage the nerve cells in human brains that produce dopamine.[49–51] Chrysanthemums are so effective at staving off insects that chemists have produced a set of pesticides that are structurally similar to pyrethrins called *pyrethroids*, which have also been linked to Parkinson's and, as discussed above, are found in many household products.

Amateur gardeners and landscapers are susceptible to the dangers of pesticides. Individuals who spent an average of 160 days with weed killers in their yard, for example, had a 70% increased risk of Parkinson's compared to the unexposed. Those who used insecticides (bug spray) in their garden had a 50% increased risk of Parkinson's, and individuals who used the insect-killing chemicals in their home had a 70% increased risk.[52] Gardeners should wear gloves, and if you work extensively with plants, you may want to adopt other protections, such as a mask or working in a well-ventilated space.

Sometimes pesticide use may be required, but regular application is usually unnecessary. If needed, consider having a professional that uses pesticides judiciously. Pesticide-free alternatives may also be available. Finally, ask your neighbors too. What they spray next door may drift your way.

18. Be Mindful of the Greens

While no studies, to our knowledge, have examined rates of Parkinson's among avid golfers, one study in 1996 looked at the death certificates of golf course superintendents.[53] They found that these workers who commonly use pesticides to keep golf courses weed-free had twice the risk of dying due to a nervous system disorder than the general population.

What are the twenty-five million golfers in the United States and sixty-seven million worldwide to do? [46,54,55] Ask your favorite course or club what pesticides they use and when they spray. Encourage them to use less. Have them consider safer alternatives. In the interim, avoid playing on courses just after they have been sprayed. And don't lick your golf ball. Swallowing pesticides is not healthy either.

19. Look Around Your Child's School

According to an analysis by the Environmental Working Group, over 4,000 US elementary schools are located within two hundred feet of crop fields.[56] In the farming state of Iowa, 90% of public school districts have buildings within 2,000 feet of a farm field, "making students and teachers susceptible to being exposed to pesticides that drift from the fields when pesticides are sprayed."[57,58]

Also check out the playground and soccer field. One of the most widely used pesticides on sports fields is a weed killer called 2,4-D.[59,60] Millions of children around the world are likely exposed to the toxic chemical, created in 1941, when they play at school or recreationally.[61–63] The pesticide is associated with a 150% increased risk of having symptoms of Parkinson's.[64] Parents can ask their school leaders about what pesticides, if any, are used on their kids' playgrounds and fields. Sports teams at all levels can reduce their use of pesticides or use less toxic ones.

20. Use Personal Protective Equipment

In addition to protecting against the harmful effects of infectious viruses and bacteria, personal protective equipment can reduce the toxic effects of chemicals.

We know PPE can protect farmers. It can also help landscapers, pesticide applicators, and those who work with industrial chemicals like TCE and PCE.[65] Long sleeves, pants, goggles, and respirators can all limit occupational exposure to chemicals. Some of these measures are uncomfortable (especially when it is hot), costly, and not always available.

PPE is also, of course, important for fire fighters, who may be at higher risk for Parkinson's due to exposure to many inhaled toxicants.[66,67] These include chemicals, like toluene, and metals, such as manganese and lead.[66,68]

If you are an employer, protect your employees by providing them the appropriate PPE for the work required. If you are a worker, use it. It may save you and your family a lot of personal suffering and financial hardship in the future.

MORE

21. Exercise

In his best-selling book *Outlive*, Dr. Peter Attia wrote, "I now tell patients that exercise is, full stop and hands down, the best tool we have in the neurodegeneration prevention tool kit."[69] Exercise may improve the function of the mitochondria, the energy-producing parts of cells, that are damaged by environmental toxicants. Physical activity also releases growth factors in the brain that protect nerve cells, including the dopamine-producing ones.

Vigorous exercise can lower the risk of developing Parkinson's,[49,70–72] and moving every day is also beneficial for those who already have the disease.[73,74] A recent study found that six months of aerobic exercise (riding a stationary bike at least three times weekly) reduced brain atrophy and slowed disease progression.[75]

Now you have more reasons to sweat.

22. Sleep Well

Improving sleep is important to maintaining brain health, and it may be important for preventing neurodegenerative diseases. Sleep is restorative and has been shown to clear toxins from the brain, including the Parkinson's-related protein alpha-synuclein. When you are sleeping poorly, these proteins and other waste products accumulate in your brain and set you up for diseases like Parkinson's.[76–78]

People who are restless or act out their dreams are at higher risk for Parkinson's,[79] and as such, some people will proactively monitor their sleep by using a wearable sensor. By increasing the number of hours of quality sleep per night, you can enhance your daily productivity and hopefully stave off the brain inflammation contributing to the disease.[80–85]

23. Avoid Head Trauma

Head trauma increases the risk of Parkinson's. A recent report suggested that the risk of Parkinson's was 57% higher in those who had experienced a concussion.[86] Head trauma may also amplify the risk of pesticide exposure. For example, the combination of traumatic brain injury and living near where paraquat is sprayed triples the risk of Parkinson's.[87]

So what to do? First, wear seat belts. Second, exercise caution with sports with a high risk of head injury, such as football, especially for children.[88,89] Modifications (for example, no heading in soccer) may make sports safer and more enjoyable. Third, wear a helmet when you bike, skate, or ski.

24. Act Locally

Much of our local environment is under our control. Palm Beach, Florida, is a thin, eighteen-mile-long barrier island full of multi-million-dollar homes, spotless yards, and immaculate golf courses. The island has long served as the home to the rich and famous, including presidents from John F. Kennedy to Donald J. Trump.

Every Monday morning, trucks cross three short bridges to enter the eight-square-mile town. While many bring food, beverages, and retail goods, an increasing number bring pesticides. Five women, who have been longtime residents of the community, have become increasingly concerned that these pesticides, sprayed on just about everything green from grass to bushes to golf courses, could be responsible for the loss of songbirds in their small slice of heaven. For the past five years, these women, who include a local councilwoman and a former reporter, have helped reduce the use of pesticides on town property, around schools, and even on golf courses.

However, you do not need to be part of an especially wealthy community to take action. In Henrietta, New York, where it snows six months a year, town supervisor Stephen Schultz is taking simple measures. He is just decreasing the use of pesticides everywhere he can—medians in roads, golf courses, schools, and parks—in the middle-class town outside Rochester. He recently remarked that he had yet to sign an invoice to purchase pesticides this year. Not only is he saving the town money, but he is making it healthier.

25. Support Our Veterans

Veterans make up 6% of the US population but 10% of individuals with Parkinson's.[90]

Veterans are at increased risk for at least three reasons—exposure to certain pesticides, TCE, and head trauma. Some of these exposures are amenable to prevention efforts. Some pesticides, like Agent Orange, have been linked to Parkinson's, and US veterans who have had such exposure and now have the disease are entitled to health benefits and compensation.[90] Many service members have been exposed to chemicals like TCE, often knowingly. Those who served at Camp Lejeune between 1953 and 1987 and have developed Parkinson's are entitled to benefits.[91] Finally, head trauma is common in the military, and 400,000 service members sustained a traumatic brain injury between 2000 and 2019.[92] Veterans who have sustained a moderate to severe traumatic brain injury during military service and are later diagnosed with Parkinson's are also eligible for benefits.[93]

The cost of service should not be unnecessary exposure to harmful toxicants. The tragedy of Camp Lejeune is that much of the suffering endured by thousands was preventable if leaders had acted when they knew of the contamination. Unfortunately, they did not.

Today, scores of military bases in the United States, especially in the Air Force where Jana Reed and Sara Whittingham trained and served, and around the world are contaminated with TCE.[94-96] Veterans who served at these bases are often not informed of their possible exposure or of steps (e.g., screening) to reduce their likelihood of adverse health consequences. Similarly, many of these bases remain contaminated. Untold numbers have suffered and continue to do so because of this pollution.

The terrible lesson from Camp Lejeune is that disease is preventable. It just requires the courage to act.

PART 3

AMPLIFY

7

AMPLIFY THE VOICES

Building a More Complete Parkinson's Universe

There is always light. If only we're brave enough
to see it. If only we're brave enough to be it.

—Amanda Gorman, the youngest inaugural poet in US history

WHEN NEIL ARMSTRONG WAS WALKING ON THE MOON, RICK JOHN-son was withdrawing from society. A former Vietnam veteran and phi-losophy major, he retreated into nature at an early age, deeply worried about the fate of the Earth. He took his philosophy from Henry David Thoreau: simplify, simplify, and simplify. He built a Seminole Indian–inspired chickee with a simple thatched roof supported by wooden posts, and at night he read his philosophy books by kerosene lantern and slept under a mosquito net. He buried his septic tank deep in the ground and composted everything imaginable in a deliberate effort to convert organic materials into a nutrient-rich, biologically stable soil. Rick had found his perfect life, until Parkinson's found Rick.

The seclusion, which supplied much of his self-worth and meaning, was challenged by his Parkinson's. When he developed the disease, he self-medicated with plants. He gradually faded until he wasn't able to care for himself. We heard about Rick from a concerned community member, and he reluctantly volunteered for our Operation Housecall.[1] The program, established at the University of Florida in partnership with the Smallwood Foundation, provided person-centered care for those in need. Young neurologists in training created action plans and secured volunteer commitments from multidisciplinary experts and community members.

Rick and five others (two men and three women) with Parkinson's took part in the project, and each was followed regularly in their home. Five could not obtain health insurance, and one could not afford transportation. Through the project, all improved in both outlook and symptoms. Most felt that they had regained some independence in daily activities, and all had improved quality of life. Despite the known Parkinson's hospitalization risk of 30% per year, none was admitted.[1] The experiment's lone casualty was a scorpion who met the bottom of a trainee's shoe.

So why did Rick and the others who enrolled in Operation Housecall enjoy such robust outcomes? Was it state-of-the-art drug therapy? Nope. Did the young trainees cure any of the participants? Not a single one. Was it the charisma of the young doctors? Unlikely. The secret sauce was changing the Parkinson's Universe. The patient was the sun, and the multidisciplinary team became the planets, all orbiting the patient to improve his or her life. Their voices were not only received but amplified.

Each person enrolled in Operation Housecall benefited from an updatable and sharable electronic medical record. The house calls they received from neurologists accomplished much more than care. Focused on the voices of the patients and caregivers, the visits pinpointed everyone's needs, which resulted in the implementation of medication changes, rehabilitation therapies, and exercise programs, as well as the identification and rapid treatment of mood disorders. At each visit, the care coordinator would ask a simple question: What services would this person benefit from? Whether the patient had shuffling steps or depression, it was up to the care coordinator to identify the appropriate specialist and meet the need. One uninsured Operation Housecall participant received a brain surgery called deep brain stimulation (DBS), an option previously unimaginable due to the astronomical cost.

Coordinated care should be an essential priority—even a right—for people with Parkinson's. When we provide coordinated care, the person experiences a substantially better quality of life. The idea is that care is the continuous process of practical, proactive, preventative assessment of needs, coupled with timely provision of services. The shocker is that many of these services, like physical, occupational, and speech therapy, are available in many health care systems. The challenge for a person with Parkinson's is to be proactive, preventative, and coordinated, because for the average consumer, accessing these services is daunting. The chances their voices will be heard and amplified in the current health care system are close to zero.

Though prevention is indisputably Parkinson's greatest treatment, there are over ten million people worldwide with the disease today, and their numbers and voices are growing. Some, like Brian Grant, grew up living off dirt roads, while others, like Michael J. Fox, have lived in large cities like Vancouver and New York. Some are being diagnosed late in life, while others, like Jana Reed and Sara Whittingham, are struck with the disease in their forties. We have introduced you to many people whose stories have highlighted the importance of prevention, and one commonality is that they all face a challenging disease, one that will affect every corner of their lives. We will now introduce you to the health care professionals, scientists, and other stakeholders who are working today on a better plan for how to live with Parkinson's. We have in many cases changed names and slightly altered patients' stories to preserve anonymity.

While we still long for the medical breakthrough that will allow us to cure this disease, there is much we can do in the meantime if we put the patient at the center of care and "flip the script," making the health care system work for us. How will we light the path? Though it would be fabulous if we could have an Operation Housecall for everyone, it is not readily scalable. We need a new model. We need to listen and to amplify the voices of persons with Parkinson's and their caregivers. We need to provide them with critical care services. We need to think bigger and to reimagine the Parkinson's Universe.

THE PARKINSON'S UNIVERSE REIMAGINED

Sun: The patient is the sun.

Mercury: The closest planet to the patient is the caregiver. Mercury orbits around the patient (the sun).

Planets: The other planets are the multidisciplinary team. They orbit around Mercury (the caregiver) and also the sun (the patient).

Mission control: This is the operations or care coordination center.

Pluto: Pluto is not quite large enough to be a planet. Pluto represents stigma, which is not always visible but always there.

Satellites: Satellites orbiting the patient (the sun) are the new technologies, like telemedicine and wearables, which improve care and bring it closer to home.

Asteroid fields: The asteroid fields are the skyrocketing costs to provide optimal Parkinson's care.

THE PARKINSON'S UNIVERSE

In 2002, we proposed a simple Parkinson's care model.[2] The patient is the sun, and all multidisciplinary care should orbit around the patient, not the doctors. The sun, though vitally important, is only one element of the universe. It is time to grow our Parkinson's care model.

The Caregivers

If we stick to the universe analogy, caregivers are represented by the planet Mercury. Mercury is the closest planet to the sun, and though the smallest in the solar system, it is vitally important. It is fitting for the caregivers to be represented by Mercury as the name represents the Roman god of commerce and communication. Mercury (the caregiver) is the messenger to the patient (the sun) and to the rest of the universe. Mercury is heavily cratered on its surface, due to the impact of many collisions. Caregivers must absorb the many challenges of living with a person with Parkinson's, and there are frequently long periods of darkness and light. Mercury (the caregiver) has the closest connection to the sun (the patient), and the planet can get hot.

Multidisciplinary Specialists

The sun's (patient's) gravity holds the solar system together. The connections and interactions drive the seasons, ocean currents, weather, and climate. In our model, the other planets beyond Mercury (the caregiver) represent the many multidisciplinary specialists who are attracted by the gravity of the sun (the patient) and who all stay in orbit to provide necessary elements of Parkinson's care.

Access and Stigma

There are many challenges to the optimal care of Parkinson's. We refer to these challenges in the Parkinson's Universe as asteroids. Asteroids are dangerous rocks or metals that are too small to be planets but also orbit the sun. Some astronomers believe they are leftover building materials from planets that were not completely formed. They can be boulder-to-city-sized, and one, named Ceres, has been referred to as a dwarf planet due to its small size (just 940 kilometers in diameter). In the Parkinson's Universe patients must avoid asteroids, which include access to and distance from care, parking, and stigma. Finally, the darker side of the universe, filled with treacherous asteroid fields, is the insurance companies.

New Technologies to Link Care

Modern care plans for Parkinson's disease would not be complete without exploiting the benefits of technology. We envision the technologies as orbiting satellites, which can be accessed anytime and anywhere by the person with Parkinson's or their caregiver. These include telemedicine, wearable devices like Fitbits and Apple watches, and artificial intelligence (AI).

Mission Control and Care Coordination

At NASA, mission control is a team responsible for overseeing and managing complex operations. Most people identify mission control with space exploration; however, the term can be applied to operations. In the Parkinson's

Universe, patients and family members need a center of operations. We consider mission control to be vital, especially when launching (new medications or therapies), orbiting (maintaining programs such as exercise, diet, and healthy living), and reentering the atmosphere (socially reintegrating into society and facing stigma). For space, mission control includes technical specialists, flight directors, engineers, and communication officers. In this

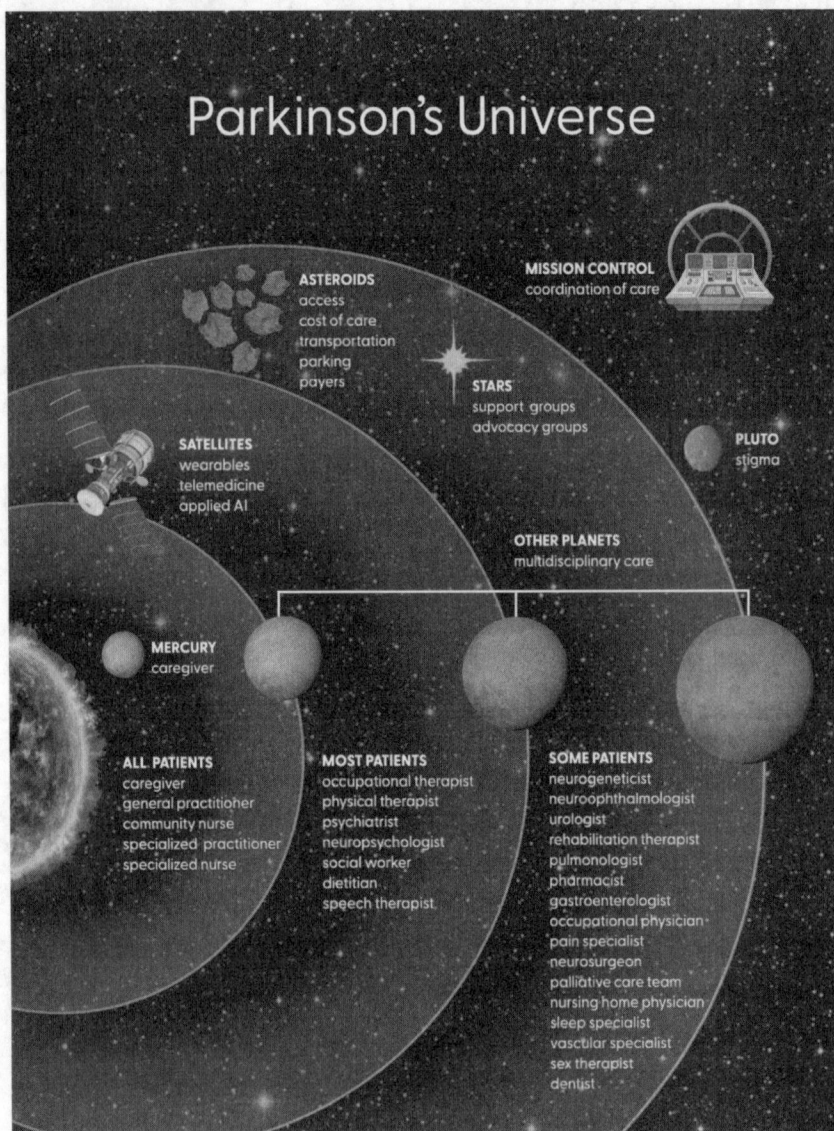

Figure 1. Parkinson's Universe.

chapter we will discuss current efforts at building mission control (the service and science hub model, ParkinsonNet, and Centers of Excellence) and challenges and opportunities for scaling these and other efforts.

Support and Advocacy Groups

The final piece in the Parkinson's Universe includes all the voices, the support networks, and the families navigating the disease. We see these support groups, networks, and advocacy organizations as the many stars in the sky. A person or family can look up at any time and find a light for their path.

The Patient Is the Sun

There are so many ways to reimagine caring for individuals with Parkinson's. The modern American health care system has been built on a primary care "gatekeeper" model. You are required to select a primary care doctor who effectively controls your care. When a medical problem escalates beyond the gatekeeper's expertise, they send a request on your behalf for evaluation by an appropriate specialist. The gatekeeper system presents a myriad of challenges for Parkinson's patients. First, there may or may not be a specialist in the network covered by the person's insurance. Second, if there is one, the wait time is often months. Third, the specialist may have little or no experience managing Parkinson's disease as it relates to their specialty. Fourth, there is usually little or no multidisciplinary discussion among the clinicians.

We don't need a gatekeeper for those living with Parkinson's. We need a care process that focuses on the person. The person with disease is the sun (**Figure 2**). If the planets are the multidisciplinary care specialists, then the challenge becomes mission control. We will present models of care, including an American "service and science hub model," the Dutch ParkinsonNet model for care, and the Parkinson's Foundation Center of Excellence.

Dan McDonald waited over a decade for Gainesville, Florida, to acquire its first Parkinson's specialist. By the time Dr. Michael Okun arrived in July 2002, Dan's situation was distressing. His primary care doctor appropriately referred him for advanced neurological care and for rehabilitation; however, the institution lacked the necessary expertise to address his disabilities.

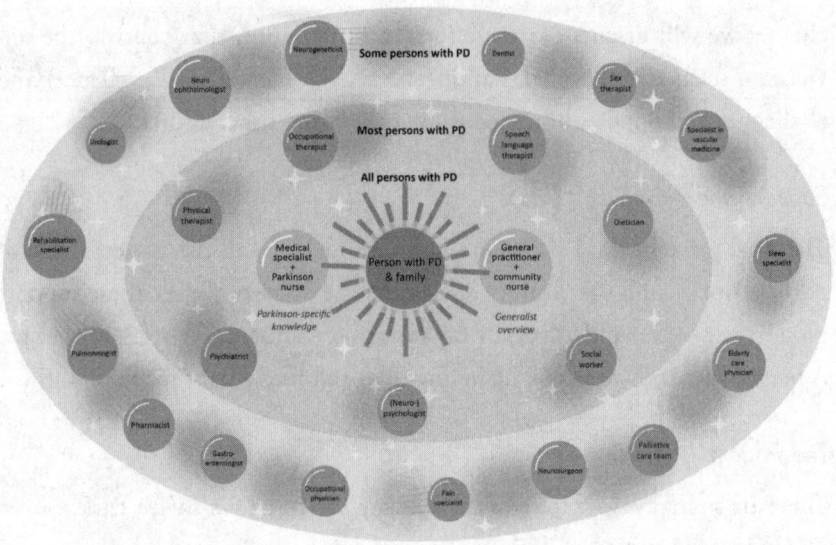

Figure 2. "The Patient Is the Sun."[2] Courtesy of Drs. Bastiaan Bloem, Christine Klein, and Michael Okun.

Dan's journey back to health was harrowing, as half the time his medications either failed to kick in, or when they did work, he would experience violent and unrelenting dance-like movements called *dyskinesia*. He was bounced like a ping-pong ball back and forth from one practitioner to another. The worst part for Dan was that each specialty was scattered across the University of Florida, which is one of the largest campuses in the country. Parking was a nightmare, and seeing two specialists in a single day was impossible.

Dan started with a neurologist and then was shuttled to a neuropsychologist, and thereafter to a psychiatrist. Next, he headed to see a physical therapist, then an occupational therapist, and finally a speech therapist. The visits uncovered that Dan required special testing to make sure that he was not swallowing food into his lungs, and of course, you guessed it, that meant another visit. Following optimization by every specialty imaginable, it was determined he required one more visit to a neurosurgeon, Dr. Kelly Foote.

When did care coordination reach its maximal impact? The moment all the clinicians assembled and discussed Dan's health. Ironically, the highest level of health care one can hope for is when a skilled team is talking and exchanging thoughts openly. Most of the time in health care you are lucky to be able to see one practitioner and find adequate parking close enough to the building to make the walk worth the effort. When you can be evaluated by multiple health care providers and they talk to each other and exchange points of view and co-create a plan, this is the best chance for success. This is also the best chance for your voice to be heard and amplified.

A consensus summary of the multidisciplinary discussion and recommendations was assembled and applied to a shared decision-making process, which included Dan and his family. This discussion is crucial to success as it is the compilation of data across multiple providers distilled into digestible language. We need to have conversations where we speak to people like Dan, not at them, and where we share with them our honest thoughts. Though this first crack at care coordination at the University of Florida was not efficient and proved a navigation nightmare, it was the beginning of process refinement. Dan would become the first person to receive DBS at the University of Florida, and his outcome was excellent. In this surgical approach, wires are placed in the brain and connected to battery packs in the chest. The procedure is like a cardiac pacemaker but designed for the brain. The birth of care coordination for deep brain stimulation was aptly named "fast track," and the process has become a standard for many multidisciplinary DBS teams across the United States and beyond.[2-7]

The delivery of specialized care for complex disorders in the United States is expensive, inefficient, and less effective than it could be. To achieve optimal care coordination, we must adopt a core philosophical principle. At the University of Florida Fixel Institute, which provides approximately 20,000 care visits a year for persons with Parkinson's disease, "the patient is the Sun and all services should orbit around them, and not the doctor."[2,8]

As the care coordination model at the University of Florida evolved to involve more than elective DBS surgery, the multidisciplinary service and science hub model evolved into an improved example for all. The hub (mission control) addressed weaknesses in process and refocused clinicians on the importance of communication, preventive care, efficiency of multiple visits, and outcome tracking.

There are four core principles to pull off implementation of a hub-based model of care for Parkinson's disease.

1. All interdisciplinary specialists who will be required to provide optimal care are **colocated under one roof**. In the case of Parkinson's disease and other movement disorders, for example, neurology, neurosurgery, neuropsychology, psychiatry, physical therapy, occupational therapy, speech/swallow therapy, and social workers all evaluate patients at a common facility. Patients can be prescheduled with multiple specialists or scheduled on demand, and practitioners can interact in real time, especially if warranted by the complexity of the case.

2. We hear everyone's voices. Each specialist develops and communicates **a patient-specific care plan** within their area of expertise, and follow-up can be accomplished in the local community if the patient lives remotely. Documentation of all subspecialty evaluations and recommendations is sent to referring care providers and any other designated local care provider, shared directly with each patient, and can be reviewed via the online medical record system.

3. **Every patient is a potential research participant**, and outcomes of all therapeutic interventions are carefully documented and tracked over time. Each patient signs an institutional-review-board-approved database consent, so that every contact with a patient becomes part of both the clinical record and the research database. Patients also specify whether they are willing to be contacted for potential inclusion in future research studies. An effort is undertaken by all specialists to perform consistent structured evaluations at regular intervals in order to maximize the uniformity of clinical data. Clinical research trials are available and conducted in the same facility.

4. The relationship between the patient and each of the care or research providers is **bidirectional**. Interactions are not solely for the patient's benefit. The hub focuses on the professional and personal needs of each provider, as well as the needs of each patient. Bidirectionality facilitates research to improve care, enhances the

education of the next generation of specialists, and fosters professional development and workplace satisfaction.[8]

So why has the United States not widely adopted or implemented the service and science hub model (mission control) for Parkinson's coordination of care? Implementation of complex coordinated care for Parkinson's disease is frequently bogged down by several critical factors, rendering it difficult to scale over large geographies, such as the continental United States. Some of the factors include poor communication, wide variations in care delivery, a paucity of outcomes data, minimal focus on prevention, suboptimal education of the next generation of care providers, failure to develop multidisciplinary care teams, and failure to achieve financial buy-in. We believe that an optimal solution to create mission control centers for those with Parkinson's will include local buy-in, state and federal policy change, and funding. The University of Florida model has started to catch on at larger academic health care centers; however, the real target is to reach everyone affected with Parkinson's disease.

Flipping Care from Reactive to Proactive with Nurses and Navigators

Care coordination is not a new concept; still, health systems and society in general have yet to fully embrace it. In Parkinson's disease, we have failed to recognize its critical importance and to widely appreciate its potential benefits. Health care experts frequently refer to this type of care coordination as the chronic care model.[9] Simply put, any time a disease fulfills the two C's, complex and chronic, this model can be transformative for the patient. In diabetes, for example, when a nurse is appointed to the role of care coordinator (mission control coordinator), care flips from reactive, without someone in that North Star role, to proactive. As neurologist Dr. Bastiaan Bloem has shown, a chronic care model shifts the role of the doctor from god to guide. Philosophers have thought of this as a shift from viewing a doctor as an omnipotent controlling figure to seeing them as a guiding presence. This alternative construct encourages supportive and productive interactions, inclusive of both people with disease and their families. It allows voices to be heard and amplified with the implementation of appropriate care solutions.

**WHAT ELEMENTS WOULD "FLIP THE SCRIPT"
FOR CARE IN PARKINSON'S DISEASE?**

- Supporting self-management
- Assisting with integrated decision support
- Delivering proactive care
- Mobilizing use of available community resources
- Exploiting the use of patient registries
- Linking specialists and generalists
- Integrating rehabilitation and mental health services
- Preventing falls and fractures
- Avoiding hospitalizations
- Employing telemedicine when appropriate

The "why" supporting major changes in Parkinson's care delivery is compelling. We continue to deliver a new diagnosis every six minutes,[10] and the Parkinson's population is on track to more than double by 2040.[11,12] Millions hope for a cure; yet we meander in our efforts to care for them. It is time we improve our command and control for Parkinson's.

LESSONS FROM HIV/AIDS

Do comprehensive care plans for chronic diseases work? You bet they do, and one of the best recent examples is HIV/AIDS.[13-18] Comprehensive care for HIV/AIDS proactively addresses the medical, psychological, and social needs of nearly all those living with the virus. The mortality for HIV/AIDS compared to other diseases has rapidly decreased. These changes have been driven by advances in treatment, prevention, and awareness, but most importantly they have been driven by a fundamental shift toward a comprehensive care strategy that didn't wait for a cure to improve the lives of the living.

HIV/AIDS emerged in the early 1980s and quickly became a leading cause of death globally. By 2005, HIV/AIDS had grown into the fourth leading cause of death. Twenty years later, the recognition of the cause and the aggressive pursuit of comprehensive care plans changed the trajectory of HIV/AIDS. The change in mortality in countries where treatment was available was driven both by the widespread introduction of antiretroviral therapy and by comprehensive care planning.[19-25]

In the world of HIV/AIDS, the introduction of care programs with intensive monitoring increased access to medications. The care programs expanded to include monitoring the blood for active levels of the virus. These programs were game changers. What was the result? A massive decline in illnesses, hospitalizations, and HIV/AIDS-related deaths. Once an HIV/AIDS global health plan was constructed, organizations jumped on board and quickly scaled up prevention, testing, and treatment efforts.[26-29] Today, HIV/AIDS is no longer among the top ten leading causes of death.

How does the HIV story compare to Parkinson's disease? HIV was first discovered in 1983. Mortality from HIV/AIDS has significantly declined over approximately forty years. Rare cases of Parkinson's first appeared in ancient Indian medical texts approximately five hundred years before the birth of Jesus; yet, despite the passage of thousands of years, Parkinson's is now an increasingly common cause of death in the United States and beyond.[30-38]

We believe that we must implement the components of the HIV/AIDS plan, which can be immediately exported to Parkinson's disease. The Parkinson's Plan will need to start with listening to the voices of persons with disease and their caregivers and providing optimal management with Parkinson's drugs, similar to the use of antiretroviral therapy for HIV/AIDS. Additionally, the HIV/AIDS plan was successful because it provided support to make sure folks stayed on their complex medication regimens. Keeping regimens "on time every time," as published by the Parkinson's Foundation, is a critical key to living well with this neurodegenerative disease.[39-43] Are we doing a good enough job of optimizing medications for those suffering with Parkinson's? No.

Further, HIV/AIDS has provided a path to psychosocial support, including mental health services and peer-to-peer support. Parkinson's, in contrast, has been spotty in addressing this challenge. Similarly, both HIV/AIDS and Parkinson's are associated with gradual weight loss.[44-49] However, progress has only been made in HIV/AIDS, where regular nutritional support, including dietary counseling and nutritional supplements, has been emphasized for all.

Perhaps the single most important lesson that can be exported from HIV/AIDS to Parkinson's has been the provision of case management, with direct, proactive care coordination provided to help people navigate the treacherous health care system.[50–57] Care managers listen to all voices. The support also includes scheduling appointments and managing referrals. HIV/AIDS has also set the bar for development of support services for spouses, care partners, and families, and Parkinson's will need to prioritize these areas and to sprint in order to catch up. HIV/AIDS has developed an effective care coordination plan (mission control). We believe that Parkinson's has lagged so far behind HIV/AIDS because of our failure to act swiftly to put together a ground game centered on the care of the person with Parkinson's.

NAVIGATORS

Dutch neurologist and epidemiologist Sirwan Darweesh has spent his career uncovering patterns and causes of disease. When Sirwan and his colleagues asked people with Parkinson's what their top priorities were, "a single point of access" consistently appeared on the list. Sirwan has become convinced that "a single health care provider acting as a personal care manager is the key." This manager listens and "either answers simple questions directly or navigates the patient towards other professionals who are better suited to address the specific issue at hand, thus ascertaining integration as well as continuity of care across disciplines and across different workplaces." It is common for persons with Parkinson's to require management of multiple challenges including tremor, use of utensils, and unsteadiness. A common misconception is that a single physician can manage all these challenges. This is flawed thinking, as an occupational therapist will be better able to address utensil use and a physical therapist to prevent falling.

The personal manager, though ideally a health care provider, could also be a spouse, care partner, family member, or friend, especially if we were to listen to them, educate them, and empower them to become part of the North Star care-coordination plan. The current health care system does not prioritize funding for care management, and we should be pivoting toward alternative pathways to meet this challenge. The transformation of care management in Parkinson's disease could be achieved by assembling the four elements of care coordination: patient navigation, provision of information, early detection of emerging symptoms, and continuous monitoring of the process. One approach would be to champion patient navigators who can be trained to identify, in real time, the individual needs of a person, and by taking a play from the Operation Housecall experience, we could match them with appropriate services and providers. A navigator (mission control) steers a person through the intricacies of health care systems. The navigator solves the access issues and collaborates with all providers.[58-61]

Though navigators have traditionally been nurses, social workers, physicians, and advanced practice providers, in some diseases like diabetes, community volunteers, family members, and patients themselves can play a key role in navigation. There is precedent for the lay community to become patient navigators and to interface with the medical community.[62-66]

AI could potentially help to fill the gap. Imagine a system where a spouse, care partner, family, or friend inputs regular, symptom-specific, and preventative care data into an automated system that is capable of providing both recommendations and care referrals, all with a touch of a button. Ideally, the solution will include a real person provided by an insurance provider, but the best way to achieve that investment would be to prove the concept works by starting with something more cost-effective and sustainable. As we imagine what care coordination (mission control) could or will look like in the near future, navigators and AI will both have the potential to improve outcomes.

THE DUTCH MODEL FOR PARKINSON'S CARE

One American Thanksgiving, Michael and his wife were on a plane to the Netherlands, wondering what spending a major holiday abroad would be like. Michael was booked to be the keynote speaker at a meeting of ParkinsonNet. The venue was inside the Royal Jaarbeurs Event & Exhibition Centre in the city of Utrecht. He slipped past the rows of bicycles and into the unmistakable building unnoticed. He was instantly transformed by the energy of the assembling crowd. There were over 2,000 physical, occupational, and speech therapists bouncing around the lobby, meeting rooms, and central theater. The energy was more like a Beatles concert than the subdued academic conferences he was used to. He stopped a young speech therapist and asked her why she was so excited. "We do this once a year, and it is energizing to be part of a group of therapists changing lives. We love it."

Though the population of the Netherlands is roughly the same as Florida's and both have similar numbers of individuals with Parkinson's, the care in the Netherlands is much better. The reason is ParkinsonNet. ParkinsonNet was envisioned about twenty years ago by neurologist Bastiaan Bloem and his good friend physical therapist Marten Munneke.[67-83] Both practiced at Radboud University Medical Center within the petite city of Nijmegen, and both were frustrated by the "unacceptable variations in the quality of care, the suboptimal health outcomes and especially the high costs" they observed around them.

In response, Bloem and Munneke created a set of multidisciplinary networks of allied health professionals spread all over the Netherlands. Over time, their initially tiny networks multiplied to cover the whole country. Therapists were excited to connect with like-minded individuals. It was not a hard sell to get these folks to a yearly meeting in the city center of Utrecht and into other major and smaller Dutch cities. Training was fun and focused on evidence-based practice guidelines. The bonus was that all of the knowledge was transferable to real people living with Parkinson's disease. Today, there are sixty-nine regional networks with about 3,000 health professionals, all readily available to patients. All the care is linked by a common medical record. If you are a person with Parkinson's in the Netherlands, you are set. You can seek care in any region and from any specialist, from a doctor to a nurse, from a rehabilitation team to a counselor, and you can do it with confidence that you are receiving the latest in evidence-based care for Parkinson's disease. Over the years Bloem and Munneke have deepened their friendship and continued to toil to identify, train, and integrate more specialties, including everything from social workers to sex therapists.[67-83]

What is the mission control concept that has made ParkinsonNet so effective? Two words provide the answer: care coordination. Instead of using a single person as a coordinator, like a volunteer with Operation House-call or an insurance-company-provided nurse, ParkinsonNet created access to care, implemented evidence-based practice guidelines, and increased the specialist experience in the quest to care for persons with Parkinson's. The network has also facilitated rapid communication between specialists.

ParkinsonNet functions with only a modest-sized coordination center (mission control), which is in Nijmegen, one of the country's oldest cities, and in most cases there is continuity in the care provider. The magic is achieved through local volunteer networks, a shared medical record, and free, patient-based decision-support tools. As Bloem and Munneke's efforts grew, they recognized that network-based data on outcomes was lacking, and they formed a National Quality Registry for Parkinson's. This databank enabled ParkinsonNet to compare and contrast outcomes across Dutch regions. Bloem and Munneke have used the registry to shine a spotlight on the data from both high-performing and low-performing regions. Detailed interviews and site visits were used to uncover the secret sauce of each region and to export the recipe to benefit other provinces. Bloem and Munneke discovered that care across their network was highly specialized and that each team innovated unique processes to enhance the quality-of-care delivery and to reach more people. In some cases, the sharing of information led to dramatic benefits such as prevention of aspiration pneumonia, the leading cause of death in Parkinson's. In other cases, it led to improved marriages, travel tips, and better sex lives. The network was important for destigmatizing symptoms and personalizing care.

SUPPORT THE CAREGIVERS

If the patient is the sun, then the caregiver is Mercury, which has the closest orbit. Being that close to the patient (sun) can be hot, and as the World Health Organization (WHO) has pointed out, specific factors contribute to increased caregiver burden, including the progressive nature of Parkinson's and the timing of onset for the patient. As the disease advances, cognitive impairment, psychiatric manifestations, and sleep disruption add to the burden. Reduced social interactions, frustrations with complex medication regimens, and limitation in their abilities to provide care emerge.[84,85]

An unspoken truth is that a caregiver's own health issues may also impact the plan. We know that effective caregiving has benefits for both the caregiver and the person with Parkinson's. If we invest in the caregiver, we can avoid or delay institutionalization and prevent costly hospitalizations.[86–88]

A recent WHO panel found that factors that reduce caregiver burden include "provision of a timely diagnosis; effective communication and education about caregiver roles, medications, and adverse effects; and rehabilitation and palliative care strategies, including governmental entitlements and discussions of decision-making capacity. Social workers, patient support groups, and community-based services can provide effective resources."[85]

The Parkinson's Plan should recognize the key role of the caregiver and should address the health of both the patient and the caregiver. If we shift our approach to both, we can recognize and treat demoralization, depression, and mood disorders earlier and have the potential for better outcomes as well as cost savings by keeping care in the home rather than in an institution or hospital. Most Parkinson's caregivers suffer from caregiver strain.[86–91] We need to wake up and realize that the caregiver is Mercury, the messenger who rules over wealth, good fortune, and commerce. If we prop up Mercury, the rest of the Parkinson's Universe will be stronger. We need to hear the voices of the caregivers, and we need to amplify their voices by providing critical care services.

WHERE TO LOOK WHEN YOU NEED SUPPORT

Any model aiming to improve care delivery for persons with Parkinson's will need to expand beyond the standard provision of medical services. A Parkinson's Plan cannot be complete without strengthening and doubling down on local, regional, national, and international support groups as well as advocacy organizations. Today a person or caregiver with Parkinson's can gaze in almost any direction and encounter the light of many stars. We must invest more in teaching persons with Parkinson's disease and also caregivers how to navigate the numerous stars, such as the Michael J. Fox Foundation, the Parkinson's Foundation, the PD Avengers, Parkinson's Africa, Parkinson's UK, Parkinson's Australia, and many others. Navigation has for centuries been a vital skill for mariners, explorers, and travelers. Since navigation is a skill, we must teach it. We must assist in finding position and direction and in the effective use of support groups and advocacy organizations. We must teach people how to listen.

As a young real estate attorney, Nathan Slewett helped turn Staten Island's potato farms into neighborhoods, and when he moved south, he pivoted his attention to developing a hub for Parkinson's disease. No one in Nathan's family was affected by Parkinson's disease; yet he was inspired by witnessing the shaking, shuffling, and stumbling of a neighbor. Nathan embarked on a lifelong quest to raise money for Parkinson's research, transforming into the most well-known lay person in the Parkinson's disease space and raising over $100 million throughout the span of his career. He became the face and chair of the National Parkinson's Foundation, a role he would hold for over forty years until his death at age ninety-seven. Nathan would be at the center of a worldwide movement to change the way we imagine care for Parkinson's disease.

Nathan imagined bestowing a prestigious designation on Parkinson's disease centers to drive improvement in both care and research. Nathan felt it was an advantage to colocate the best clinicians next to the best researchers and to partner with patients to drive the research. Centers of Excellence for Parkinson's disease, the first step toward a service and science hub model, were born under Nathan. This idea for a center did not exist for any other neurological disease at the time. Now it is commonplace.

Nathan used his skills as a real estate developer to pedal his idea from center to center until it caught on. Four university centers, including two Ivies, agreed to sign on. All were delighted by the money and, of course, the prestige. However, all resisted the idea of standardization, because every center inherently believed the way it provided care was best. Today we now appreciate that sharing outcomes from different centers and approaches has led to advances in care for Parkinson's. The answer was not a "one-size-fits-all" model. There are fifty-four medical centers around the world holding the Parkinson's Foundation designation; however, there are dozens of other Centers of Excellence sponsored by other organizations, such as the Veterans Administration's Parkinson's Disease Research, Education, and Clinical Centers (PADRECCs), the American Parkinson's Disease Association Centers of Excellence, and the European Parkinson's Disease Association Centers of Excellence. There has also been a recent movement to designate dozens of comprehensive care centers, focusing on the person rather than on a dual role for care and research. The Parkinson's Plan will benefit from expansion and partnerships with such centers.

Sarah Johnston called the Parkinson's Foundation helpline because she was confused about the different options for deep brain stimulation surgery. She wanted to understand which brain target and approach would provide her the most short- and long-term relief, given that she was now experiencing hallucinations. They listened, and the call may have saved her life, as undergoing DBS surgery with active psychosis could have been dangerous. Sarah was not aware of the importance of multidisciplinary DBS-candidate screening and that patient selection is the first and most important step toward the potential success of the procedure. For Sarah, DBS was not the right option; however, changing her medications was transformative.

Access to specialized education and support tools is critical for those living with Parkinson's disease. We believe that AI-based systems will one day play a part in care coordination. However, it is hard for us to imagine best Parkinson's care without a human element in some form listening to the voice of the person with disease.

NO PERSON WITH PARKINSON'S LEFT BEHIND

Jim Jones was a seventy-six-year-old retired engineer eager to volunteer for the latest drug available for Parkinson's disease, whether approved or in clinical trial. He was faithful in regularly visiting not only his neurologist but also his physical, occupational, and speech therapists. Jim embraced new exercise regimens and learned "brain games," which he found bulked up his cognitive muscle. Over the years, however, Jim became more and more forgetful, and one day he disappeared from our clinic schedules. His family had pulled the trigger and moved Jim into a nursing home. His care became disconnected, and had there been a navigator and North Star coordination plan, this would not likely have happened. Jim and his family lost their connection to the Parkinson's care universe. Tragically, Jim's brightness disappeared, and he died within a year.

Sol De Jesus, a neurologist at Penn State University, has been interested in what happens to the "Jims." She estimates that approximately 20% of the current Parkinson's population is made up of Jims, or people who are managing well with their Parkinson's until they become unplugged from their medical network. Sol and her colleagues believe it is time to reconnect the Jims to care, but how?[92]

The answer may be in the growing palliative care movement. Benzi Kluger, a neurologist at the University of Rochester, was a behavior and movement disorders neurologist before he fully embraced the palliative care revolution. Benzi performed a randomized clinical trial of 210 people with Parkinson's disease and related disorders. What he found was eye-opening. If you were diagnosed with Parkinson's disease and received palliative care, you experienced a better quality-of-life outcome and had an overall reduction in your symptom burden.[93–95]

When folks hear the term *palliative care*, their minds jump to hospice. But palliative care for Parkinson's disease is not hospice. Neurologists on palliative care teams work side by side with a pharmacist, a nurse, a chaplain, and a social worker.

WHAT IS PALLIATIVE CARE FOR PARKINSON'S DISEASE?

- Palliative care is not the same as hospice for cancer.
- Palliative care is an approach aimed to improve quality of life for both persons with disease and their families.
- Palliative care addresses physical, emotional, and psychological aspects of a Parkinson's journey.
- Palliative care focuses on relief from symptoms and stress.
- Palliative care does not focus on cures.
- Palliative care focuses on symptom management, emotional support, advanced care planning, and addressing more than physical symptoms.
- Palliative care emphasizes social, spiritual, and psychological domains of living with Parkinson's.
- Palliative care provides support for caregivers.

STIGMA IS ALWAYS THERE

Though Pluto is not quite large enough to be a planet, it is always present and in continuous orbit around the sun (the patient). In the Parkinson's Universe, Pluto represents stigma. Pluto is the ninth-largest mass to orbit the sun. Pluto is a perfect representation of stigma as it is dark, icy, isolated, and rocky.

The stigma of a Parkinson's diagnosis is huge. Stigma comes from the negative perceptions and stereotypes that those diagnosed encounter in society. Believe it or not, stigma can even be propagated by health care providers themselves. Since stigma impacts emotional, psychological, and social well-being, we believe strongly that persons with disease, caregivers, care partners, and family members all need to be educated on the effects of stigma and how to actively address it.[96–102] There are many solutions, which can lead to empowerment; however, until stigma is recognized and appreciated, it cannot be mitigated.

Dr. Indu Subramanian, a professor at the University of California, Los Angeles, and director of the Los Angeles Veterans Affairs PADRECC, has traveled the world lecturing on appreciating and addressing stigma in Parkinson's. Stigma not only affects an individual's sense of self but is also considered a significant social determinant of health that contributes to morbidity, mortality, and health disparities. Stigma is among the most frequently discussed major public health concerns by leading health officials, epidemiologists, and physicians like Indu. Neurological disorders such as Parkinson's are among the most highly stigmatizing diseases in the world; yet we do little to identify and address that fact.[103]

Although motor symptoms caused by Parkinson's are impactful on the experience of stigma, the mediating role of depression and the burden of this disease should not be underestimated. Research suggests that treatments focused entirely on alleviating motor symptoms that do not target the emotional response to Parkinson's disease are inadequate. We must also focus on mental health issues. Physicians or other members of the medical team may be able to help manage the deleterious effects of stigma by addressing not only the physical symptoms but also psychosocial pressures. If the physician does not initiate a conversation, patients must feel empowered enough to bring these issues to the attention of their medical team. Patient empowerment is key.

At the individual level, interventions directed at knowledge, self-concept, self-esteem, and developing coping skills may be helpful. These goals can be achieved through individual counseling and focus. The more structured approach of cognitive behavioral therapy can also be helpful as it provides stress-management strategies, challenges negative beliefs normalizing stigma, and helps patients feel that they are not alone. Support groups are also valuable in helping those living with Parkinson's disease to improve their self-esteem and coping skills and lessen social isolation. Support groups are an example of a disease self-management strategy that has garnered increased research attention as a way of helping those affected to navigate the unknowns. Mentors and "Parkinson's disease buddies" can play a role in educating their peers about their disease through sharing experiential knowledge and normalizing the stigma experience. The sharing of challenges, which includes the exchange of lived experience, emotional issues, and coping strategies, can be an essential resource to overcome fear and stigma. This type of exchange can lead to feelings of peer acceptance, energize those living with chronic illness, and foster empowerment and hope. Among the potential treatments demonstrating effectiveness in attenuating the negative effects of stigma and improving a variety of positive outcome measures (e.g., depression, emotional well-being) is social support. A recently described way to improve social support and connection is social prescribing, which is one way for clinicians to help patients increase community connections, thereby improving health outcomes.[16,96–103]

HOW CAN STIGMA AFFECT A PERSON WITH PARKINSON'S DISEASE?

- Physical symptoms can be mistaken for intoxication or other conditions, and this has been shown to lead to social isolation

- and other challenges. People may also get impatient with a person for slowness to complete a task.
- Internalized stigma may lead to shame or embarrassment and reduced social interaction. Some cases can even progress to depression.
- Mental health may be worsened by stigma, leading to anxiety, depression, and a lower quality of life.
- Fear of being judged or misunderstood can lead to serious consequences, such as lack of medical attention or compliance (e.g., an assistive device for walking is not used, putting the person in danger of falling).
- Workplace stigma may lead to feeling misjudged and mistreated.
- Avoidance of social situations may lead to increasing isolation.

CREATING CONNECTIONS TO BRING
CARE BACK TO THE HOME

Guo Hu lived in Beijing and had just been implanted with a deep brain stimulator. He was sent home to recover and was to return a few days later for his device activation. Then Covid-19 hit, and he was stuck at home, unable to activate his new devices. His doctors scrambled to employ a Bluetooth-enabled telemedicine programming system to activate devices and manage Guo and many other bionic people with Parkinson's in their homes.[104] The Parkinson's Plan should include provisions to use telemedicine, neurotechnology, and AI to bring care to those who need it. In our Parkinson's Universe model, we refer to these technologies as satellites. In this case we suggest that the satellite should orbit the sun (the patient).

In the span of a few weeks, the Covid-19 pandemic changed the way we care for individuals with Parkinson's disease. Telemedicine, the delivery of health care at a distance, instantly transformed from a niche practice into the dominant means of providing care. Telemedicine offers four C's: care, convenience, comfort, and confidentiality. Technology can bring care into the home and make it more accessible to individuals with Parkinson's.

Many, if not most, individuals with Parkinson's disease lack access to care due to distance, disability, or simply the absence of doctors.[85,105–107] In 1993, Dr. Jean Hubble and colleagues demonstrated the ability of tele-medicine in the setting of satellite clinics to deliver care to rural Kansas residents.[108,109] While traditional clinics are accessible to individuals with early or mild Parkinson's, they are often inaccessible to those in the later stages of the disease. Several programs have demonstrated the ability to reach individuals with advanced Parkinson's, including those in US-based nursing homes, who account for up to a quarter of older adults in this coun-try. Many individuals with Parkinson's remain undiagnosed, especially in parts of the world where the demand for care far exceeds the supply of specialists. In Beijing, for example, nearly half the people with Parkin-son's are currently undiagnosed, and China has the fastest-increasing rates of Parkinson's disease. Smartphones, which are ubiquitous, could greatly expand access to care by connecting those in need to a wide range of global clinicians.

In addition to increasing access, telemedicine can transform care. Studies have demonstrated that a typical thirty-minute office visit for Parkinson's disease consumes over four hours for patients and caregivers, door to door. The vast majority of that time is spent traveling and waiting. Telemedicine visits save money, save patients many miles of difficult travel, and reduce the risk of falls and accidents.[105,107] The economic costs of travel and parking can exceed an insurance copayment and can become a major barrier limit-ing access to care.

Telemedicine allows patients to be evaluated from the comfort of their own homes. In many ways, telemedicine represents the second generation of the classical house call. In the 1930s, 40% of physician-patient encounters occurred in the home. Telemedicine enables physicians to reenter the home and to examine the patient in their own natural setting. This setting may provide better insights into how individuals function in their daily lives. Telemedicine offers enhanced understanding of social circumstances and the possibility of a more patient-centered experience. The "power asymme-try" between patients and clinicians can be reduced, because in telemedicine both parties are seated at eye level and patients are operating in their homes and clinicians in their office environments. Additionally, most patients and families prefer the comfort and convenience of telemedicine visits.

While the privacy and security of video visits have been raised as potentially serious concerns, in many ways virtual visits do offer a different form of confidentiality. In-person attendance at a movement disorders clinic broadcasts to everyone present "I have a neurological disorder." The confidentiality offered by telemedicine may be critically important to asymptomatic individuals at (genetic) risk for Parkinson's disease.

Despite these advantages, it took contagion to tip the scales toward a wide global embrace of telemedicine.[105,107] Covid-19 forced many ambulatory clinics to close, and a large proportion of visits transitioned to phone calls or video conferencing. This rapid transition was necessary to minimize the spread of the infectious disease and to preserve personal protective equipment and resources for those in the most need. As a result of this change, many clinicians and patients experienced telemedicine for the first time. At many medical centers, telemedicine visits have increased 100-to-1,000-fold, and during the pandemic they represented the majority of clinical encounters for persons with Parkinson's disease.

Telemedicine does have well-established limitations. Many elements of the physical examination, like assessing eye movements, evaluating rigidity, and testing reflexes, are difficult, if not impossible, to do remotely. Despite these limitations, numerous parts of the examination can, with some creativity, be conducted remotely. For example, with the help of a family member or friend, asymmetries in rigidity can be assessed remotely in a seated patient by observing how the legs—when passively swung by the care partner—gradually come to a standstill. While the examination is important, 80% of medical diagnoses are based on history. Moreover, Dr. James Parkinson's original description was largely based on observation, and Sir William Osler wrote in 1892, "When well established, [Parkinson's disease] is very characteristic, and the diagnosis can be made at a glance."

The digital divide—the differential access to the internet based on geographic, social, and economic factors—is another real concern, representing a serious barrier for many people to realize the benefits of telemedicine. For example, in the United States, 20% of households lack broadband access at home or have no access to a smartphone. Increasing global access to these technologies will be necessary for telemedicine to grow and to address existing disparities in care.[105,107] And telemedicine itself doesn't solve the problem of the relative scarcity of Parkinson's specialists.

But video visits will expand beyond neurologists to include many other clinicians on the multidisciplinary care team, including physical, occupational, and speech-language therapists, nurses, dieticians, psychiatrists, psychologists, and genetic counselors. This expansion will be accompanied by an increasing chance that a patient's voice will be heard and that appropriate care will be amplified. Video visits can also include family members who may be in different cities or even different countries. Multidisciplinary care may be easier to deliver remotely and could potentially be family-centric. Many teams in the world now have the positive experience of performing multidisciplinary team meetings remotely, as video visits no longer require all team members to be present in the same room at the same time. Some of these telemedicine efforts will involve group visits, nonclinicians like exercise coaches, and even digital therapies like speech-language therapy. Telemedicine postpandemic has begun to merge more with traditional care, where infrequent in-person visits may be combined with more frequent telemedicine appointments. Clinical research, including both observational and interventional studies, has been rapidly adopting remote visits.

While telemedicine may be enjoying its finest hour, its future is not completely certain. Many of the changes in the United States that enabled telemedicine use during the pandemic, including insurance coverage by Medicare and reduced licensing restrictions, were only temporary, and despite individuals around the country sending thousands of red cards to the White House after publication of our book *Ending Parkinson's Disease*, which advocated for renewal, telemedicine access has been more recently reduced. People with Parkinson's have the right to telemedicine. We should also be investing in wearable technologies that have the potential to monitor people at home (satellites) and to send vital information to care coordination centers (mission control), which can monitor and, when necessary, change course in real time. Wearable technologies may one day provide the information necessary to pick up urinary and other infections early and to prevent sepsis (a potentially deadly infection in the blood). These technologies will be able to monitor symptoms and suggest appropriate changes in medication and device settings to optimize outcomes. Finally, imagine if we could prevent folks with Parkinson's from falls, fractured hips, and treacherous admissions to the hospital, which is not a safe place for those with this disease.

ADDRESSING COST

The cost barriers to accessing appropriate care for Parkinson's disease are formidable, and getting around them can frequently feel like navigating an asteroid field. When Han Solo and Chewbacca flew into an asteroid field during the iconic movie *Star Wars*, the possibility of successful navigation was 3,720 to 1. When a person with Parkinson's and their caregiver enter the disconnected health care system, their odds of success are similar.

Although growing evidence strongly supports a multidisciplinary approach for a proactive, preventative care plan for people with Parkinson's disease, right now there's no way to do it. No mechanism in the American or other health care systems can widely facilitate it. Implementation of multidisciplinary care will provide billions of dollars in economic and societal savings, reducing falls, fractures, nursing home placements, and countless other costs.

Implementation will keep us out of the asteroid field. How can we get there? The total accrued expenses of Parkinson's disease will cripple Medicare and devastate private insurance. Parkinson's is the fastest-growing neurological disease and one of the most expensive. A recent study revealed that the economic burden of the estimated one million Americans with Parkinson's is $52 billion.[110] Future costs will continue to mushroom.

Many critical services are not covered by insurance, and many others are not accessible for persons with Parkinson's disease living with mobility challenges and without adequate transportation. These services include licensed clinical social workers, mental health professionals (including counselors), personal trainers, and dieticians. One way to make these critical services and their integrated benefits affordable and accessible would be a tax benefit.[111]

The system would provide a yearly tax refund for those with Parkinson's in order to provide the necessary services to navigate and thrive with the disease. Under such a system, licensed clinical social workers could be part of the North Star plan for each individual and provide the necessary coordination of care. Regular consultations with social workers would connect people with Parkinson's disease and their families to current and emerging local, state, and federal programs. Social workers could then facilitate wellness and aid in navigating both the health care system and the disease. Additionally, many licensed clinical social workers could provide counseling, similar to counseling psychologists.

Providing a benefit to cover the expense of a licensed clinical social worker once a month could be a game changer. Regular access to a social worker will facilitate early and more timely referrals to neurologists and psychiatrists. Earlier referrals will translate into proactive identification and treatment of severe depression, anxiety, and demoralization, all of which commonly contribute to Parkinson's hospitalizations, morbidity, and, in some cases, even death. Additionally, research strongly supports that caregiver strain occurs in the majority of Parkinson's cases[87,112–114] and largely goes unaddressed. More frequent hospitalizations and emergency room visits are highly dependent on the skillset and disposition of the caregiver, so it is appropriate that we focus attention on their empowerment and well-being. A tax benefit could close the gap in addressing caregiver strain.

Providing a tax benefit could also incentivize persons with Parkinson's to integrate an alternating-week personal-trainer strategy. Many personal trainers will meet people with Parkinson's disease in their homes, which of course improves access. Additionally, regular visits with certified personal trainers will reinforce the crucial importance and benefits of continuous exercise for Parkinson's, which is preferable to bursts of therapy. Personal trainers can provide a link to physicians and to rehabilitation services and could be utilized to facilitate more timely referrals. Timeliness in addressing emerging issues will reduce falls, fractures, hospitalizations, morbidity, and in some cases mortality.

The current health care system does not provide access to and reimbursement for dieticians, though emerging evidence has revealed that diet impacts medication absorption, the microbiome, and many Parkinson's symptoms. Absorption of Parkinson's medications may be enhanced by reducing protein intake and slightly adjusting medication timing. Timing and coordinating nutrition with medication is important and underappreciated. There is emerging evidence that the Mediterranean and other diet plans may impact Parkinson's symptoms beyond their benefits for general health and wellness.[115–118]

Weight loss is another challenge for the entire population of folks living with Parkinson's disease. We know that there is a slow, continuous weight loss contributing to frailty and to a higher risk for bone fractures.[47] Dieticians can address these issues proactively, neutralize weight loss, and facilitate appropriate referrals for bone health. Finally, constipation is one of the most common, disabling, and undertreated symptoms of Parkinson's disease.[119–123] Access to a dietician has the potential to improve quality of life and promote healthier living.

A tax credit or incentive to access and fund regular psychological counseling services through telemedicine will reduce the burden of depression, anxiety, and demoralization. Frequent visits to therapists will also serve as a monitoring tool for triggering earlier referrals to psychiatrists and neurologists. Earlier treatment translates into an opportunity to reduce hospitalizations, attempted suicides, and deaths.

If we made a tax credit available and 75% of the one million Americans with Parkinson's cashed in the full tax credit of approximately $6,200 a year to provide all of these critical services, the total cost could reach $4 billion to $5 billion. The current cost of Parkinson's disease each year in the United States is $52 billion. The tax benefit would pay for itself. Hip fractures alone cost the American health care system about $50,000 per person. About one-third of persons with Parkinson's will experience at least one hip fracture within ten years of diagnosis.[124–128] The opportunity for improvement each year could translate to billions of dollars of savings for the system.[111] A tax benefit of approximately $6,200 for those diagnosed with Parkinson's disease in the United States will translate into more fall prevention, more care provided in the home setting, fewer hospitalizations, less depression, less anxiety, less demoralization, better diets, and fewer placements in nursing facilities. If those benefits are not enough to convince you of the merits of a tax benefit, then consider the billions of dollars in savings to the health care system.

And American taxpayers shouldn't be the ones to foot the bill. Pesticide and chemical companies should be legally required to contribute, given their generation of billions of dollars in profits through the manufacturing and distribution of products associated with Parkinson's disease.[111] We must amplify voices, lift the living, and light the path together.

DOPAMINE FOR ALL

In July 2022 a group of us got together with the World Health Organization to outline six action steps to address global disparities in Parkinson's disease. We believe that one of the most important is providing dopamine replacement therapy (pills) for all who have been diagnosed with Parkinson's. We identified a huge global gap, with many areas revealing reduced access to effective medications and, when they are available, high cost. According to the WHO Atlas for Neurological Disorders, only 37 of 110 countries had dopamine-replacement pills (levodopa/carbidopa) consistently available in primary care settings. A continent-wide survey of twenty-eight African countries revealed serious challenges with availability and high cost.

One proposed solution has been the use of *Mucuna pruriens*, also known as the velvet bean, and *Vicia faba*, known as the broad bean.[129–131] These legume plants contain measurable and clinically active dopamine (levodopa) and could serve as a substitute in resource-limited countries. The preparation of dopamine from these plants has proven tricky as there can be production of toxic chemicals and variable concentrations. This is an area of the Parkinson's Plan we should be investing in.[85] We believe it is unconscionable for anyone diagnosed with Parkinson's disease to be denied levodopa. If we can get HIV/AIDS drugs to the world, we can get dopamine out there too. Low- and middle-income countries face economic barriers, supply chain issues, and less developed health care systems. We have options, including the production and delivery of generic medications as well as the development of new, safer, and easier-to-prepare legume plants. We can promote international health organizations and nongovernmental organizations to improve access across regions for those lacking dopamine-replacement pills. Levodopa (dopamine replacement) is on the WHO List of Essential Medicines, which means it is considered a critical treatment that should be available to all people who need it across the globe. This listing encourages governments and health care systems to prioritize access to levodopa.[85] We need to lean in and get this done.

DO YOU KNOW THE SIX ACTION STEPS SET BY THE WORLD HEALTH ORGANIZATION TO ADDRESS GLOBAL DISPARITIES IN PARKINSON'S DISEASE?

1. Address the burden of disease with more spending in this area
2. Increase advocacy and awareness about disability, workplace rights, and improved governance of financing and insurance
3. Augment prevention and risk reduction, including by studying the environment and removing relevant pesticides and chemicals
4. Improve diagnosis, treatment, and care; ensure availability of essential drugs, diagnostics, and interdisciplinary therapies, including dopamine (levodopa) for all
5. Provide caregiver support, address caregiver burden, and provide appropriate social workers and care navigators
6. Conduct research into the epidemiology of the disease and ensure countries have appropriate funding to do so

---

LISTENING AND LEANING IN TO THE PARKINSON'S UNIVERSE EXPANDED MODEL

Promoting a practical preventative and proactive Parkinson's Plan to cover the costs of care will advantage both this generation and the next. Beyond the ten "must-do" care items (see below), expanding the Parkinson's care model from the "patient is the sun" into a larger and more coordinated universe of care is the right direction. We must listen to the voice of the caregiver (Mercury) and set up systems with care-based operations centers (mission control) that can monitor the specialists (the planets), combat stigma (Pluto), and utilize technology to monitor and enhance care (through satellites). We can make dopamine available to everyone on the planet by following the script set by HIV/AIDS drugs. We already have much of the knowledge that will be necessary to improve the care of individuals with Parkinson's disease. We can shift the broken and fragmented model to one that is comprehensive, coordinated, and proactive. How we create the Parkinson's Universe is up to us. We must listen to the voices of patients and caregivers and amplify them by providing the care services they need. All we need is the will to implement and the courage to light the path, and we can lift the living.

TEN "MUST-DO" CARE ITEMS IF YOU ARE DIAGNOSED WITH PARKINSON'S DISEASE

1. Take one multivitamin a day, since dopamine replacement therapy depletes important factors and may lead to neuropathy and other nutritional deficiencies.
2. Apply sunscreen, wear hats, and arrange to see a dermatologist once a year, as Parkinson's is associated with twice the risk of skin cancer.
3. Exercise every day, and ideally complete 7,500 steps or step equivalents (about 1.5 hours of exercise per day), as this has been shown to improve symptoms. Ride a recumbent bike or do alternative exercise if you can't walk.
4. Make stretching part of your daily routine as rigidity can gradually impinge on your flexibility.
5. Fight frailty by staying above your ideal body weight.
6. Keep your bones strong by having a bone scan for osteoarthritis or osteopenia every two years (both males

and females with Parkinson's commonly have soft bones).

7. If you are coughing when eating, see a speech-language pathologist and consider using an expiratory muscle strength trainer to reduce the risk of aspiration pneumonia.

8. Get evaluated at least once a year by physical, occupational, speech, and swallow therapists.

9. Have neuropsychological testing once every two years, and stay engaged, exercising your brain muscle (crosswords, cognitive apps).

10. Monitor your sleep with a wearable device and work to get six to eight hours of sleep every night, as this will improve your symptoms the next day and improve stamina.

PART 4

NAVIGATE

8

NAVIGATE THE FIRST FRONTIERS
OF NEW TREATMENTS

The comeback is always greater than the setback.

—**Winston Churchill**

WHILE WE SEEK TO BETTER UNDERSTAND THIS RELENTLESSLY PRO-
gressive disease, we will need a comprehensive plan to navigate our path
toward new treatments. There are three treatment frontiers. The first is
what can be deployed now. This includes expansion of the Parkinson's care
universe along with repurposed drugs, electrical stimulation, pumps, and
behavioral interventions. All can alleviate symptoms in the near term. There
are currently over ten million people with Parkinson's who may benefit from
such a strategy.

The second frontier includes new drugs, diets, stem cells, vaccines, and
immunotherapies. These treatments are designed to address symptoms and
to slow disease progression. They will take a little longer to develop, but the
payoff will be much greater. In this chapter, we will navigate the first two
frontiers of the near-term and mid-term therapies. In the next chapter, we
will look ahead to what is possible, but perhaps further in the future.

Navigating the Frontiers of
New Treatments

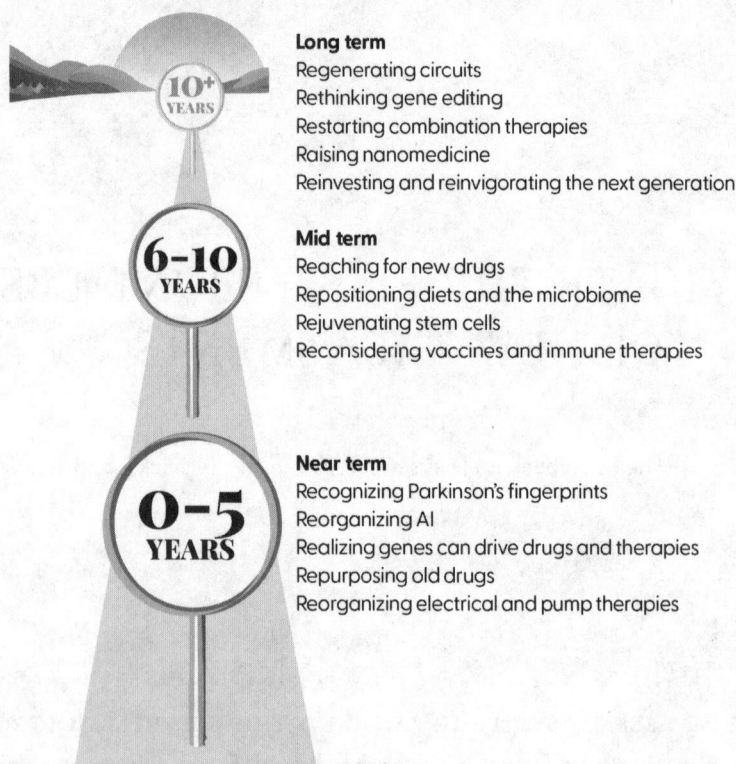

10⁺ YEARS

Long term
Regenerating circuits
Rethinking gene editing
Restarting combination therapies
Raising nanomedicine
Reinvesting and reinvigorating the next generation

6–10 YEARS

Mid term
Reaching for new drugs
Repositioning diets and the microbiome
Rejuvenating stem cells
Reconsidering vaccines and immune therapies

0–5 YEARS

Near term
Recognizing Parkinson's fingerprints
Reorganizing AI
Realizing genes can drive drugs and therapies
Repurposing old drugs
Reorganizing electrical and pump therapies

Figure 1. Navigating the frontiers of new treatments.

A TREATABLE DISEASE

In the twentieth century, two treatments transformed Parkinson's disease. The first breakthrough arrived in the 1960s with a pill to replace the brain's supply of dopamine. The medication (levodopa) rapidly transformed reality for people living with the disease.[1-4] The transformation from frozen to functional stunned even the most expert of physicians and scientists. Adding a little bit of dopamine to the brain reduced tremors, eased stiffness, and sped people up. A single pill put an end to the many hospital-based wards and asylums for Parkinson's disease. The medication decreased death rates and transformed a way of life; however, it didn't dent disease progression. Patients felt relief, but over time their function continued to deteriorate.

The second breakthrough therapy appeared when scientists and clinicians joined forces to electrify the brain. American neurologist Mahlon DeLong and French neurosurgeon Alim Benabid worked in the 1970s and 1980s to better understand the brain's circuitry and to develop and deploy deep brain stimulation (DBS).[5–10] The electrification of the brain calmed Parkinson's symptoms for hundreds of thousands of people already on dopamine who still needed an additional boost for emergent symptoms. The neurologist-neurosurgeon pair would share the 2014 Lasker-DeBakey Award for their pioneering work.[11]

Two additional advances in science have opened the floodgates to other discoveries in the field. The first landed in 1982 when neurologist Bill Langston encountered a flurry of young people with sudden-onset Parkinson's disease. Bill played detective and tracked down the cause to a synthetic heroin that was contaminated with a chemical called MPTP (1-methyl-4 -phenyl-1,2,3,6-tetrahydropyridine). When he offered dopamine replacement pills, patients rapidly and temporarily recovered, until of course the medication wore off.

The toxicant contained in the recreational drug was found to selectively destroy dopamine-producing brain cells in an area of the brain important for the control of movement. This new information was critical, and the Langston moment was an inflection point. Scientists now possessed a compound that, when given to an animal, resulted in a form of Parkinson's that could be reversed by administering dopamine. This serendipitous discovery provided a new animal model for the study of Parkinson's disease and opened a window into the degenerative process. The MPTP animal model accelerated the development of new therapies.[12–17]

The other big scientific advance came in 1996 when Mihael Polymeropoulos and colleagues discovered a large Italian American family with Parkinson's disease. Most of the members of the family lived in the small town of Contursi, located in the Salerno province of Italy. There were sixty of them in total, spread over five generations across Italy and Greece. The family turned out to possess a unique mutation in the gene that encoded for the protein alpha-synuclein. In simple terms, something in this family's DNA was causing their Parkinson's.[18,19]

Polymeropoulos's discovery triggered a surge of research, which led to the identification of the Parkinson's-related brain protein (alpha-synuclein) as the principal component of the enigmatic brain clumps present in autopsies. Before this moment, genetic forms of Parkinson's, which are today known to comprise approximately 15% of cases, had not been fully accepted, even by leading experts. Though genetics make up a small minority of cases, the study of the pathways involved has provided important breadcrumbs for us to follow in the development of new treatments.

So, as we work to develop a new Parkinson's treatment for Jana Reed, Sara Whittingham, and all those on the planet who are rightfully seeking to improve their lives, the "perfect" treatment will have five characteristics. It will be (1) inclusive of everyone, including both those at risk and those with disease; (2) noninvasive and practical (a pill, for example); (3) low risk in the short and long term; (4) accessible to everyone on the planet; and (5) cheap, especially if chronic therapy is necessary. As we embark on a journey to uncover new treatments, we should remind ourselves of these five characteristics and remain humble, as most therapies will not reach perfection. The frontiers of exciting therapies like gene editing and regenerative medicine could be transformative, but many will fall short in one or more of these five critical categories. We must take our wins where we can but also keep striving for a clean "five-characteristic" sweep.

WHY ARE WE FAILING?

Chuck Adler was born in the Bronx and raised in Philly. He idolized his grandfather, who was a self-made man living in the largely Jewish immigrant neighborhood of Washington Heights, New York. Jack Adler owned a luggage shop and was kind to all his patrons. His death just after his grandson's bar mitzvah was a devastating blow. Jack had Parkinson's disease, and though he received levodopa in 1971, he died soon after. It was unclear whether the medication was too late for Jack or the doctors did not appreciate how to use the new miracle drug.

Chuck vowed he would dedicate his life to finding a cure for Parkinson's disease, and in an essay written while he was in ninth grade, he asserted his goal. He made a promise that he would not retire until he had checked Parkinson's off his list.

The path for Chuck up the ladder was not easy. He worked summers in the library stacks pulling and xeroxing articles for his father, who was a pharmacologist. Chuck eventually earned enough stripes to join laboratory studies; he then completed a six-year combined program at New York University and received both his MD and PhD. When he was interviewing at Harvard, a comment about needing to focus on either research or care made him rethink his path. He attended the University of Pennsylvania for his Parkinson's fellowship and then took a job at the Mayo Clinic in Scottsdale, Arizona, where he felt he could both see patients and perform important research into the disease that had robbed his grandfather of many years of his life.

Adler went on to perform dozens of clinical trials and to examine hundreds of brains in the laboratory over a lengthy career.[20–31] This year, 2025, will be Chuck's final lap around the track before he retires. His promise to himself, and to his grandfather, remains unfulfilled.

The senior gods of Parkinson's disease were wrong. They told Chuck we were on the cusp of breakthroughs. Tens of millions of dollars were spent searching for disease-modifying drugs, and we are left to wonder if these dollars may have been better spent on nailing down *biomarkers* (measurable indicators of some biological state or condition), developing tools, and learning "why" (why a disease starts, spreads, and progresses).

Anthony Lang, a professor at the University of Toronto and one of the most prominent and prolific clinical trialists in Parkinson's disease, put it simply. "We lack disease state and progression biomarkers. We are struggling to identify brain cell dysfunction versus brain cell degeneration. If you give us a boost in these areas, you will see more positive clinical trials." In medicine a *disease state* is the condition or status of an individual at any given time. This state may include disease characteristics, symptoms, progression, and severity. Most experts think understanding disease state will improve diagnosis and treatment. Tony emphasizes that our ability to monitor the effectiveness of any therapy will be critical to the development of future ones.

Why have all the major clinical trials aimed at slowing progression stalled or failed? Chuck's answer is that we haven't yet understood enough about the disease. Chuck cautions the next generation of researchers searching for therapeutics that Parkinson's is tricky and has multiple causes. It is not one Parkinson's disease; it is many Parkinson's diseases.[32] We need to develop and deploy technology to create new treatments, understand pathology, and decode genetics, and we need to pay attention to the environment. We need to understand why a normal brain develops Parkinson's disease. Chuck reflects, "Once we have the why, the treatments will gush."

FRONTIER 1: THE NEXT FIVE YEARS

The Fingerprints of Parkinson's

Sally Johnston was in her early sixties and a successful accountant. She knew she had a *LRRK2* gene mutation and a strong family history of Parkinson's. Though her gene test was positive, a blood test for alpha-synuclein was negative, and she died of breast cancer at age seventy-three without ever manifesting a single symptom of Parkinson's. Simon Schuler, a computer repairman in his early fifties, had a mother with Parkinson's. He rushed out to get himself a blood test, and when it was abnormal, he confirmed his fears with a follow-up skin biopsy. Though both tests were abnormal, for the past five years he has yet to reveal any symptoms of Parkinson's disease. Darla King is a yoga instructor in her early sixties; she has been acting out her dreams, talking, shouting, flailing, and jumping out of bed for about twenty years, and she fears that she may have a degenerative brain disease. Darla has been carefully checked by her neurologist every year, and she has yet to develop a diagnosis of Parkinson's. Sally, Simon, and Darla are not in the same family. All three have an *LRRK2* mutation, and all three are devoid of any symptoms of Parkinson's.

These cases demonstrate how limited we are in our understanding of "Parkinson's genes" and that we are missing a key component of understanding an individual's status with or without the disease. Biomarkers will help address this shortcoming. Biomarkers are biological materials that can be found in the body (e.g., blood, urine, spinal fluid, skin) and reveal the presence of a disease. For example, cholesterol in the blood is a biomarker alerting us to potential cardiovascular disease.

There are many challenges for the next generation of Parkinson's biomarkers, but none larger than the realization that Parkinson's is not a single disease. It is possible to have one or more biomarkers without ever developing the disease. We must be sensitive to Sally, Simon, and Darla's situation, no matter what biomarker path we ultimately travel. Biomarkers for Parkinson's could allow us to monitor health, diagnose disease, and one day evaluate the effectiveness of treatments. These approaches are on the way. However, for Parkinson's, it may not be a single biomarker like in diabetes (blood sugar) or heart disease (cholesterol level).

The best biomarkers give us all three legs of a disease stool: diagnosis, prognosis, and treatment response. Most only achieve one. The most common and easiest leg is a diagnostic biomarker. It is a simple test that detects or confirms the presence of a disease. For Parkinson's, the diagnostic biomarker has been challenging to pin down, since not all cases have detectable Parkinson's protein (alpha-synuclein). The answer will likely be in combining two or three biomarkers together into one mega-marker for diagnosis. Currently, the leading contenders include blood and spinal-fluid levels of the Parkinson's protein (alpha-synuclein), skin biopsies, and a variety of brain-imaging scans, ranging from specialized MRIs, to the use of radioactive PET (a nuclear medicine study that uses glucose and other chemicals to evaluate brain function), to DaT scans (a nuclear medicine study that examines the dopamine transporter compound in the brain). In neurodegenerative diseases, we can and should expect updates as technology is refined. We must embrace new technologies and real-time discoveries to continue the momentum toward finding biomarkers.[33] People with Parkinson's should ask their doctors whether any biomarkers can be used to enhance their care.

The other two legs of the biomarker stool are much further from our grasp. We need, but do not possess, prognostic biomarkers, which will closely align with the disease course, and we will benefit from predictive biomarkers to measure how a person will respond to a particular treatment. Those two legs seem as distant as stars in the sky, but they are not out of reach and could be achieved in the next five years.

Biomarkers are a perfect example of the importance of nurturing novelty and changing the way we view a disease. Modern digital biomarkers, such as those collected by wearable devices like smartwatches and fitness trackers, have recently proven effective for monitoring motor symptoms, including tremors, gait disturbances, and slowed movement.[34-49] About ten different fitness trackers have been pressed into use to monitor different aspects of Parkinson's disease (Verily, Emma Watch, Global Kinetics GKC Wearable, and others). We have learned that large amounts of data can be rapidly analyzed to detect subtle changes and possibly even early warning signs of disease progression. The data from these devices can be transmitted to a health care professional or utilized directly by the person. There are now several mobile applications that track voice, movement, and behavioral patterns in Parkinson's, and more will come. We are now recommending that people consider using tracking devices for exercise and sleep, and soon the approach will provide even more actionable information.

Another approach will be to focus on understanding the molecules in our body. In the TV series *Star Trek*, a device could quickly scan a person's health. It was called a tricorder, and Starfleet personnel could use it to detect physical conditions, diagnose diseases, and recommend treatments. The tricorder could understand health without invasive procedures. In Parkinson's, the next five years will bring us closer to this reality by employing a tool called *mass spectrometry* to study individual patients in an expanding new area of science called *multi-omics*. Multi-omics allows scientists now, and one day doctors, to examine protein expression patterns in blood and to identify a fingerprint of Parkinson's disease.[50-56] Could a fingerprint serve all three legs of the biomarker stool: diagnosis, prognosis, and prediction? Maybe.

Reorganizing the Way We Use AI

Can artificial intelligence (AI) and machine learning provide a pathway to strengthen the three legs of the Parkinson's disease biomarker stool and achieve a Parkinson's fingerprint? The answer is yes. However, in the next five years we will need to reorganize our approach to AI and retreat from the inflated expectations for this technology. AI is only as good as the questions we ask it and the data we provide it. If we ask better questions and provide more data, it will help us to more rapidly identify biomarkers and possibly one day, even treatments. If we refine how we use the tool, our return on investment will be much greater. For example, instead of simply asking or expecting AI to find a cure for Parkinson's, we could ask it to solve specific questions that will light the path toward more treatment opportunities.

Cornell University scientist Chang Su and colleagues recently took a first step toward addressing the differences of Parkinson's disease by using both AI-based machine learning and deep learning to characterize subtypes and progression trajectories. They asked AI to look for a solution that could characterize Parkinson's into more discreet subtypes, which could be used later in clinical trials. His team was able to characterize an "Inching Pace" subtype with mild baseline severity and mild progression speed; a "Moderate Pace" subtype with mild baseline severity but advancing at a moderate progression rate; and a "Rapid Pace" subtype. Put another way, AI could predict the speed of progression of Parkinson's disease, and this information could be used to select the right person for the right treatment. The scientists also looked at blood markers, genes, and even drugs already on the shelf to try to individualize treatment decisions.[57] Chang Su's work is just one example of the power of data integration, which can be achieved through the use of AI and machine-learning algorithms, which are capable of integrating a ton of data from multiple sources. If we ask AI the right questions in the next five years, we will likely better predict disease onset and progression and possibly a treatment response.

When it comes to Parkinson's biomarkers, we have to stop thinking small. We need to pivot and use technology to combine advanced digital, biochemical, genetic, imaging, and omics technologies (omics are like the *Star Trek* tricorder) into an integrated AI-based Parkinson's fingerprint. We must be humble as we pursue a Parkinson's fingerprint. Anthony Lang reminds us that Parkinson's is not one disease and does not have one cause. Pursuing a one-size-fits-all fingerprint approach, if looked at as a magic bullet, has a high potential for failure. Parkinson's is a whole-body disease involving the skin, gut, brain, peripheral nerves, and other organs.

Will a *Star Trek* body scanner tricorder approach be sufficient, or are we looking for a "Holy Grail"? Lang reminds us of an important "what if" scenario. What if the inciting event for Parkinson's occurred during childhood or decades before the development of the disease? A tricorder approach will tell us something but not everything. Despite the challenges, the fingerprint could enhance our understanding of the causes of Parkinson's and has the potential to reveal individual differences in genetics, environment, and lifestyle. AI and fingerprints are on the near-term horizon.

Realizing That Genes Can Drive Drugs and Therapies

The most common Parkinson's genes include *LRRK2* and *GBA*, and since these were discovered, scientists and pharmaceutical companies have been trying to develop therapies that target these genes or their corresponding proteins in order to slow disease progression. A powerful example is how Biogen and Denali Therapeutics teamed up to develop a new class of drugs called LRRK2 kinase inhibitors. These companies worked with scientists to bring a new personalized therapy to clinical trials for those with *LRRK2*-associated Parkinson's disease. We can do more of this in the next five years.

Scientists have yet to elucidate the exact mechanisms of how a mutation in someone's *LRRK2* gene actually causes Parkinson's. One simple approach targets the precise location of the key enzyme in the LRRK2 protein. Drug designers have engineered a pill that will block the addition of a common element called phosphate. By blocking this process, these drugs can drop abnormally high levels of the brain enzyme and hopefully improve symptoms. What we do not know, however, is whether the disease may be slowed by this approach, which is currently in human trials.

Another approach to treat folks with *LRRK2*-related Parkinson's will be building drugs to target waste removal within brain cells. This approach will modulate the waste-removal process called *autophagy*. The word has a Greek derivation. *Auto* means the cell does it without help, and *phagy* refers to eating or chewing up the waste. Though it may seem counterintuitive, for a human to survive, cells must possess a "self-eating" capacity. Without the ability to remove waste or to eat our own cells, we would risk toxic brain waste piling up and contributing to disease. Drugs that can help to remove damaged parts, misfolded proteins, and debris could be helpful for Parkinson's and are all on a potential five-year testing frontier. There are several candidate drugs already on the shelf.

Finally, many groups have been interested in how *LRRK2* may impact the immune system and inflammation. If we block the LRRK2 protein, this may reduce neuroinflammation, which could have positive benefits. Fascinatingly, scientists have shown that the LRRK2 protein is highly expressed in immune cells and especially the microglia, which are the brain's vacuum cleaners. We are poised to test whether reducing inflammation is a good bet, and we have several drugs ready to trial.

The idea of LRRK2 inhibitors sounds promising; however, many scientists are concerned about unwanted "off-target effects."[58–64] What is an "off-target effect"? If a drug we administer in a clinical trial binds to an unintended receptor, enzyme, or protein, this could lead to an off-target effect. Some of the off-target effects can be so severe that they may limit or prevent the use of the new medication. One of the most famous off-target drug effects was in thalidomide, which was used for nausea during pregnancy. The off-target effect caused severe birth defects, including limb deformities in thousands of babies. We must be sure that when we design new drugs, no intended off-target effect sours their benefits. With LRRK2 drugs, there has been a concern about off-target effects impacting lung function.

The other common genetic mutation associated with Parkinson's disease is in the *GBA* gene, which codes for a specific enzyme called glucocerebrosidase (GCase). GCase drugs have recently emerged as a therapy target. Glucocerebrosidase is essential for maintaining the health and homeostasis of your cells and for clearing out waste and debris. In Parkinson's, mutations in the *GBA* gene reduce GCase activity, and scientists believe that this is bad, as unwanted debris can begin to accumulate and disrupt normal cell function. Intriguingly, reducing the action of the enzyme leads to the clumping of the Parkinson's-related protein alpha-synuclein. This gave scientists an idea for a potential treatment.

Professor Anthony Schapira has been testing a common component of a cough syrup called ambroxol at the University College of London. Ambroxol is a tiny molecule that enhances GCase enzyme activity. It is widely available and is cheap. Schapira and colleagues have published a small preliminary study and are currently studying ambroxol in a larger effort as part of a Cure Parkinson's Trust study that will test the effects of raising the enzyme. They aim to test this approach in folks with and without *GBA* mutations to see if there is a common pathway that may benefit all.[65–71]

An approach that has been quickly gaining traction has been to identify a gene underpinning a disease and to use something called antisense oligonucleotides, or RNAi, to silence that gene. Recently, scientists have begun making these molecules and inserting them into people in an effort to treat human disease. Oligonucleotides provide only short-term benefit, so regular readministration of these therapies may be required. There are some early-stage clinical trials underway; however, the recent failure of this form of therapy for Huntington's disease[72–75] has led many scientists to rethink the approach, and this frontier of using genes to guide treatments may fast be disappearing from the near-term horizon unless we can rethink how to approach this type of therapy.

Repurposing Old Drugs

The Food and Drug Administration has approved more than 20,000 prescription drugs, and there are now thousands of over-the-counter medications available to be repurposed or reused for Parkinson's disease. Recently, a diabetes drug called semaglutide has zipped to the top of the list of those that may be repurposed for Parkinson's disease. The recent 2024 French trial with a diabetes drug called lixisenatide was published in the *New England Journal of Medicine* by Wassilios Meissner and colleagues.[76–80] Along with semaglutide, the drug belongs to a class of compounds called GLP-1 (glucagon-like peptide) agonists, which have commonly been used to treat obesity. The investigators thought that GLP-1 agonists may have the added benefit of protecting the brain cells and surrounding connective tissue. In a study of 156 persons who received either lixisenatide or a placebo injection, the group who received lixisenatide had slightly better motor function than those who received a placebo. There are several other ongoing studies of GLP-1 diabetes drugs for use in Parkinson's, like exenatide, and these data will help us to determine whether this is an avenue worth pursuing over the next five years.[77,81,82]

There are many other repurposed drugs under study, ranging from cough syrups to drugs for bone health and antibiotics. The challenge with repurposing drugs is figuring out whether "the juice is worth the squeeze," as the cost of a single large-scale clinical trial can easily climb to tens of millions of dollars. Professor Joaquim Ferreira and colleagues at the Campus Neurológico in Torres Vedras, Portugal, recently reviewed 152 potential drugs for use in Parkinson's disease. New compounds fared better, with 21% eventual approval, compared to 7% for repurposed compounds already on the shelf.[83] We must do better. Below is a list of some of the drug repurposing we will be working through in the next five years.

- **Ambroxol:** A medicine for cough and colds that reduces activity of an enzyme in the brain, which may in turn reduce the protein alpha-synuclein.
- **GLP-1 agonists:** Diabetes drugs that act on a brain receptor and may improve Parkinson's symptoms and/or slow disease progression.
- **Tyrosine kinase inhibitors (c-ABL inhibitors):** Leukemia drugs that may benefit Parkinson's. Even though there was a recent failure of nilotinib, others are being studied.
- **Terazosin:** A drug used to treat an enlarged prostate gland and high blood pressure. It may increase energy within brain cells and protect them from dying.
- **Metformin:** A common treatment for type 2 diabetes that may reduce inflammation and improve function of the muscle of the brain cells (mitochondria).
- **Raloxifene:** A selective estrogen receptor modulator used for bone thinning (osteoporosis). This medicine may have a positive benefit on dopamine brain receptors and may possibly slow disease progression.
- **Ceftriaxone:** A common antibiotic used to treat bacterial infections that may increase levels of a protein called GLT-1. This protein removes a potentially damaging chemical from the cell called glutamate.

- **Tacrolimus:** A drug used to suppress the immune system in organ transplant patients. This drug may reduce inflammation, possibly slow down disease progression, or improve symptoms.

Reorganizing Electrical and Pump Therapies

Diane Waxman was diagnosed with Parkinson's at the age of forty-seven, and by age fifty-two, she was made bionic by the addition of brain implants. Her deep brain stimulator, or DBS device, turned her life around as her tremor melted away, her stiffness receded, and her dyskinesia disappeared. However, by age sixty she had developed shuffling steps and a soft voice and had turned over the finances to her husband. Diane kept returning to her doctor for adjustments to her device, but nothing addressed her new symptoms. She wondered what was next.

The introductions of levodopa and later DBS have been heralded as the two largest and most important advances in the treatment of Parkinson's. Applying a tiny amount of electricity into one node within a complex brain circuit has resulted in life-changing improvements in motor fluctuations, dyskinesia, and tremor. However, as Dr. Jill Ostrem, a neurologist and expert at the University of California, San Francisco, points out, frustratingly, the disease progresses despite DBS therapy, particularly in the worsening of walking, talking, thinking, and falling.[84]

We must improve the next generation of DBS[85-87] and focus over the next five years on improvements in how we can apply electricity, how precise we can be, how adaptable we can make the devices to human symptoms, and how many of the symptoms we can alleviate for patients like Diane who received the first generation of DBS devices.

One advance that is already being trialed in humans today is adaptive DBS. Previously, we implanted wires into the brain and activated them by delivering continuous electrical stimulation 24/7. Adaptive DBS systems, in contrast, use a signal recorded from the brain to provide real-time feedback, which the device can use to adjust and readjust settings. The implanted mini-computer does all the work in the background. The adaptive DBS approach has been useful for motor symptoms and sleep dysfunction;

however, it still falls short in addressing walking, talking, thinking, and falling. Jill and her colleagues were part of a large, first-of-its-kind adaptive DBS trial sponsored by the company Medtronic, and the preliminary results have been promising.

Recently, an adaptive DBS device manufactured by Neuropace has been used to detect seizures before they occur and to provide a train of stimulation to prevent disabling spells. Why are we talking about seizures in a book about Parkinson's? It is because AI algorithms have used the mountain of data collected in seizure patients to personalize stimulation settings and make critical suggestions in the timing of medications.[88-95] We are now gaining momentum by moving toward data-driven personalization, and this can be achieved as a near-term frontier. Optimizing medical management and rehabilitative therapies may also one day soon be guided by AI.

Today, DBS devices are large and require that a wire be implanted under the neck and connected to a power pack placed under the collarbone. Tomorrow, devices will be smaller, less invasive, and powered without wires. These changes can reduce surgeries required for battery changes, infections, and fractures in wires continuously stressed by neck movement.

The excitement of applying optogenetics to dissect the relevant brain circuitry for Parkinson's has also been exploding over the last decade.[96-100] *Optogenetics* is a Greek word derived from *optós*, meaning "light," and *genesis*, translating to "birth." The advantage to applying a light-gene therapy combination is that the approach will provide exquisite control of brain cell firing. Unfortunately, optogenetics is unlikely to be applied to humans any time soon due to challenges with both gene and light delivery, as well as human safety issues, but a new generation of researchers like Aryn Gittis at Carnegie Mellon University has been part of a revolution called "optogenetics-inspired DBS."[98] Researchers have employed optogenetics to choose brain targets for DBS therapy. The Gittis laboratory has recently taken the field one step further and shown the intriguing possibility of cell-specific deep brain stimulation. By selectively targeting specific populations of neurons within a structure called the pallidum, Gittis was able to modulate abnormal brain activity more precisely than traditional indiscriminate DBS therapy.[87,96,101-104] Gittis thinks these methods may also be important for reducing common DBS side effects such as dyskinesia; however, translating them into humans remains an unmet challenge. Recently Gittis teamed up with neurosurgeon Nader Pouratian at University of Texas Southwestern for an early human trial using a novel form of burst stimulation inspired by animal work.[104] Optogenetics-inspired DBS will be a reality in the next five years.

Tomorrow, neurosurgeons will perform operations on patients with Parkinson's disease in a virtual 3-D environment before ever stepping foot in an operating theater.[105–107] These environments have already been built by Cameron McIntyre at Duke University. Neurosurgeons will no longer choose a conventional brain target but instead will find and tap the optimal superhighway to maximize benefits and minimize side effects. Andreas Horn has perfected this technology and made a public tool available called "Lead DBS," and neurologists like Michael Fox at Massachusetts General Hospital are using this tool along with advanced imaging techniques to map a new future path for optimizing DBS devices.[108–111] More-advanced electrode designs will continue to evolve, and we will begin to pivot toward combination therapies: DBS plus drugs, nanoparticles, optogenetics, or gene therapy. Finally, DBS has become too complex for the general practitioner and even for the specialist neurologist. Telemedicine and AI-robotic-assisted programming will play a larger role in the near term of the next five years.

Less-invasive therapies such as transcranial magnetic stimulation and transcranial direct current stimulation have been useful for research but have been less impactful than DBS for treatment. There is, however, hope that newer treatments such as Ed Boyden's temporal interference may one day eliminate the need for opening the skull and brain to deliver neuromodulation therapies. Several groups have begun to test early temporal interference techniques on human subjects.

There has also been a movement to consider a return to making brain lesions with an instrument called focused ultrasound. Although it has been around since 1958 in neurosurgery, recent methodological improvements have driven its recent reintroduction into the treatment armamentarium.[112–116] Also, scientists are hard at work developing dopamine-pump-based therapies, which will work by delivering the drug under the skin. To date, the results have been impressive, though not at the level of DBS therapy. This approach is safer than brain surgery and has already arrived.[117–124]

FRONTIER 2: SIX TO TEN YEARS INTO THE FUTURE

Reaching for New Drugs

The alternative approach to repurposing drugs will be to reach for new ones. This is a multistep process. Researchers like Ted Dawson at Johns Hopkins University must identify a brain target and then perform a series of experiments to make sure that the target is involved in the process leading to Parkinson's. If a reasonable brain target is identified, then we must use libraries of existing compounds to determine what may or may not tickle that target. Scientists must optimize the compound and make sure it can reach the area of the brain efficiently and realize its potential to improve symptoms without unnecessary side effects. Finally, and in most cases, testing must be performed first in cells, then in animals, and finally in humans. This process can take about fifteen years, and we and other experts believe that one key to developing new therapies will be to reduce the time for reaching new drugs from a longer-term frontier of more than a decade to a mid-term frontier of six to ten years.

Repositioning Diets and the Microbiome

Two and half hours north of Philadelphia in the Lehigh Valley sits the steel town of Bethlehem, Pennsylvania. Growing up the son of a special education teacher, Tim Sampson was a second-generation Italian-German American who loved gazing endlessly into a microscope at anything living that he could fit onto a slide. His favorite was the pond water collected from tributaries of the Delaware River, which, as he appreciates today, were heavily polluted by the steel industry. The town of Bethlehem is known for several major achievements, including being the first to decorate an American Christmas tree, delivering the I-beam to enable skyscrapers, and manufacturing over 1,000 ships in World War II. But Sampson was not focused on the big things in his small town. His eyes were fixed on the small organisms, which were too large to ignore.

Tim became a microbiologist, and it was a lucky break that when he started his postdoctoral fellowship at Cal Tech in Sarkis Masmanian's laboratory, Sarkis and his colleagues had turned their attention toward neurodegenerative diseases like Parkinson's. They were interested in how the gut affected the brain. They wanted to produce a germfree animal model of Parkinson's disease. A germfree animal has no microbes or invisible organisms present, so the starting point for every experiment would be a gastrointestinal tract (normally filled with bacteria) scrubbed completely clean. Tim could use such an animal to shape the microbiome—the collection of tiny organisms living in the gut—and to learn what effect changing these organisms might have on Parkinson's.

Creating experimental animals in a germfree environment was not new to science. Professor James Arthur Reyniers from Notre Dame pioneered the first germfree animal,[125–129] which was hailed in *LIFE* magazine as a triumph of science on November 10, 1941, just a month prior to the Japanese invasion of Pearl Harbor.

In genetics, scientists will knock out or remove a gene and then examine the behavior of an animal. In a germfree animal, the scientist knocks out the microbiome and then studies the behaviors by reintroducing specific organisms. Scientists like Michael Fischbach and colleagues at the University of California, San Francisco, are building on this work by mixing and matching common microbes to unlock the basic enigma of what all of the creatures in your gut are actually doing there and how their presence may be important to human health.

If you switch to a plant-based diet, your microbiome will shift. If you begin eating meat again, it will shift back. Developing a disease like Parkinson's will cause your microbiome to shift. We don't yet understand how long that shift takes. The current best guess from experts like Sampson is about two to three years. Experts believe that the composition of the microbiome normally stays relatively stable; however, the activity of certain microbes seems to change in response to Parkinson's disease.

The microbiome can be modified by diet and most recently by a procedure called fecal microbiota transplantation, where healthy bacteria from a donor's stool are transferred into a patient's gastrointestinal tract. Neither seems to result in sprouting new brain cells or slowing disease progression. There are potential health benefits of shifting the microbiome, whether or not you have Parkinson's, and it is possible that one day a microbiome approach could change symptoms or slow disease progression.[130,131]

How should we begin to reposition Parkinson's diets and the microbiome over the next five years? Should everyone with the disease get their microbiome checked? Maybe. Would knowing the results of your microbiome currently change treatment? No. Are there a bunch of commercial companies offering to perform a microbiome analysis for cash? Yes. There may, however, be a day when everyone with Parkinson's disease has their microbiome checked and tracked; however, we are not there yet. A ton of books and articles purport to have discovered "the diet" for Parkinson's disease and the path to the perfect Parkinson's microbiome, but most experts advise not following them. Most of the data we have supports the use of a Mediterranean diet (high in fruits and vegetables and low in animal products); yet we do not know what we do not know. People with Parkinson's should be cautious of nutritional overreach, which is the practice of selling an idea or product without much, or any, clear supporting data.

If you decide to have your Parkinson's microbiome checked, it might show reduced diversity in the organisms of the gut compared to healthy folks. It may reveal increased levels of the bacteria called Enterobacteriaceae, and recently studies have been trying to link these changes to motor impairments in actual people with the disease.

Another finding has been decreases in a different type of bacteria (Prevotellaceae), which may be important in producing short-chain fatty acids, important to both gut and immune health.[130,132-137] How inflammation in the gut connects to the brain remains a Parkinson's mystery, and we hope from a diet standpoint to begin to sort this out over the mid-term frontier of six to ten years.

One intriguing idea would be to combine screening tests, such as of the microbiome, with a class of drugs called inflammasome inhibitors. Anthony Lang sees these drugs as an emerging and untested strategy in Parkinson's. Your cells contain inflammasomes, which are multiprotein complexes important in your immune system. Inflammasomes detect pathogens and stress, and to protect the cell, they activate an inflammatory response. The big question is whether, by the time symptoms manifest, it will be too late if we act by blocking the brain's inflammasomes. There are common drugs like colchicine (used to treat gout) that can do this, and newer drugs are in clinical trials. We do not know if blocking the inflammasome will be of benefit; however, the next six to ten years will likely give us the answer.

There is no one single microbiome signature for Parkinson's disease. If testing is one day pressed into clinical practice, it will be important to examine the microbiome before and after adding probiotics or making changes in a diet. If we boost the wrong bacteria or gut organisms, we risk worsening the situation for anyone with a neurodegenerative disease such as Parkinson's. Alternatively, Tim hopes that one day we will be able to regulate the gut for health and other benefits for those with Parkinson's.

Rejuvenating Stem Cells

A stem cell has the unique ability to develop into many different types of cells. For example, stem cells can divide and renew themselves and decide to become virtually any cell type in the human body. Though there has been general disappointment in stem cell use for Parkinson's, certain areas may lead to a rejuvenation of the field in the mid-term frontier.

Roger Barker, a professor at Cambridge in England, marvels over the capacity of the "relatively" simple approach of using transplanted dopamine cells that can survive, grow, and replenish areas where there is no dopamine. A dopamine stem cell is great for the laboratory, but it may not be the limiting factor for Parkinson's stem cell transplantation.

Stem cells and other transplants have depended largely on the delivery technique. The cell itself may be fine; however, it will need to be delivered to the right region, connect to other brain cells, and survive. Transplanted cells are also frequently seen as foreigners to the brain and body and must escape destruction by the immune system. So what good is the perfect stem cell if it doesn't integrate into the brain, stay healthy, and contribute to rebuilding the circuit? Delivery and integration may be as important as the actual cell, and this may partially explain the many failures in Parkinson's transplant therapies. Engineering a technique to more efficiently deliver and integrate stem cells (as brain cells) remains an unmet challenge, and one that could help us develop new therapies.[138–147]

Perhaps the biggest surprise in regenerative medicine is that if you ask most of the experts what their goal is, it is not to "cure the disease." As with deep brain stimulation, they are aiming to add years of meaningful life. Regenerative medicine researchers appreciate that the field is getting better and better at treating motor dysfunction. However, memory, hallucinations, and dementia have challenged the regenerative medicine folks to look for outside-the-box and novel approaches.

Roger Barker and the founding father of brain repair for Parkinson's, Anders Björklund from Stockholm University, have been among a group of regeneration experts who have renewed interest in targeting a region called the basal forebrain system. This region of the brain is thought to under-pin some of the cognitive and thinking deficits in people with Parkinson's. The nerve cells here use not dopamine to communicate but a different brain chemical called acetylcholine. Recent technological advances have allowed us to create memory-related brain cells from these stem cells.

Why are Barker and Björklund high on this idea? Research has shown that if you have Parkinson's and you develop dementia, this is linked to the loss of basal forebrain cells. Many of the nerve cells in this region are lost, and the amount of cell loss has been correlated to the amount of cognitive impairment. Their approach represents a pivot in regenerative medicine for Parkinson's toward the unmet need of treating cognitive impairment. Cell therapy aimed at replacing the lost cells important for memory represents an interesting strategy to combat Parkinson's disease dementia.[145] Barker's wisdom is that we need a clear rationale for what we do. If it does not work, we should ask why rather than simply give up. This approach for rejuvenat-ing the stem cell treatment for Parkinson's could be prime for a mid-term frontier.

Reconsidering Vaccines and Immune Therapies

William Foege was a towering figure in the history of vaccines who worked with the Centers for Disease Control and Prevention and the World Health Organization in the late 1960s and early 1970s to eradicate smallpox. He famously said, "Vaccines are the tugboats of preventative health."[148–153] Foege won the Presidential Medal of Freedom in 2012. If we are to move vaccines to brain diseases, we will need to reconsider our approach and invest more dollars in refining it.

We have successfully used vaccines to control smallpox, measles, diphtheria, tetanus, pertussis, polio, and, most recently, Covid-19. We have all received many of these vaccines ourselves. Why not reconsider the possibility of a vaccine for Parkinson's? Admittedly, Parkinson's is not thought to be infectious; however, vaccines may have utility beyond diseases caused by bacteria and viruses. The Covid-19 pandemic demonstrated that we can rapidly develop vaccines if the need arises. Can we apply that knowledge? Can we deploy an Operation Warp Speed for Parkinson's disease? In an op-ed for *The Hill*, we advocated for just that and discussed the urgent need for accelerated research and development efforts to address the Parkinson pandemic.

Vaccines are not new for Alzheimer's and Parkinson's, but they have met with limited success. Perhaps the failures can serve as guideposts in the reconsideration of a new Parkinson's vaccine.

Instead of directing a vaccine against a virus like Covid, a vaccine for Parkinson's could be directed against the misfolded protein alpha-synuclein. This might allow the body's own immune system to clean up damage or to prevent the future spread of the disease. Even if a vaccine does not work, other immune therapies that have provided breakthroughs in cancer may. Alternatively, we could turn the tables and enhance the function of existing proteins that are vital for human functions such as memory. Maybe a winning approach will not be a vaccine but a more selective immune therapy. Cancer has built a road for immune therapies with the development of monoclonal antibodies and more. So far in Parkinson's, immune therapies, including monoclonal antibodies, have been effective only in animal models, but never say never.

The target for the current Parkinson's vaccines has been the accumulation of alpha-synuclein plaques in the brain. The company Affiris AG has developed a peptide-based vaccine with the simple idea of triggering the immune system to generate antibodies to target and clear Parkinson's-related protein (alpha-synuclein) clumps. The company produced short peptide imposters of alpha-synuclein to fool the immune system into overreacting. A second peptide-based vaccine recently produced by the company Vaxxinity is undergoing clinical trials. A third vaccine targets specific markers on alpha-synuclein called epitopes. All of these approaches have been shown to be reasonably safe and have produced an immune response.[154-161] It is unclear if any will improve symptoms or slow disease progression, because clearing the clumps may happen too late in the process; the damage may be done. We will, in the next six to ten years, uncover whether this approach will be viable for Parkinson's.

Another approach has been to simply "rev up" the immune system to clear the Parkinson's protein by directly infusing antibodies through an intravenous therapy. Vaccines generally work by stimulating the body to produce antibodies to fight off infection. If the body cannot generate antibodies itself, sometimes the antibodies can be directly administered. This approach has been applied to a wide variety of conditions, from polio to rabies. It has even been studied for Alzheimer's. Two recent attempts have fallen short, with both results published in the same issue of the *New England Journal of Medicine*.[162-164] Some of the data supporting one of the therapies may have been falsified, as recently reported by investigative reporter Charles Piller.[165] A National Institutes of Health neuroscientist is under investigation for "doctoring images" and data in papers that have been cited in 238 drug company patents. Though Piller comments that this must "provoke anxiety among multiple drug companies," it does not invalidate the work of many other credible scientists in the field. This antibody approach in its current form has been disappointing, and if it is to make a comeback, a new approach will need to be considered.

Alberto Espay, a neurologist at the University of Cincinnati, is not convinced that targeting clumps of misfolded alpha-synuclein is the right approach for Parkinson's disease. Alberto's father was a calculus teacher, a political exile from Chile, and a deconstructionist. He taught his son the value of challenging traditional ideas and dogma. Alberto does not believe that Parkinson's is caused by a toxic protein accumulation (also known as a proteinopathy). He has proposed that the cause is *proteinopenia*: that the loss rather than the clumping of alpha-synuclein is the crux of Parkinson's and a critical factor in disease progression.[166,167] He has taken a lot of heat over his view, but he says he does not take it personally. He knows that his colleagues and scientists have the best intentions when criticizing him. But if Alberto is right, we will need to rethink vaccines and antibody therapy approaches and consider shifting to protein-replacement therapies. This question can be resolved in the second frontier.

Looking Forward

Investing in the near- and mid-term frontier for new therapy development will be a critical component in a successful Parkinson's Plan. Reaching biomarkers, reorganizing AI, realizing the potential of genes, repurposing drugs, and refining our approach to electrical and pump therapies can all happen now. The mid-term frontier of reaching for new drugs, repositioning diets, rejuvenating stem cells, and reconsidering vaccines should be emphasized. In the next chapter, we will address the planning required for a longer-term frontier. This frontier will require great levels of creativity and innovation. As Sam Walton, founder of the Walmart empire, once advised, "If everybody is doing it one way, there's a good chance you can find your niche by going exactly in the opposite direction." Our success in the final frontier for Parkinson's treatment development will be limited only by our imaginations and our will to persevere.

9

NAVIGATE THE FINAL FRONTIER

New discoveries in science will continue to create a
thousand new frontiers for those who still would adventure.

—Herbert Hoover

THE LONG-TERM FRONTIER FOR NEW TREATMENTS WILL REQUIRE A
bold vision. We will need to initiate the plan for the future today. What
new tools and delivery systems should we be investing in to catapult discoveries from journal articles to real people? Are we ready to take chances
and learn from our failures? Are we prepared to meet the challenge of
developing a plan for Air Force Academy graduates Jana Reed and Sara
Whittingham, who are part of a growing younger generation of people
with Parkinson's? Will we meet the need of creating a plan for the more
than ten million people like Dan Kinel who already have Parkinson's?

The long-term frontier should include both in- and outside-the-box
therapies. Regenerating circuits, gene editing, combination therapies, and
nanomedicine should all be part of our vision and plan. Our long-term plan
needs to expand our resources and launch a new generation of researchers. This new generation of doctors and scientists must be encouraged and

Navigating the Frontiers of
New Treatments

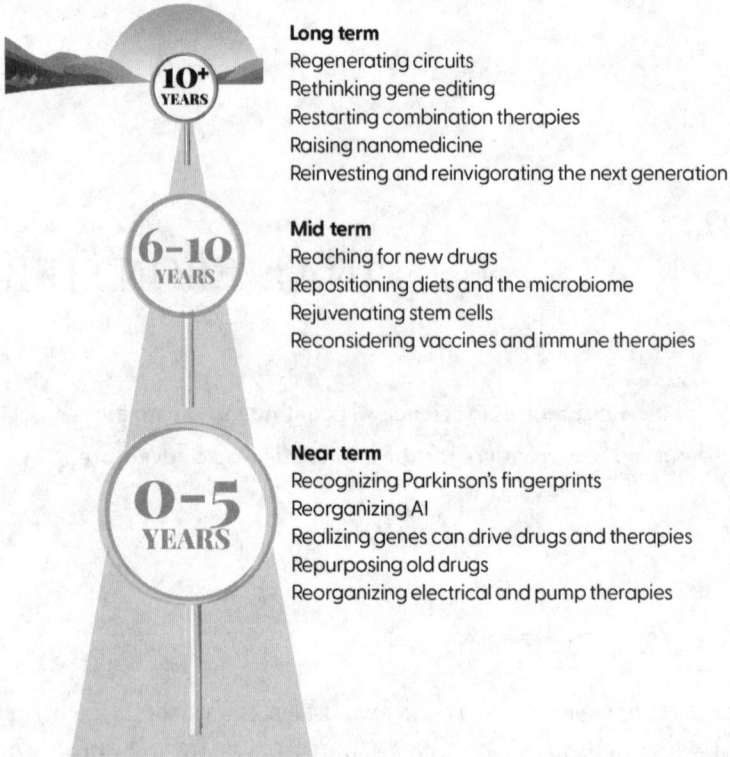

Long term
Regenerating circuits
Rethinking gene editing
Restarting combination therapies
Raising nanomedicine
Reinvesting and reinvigorating the next generation

Mid term
Reaching for new drugs
Repositioning diets and the microbiome
Rejuvenating stem cells
Reconsidering vaccines and immune therapies

Near term
Recognizing Parkinson's fingerprints
Reorganizing AI
Realizing genes can drive drugs and therapies
Repurposing old drugs
Reorganizing electrical and pump therapies

Figure 1. Navigating the frontiers of new treatments.

resourced to dream big and be ready to embrace discovery. They should also be on the lookout for serendipity in case it strikes again.

Steve Case, the former CEO of AOL, encapsulates staring down a new frontier. "There are no road signs to help navigate. And, in fact, no one has yet determined which side of the road we're supposed to be on." This longer-term frontier is the most exciting; however, to realize it, the planning must start now. This chapter, though written primarily for doctors, researchers, and funders, will be useful for everyday readers. They too can be informed about the longer-term frontier and advocate powerfully for it.

REGENERATING CIRCUITS

Gene therapy has improved and is reemerging as a promising treatment approach. By delivering genetic material into brain cells, gene therapy can restore dopamine levels, protect dying brain cells, and even regenerate new ones.[1] An early gene therapy trial successfully replaced the activity of a key enzyme in Parkinson's and improved patient symptoms.[2–6] Other gene therapy approaches have reduced Parkinson's-related proteins (alpha-synuclein) in the brain and rebuilt circuits, especially motor ones. In one impressive experiment, Michael Kaplitt and colleagues at Cornell University used gene therapy to change a critical region of the brain to use inhibitory chemicals instead of the native excitatory ones. In their trial, the patients who received the gene therapy in the subthalamic nucleus experienced improved motor symptoms.[7,8] Several early gene therapy trials are ongoing, and this approach will likely evolve rapidly as a treatment for select individuals with Parkinson's gene mutations.

Some scientists have pursued brain growth factors like Miracle-Gro®. However, Roger Barker and other experts believe the future is not in growth factors but rather in driving stem cells into different destinies and in building and testing models of brain neurodegeneration. If we can lean in and develop the tools that Texas-born Massachusetts Institute of Technology scientist Ed Boyden believes are necessary to understand the cellular environment, we will have a much better chance of engineering the solution.

Barker is adamant that we don't need trials with huge numbers of people to drive regenerative medicine. Small, well-designed studies conducted through a diverse consortium of younger and more seasoned researchers offer a potentially fruitful path. Since animal models have failed to recreate and capture the human condition, he is interested in going directly to humans. Barker believes that if we test just five patients over five years, this can be as meaningful as using hundreds of patients and possibly safer. This strategy for regenerating circuits is feasible and could show successes in the long term.

RETHINKING GENE EDITING

Claire Clelland was born in Oakland, California. She spent most of her upbringing in small towns. When she was a child, Claire, her mom, and her brother moved to Truckee, California, a town of less than 20,000 residents and later settled in Gold Hill, Oregon, with a population of less than 1,000. The teachers proved exceptional for Claire in an otherwise lackluster public school system. Claire excelled at science and loved asking questions such as "what really is consciousness?" This led her to study both philosophy and biology in college. The former honed her critical-thinking skills, and the latter taught her how the natural world works.

Claire considered herself lucky to graduate during the stem cell age, when leading scientists were talking about repairing the brains of those with disease. She joined Rusty Gage at the University of California, San Diego, and the Salk Institute and quickly landed a life-changing opportunity that provided her the best of two worlds. She learned brain repair from Rusty to earn her PhD and snagged a master's degree from the University of Cambridge by studying with rising regenerative medicine star Roger Barker. Claire knew that she wanted to help patients, and after her PhD, she completed medical school at the University of California, Los Angeles.

Across the bay, during her residency at the University of California, San Francisco (UCSF), a new technology named CRISPR was being developed in Berkeley. At the same time, next door in UCSF's Gladstone Institute, Shinya Yamanaka had just won the Nobel Prize in Physiology or Medicine for pioneering techniques to make induced pluripotent stem cells. Claire was in the Fertile Crescent for brain repair.

Claire realized early in her career that animal models could never faithfully replicate human disease. Her strategy was simple: use CRISPR gene editing and stem cell technology to model human disease in a dish.[9-11] The word *CRISPR* is an acronym for "clustered regularly interspaced short palindromic repeats." The idea behind CRISPR was brilliant. Use an enzyme to act as a pair of molecular scissors to precisely cut DNA at a prespecified location to disable a gene or even insert a new one.[12-24] Claire would like to rethink CRISPR and to move it to treat diseases of the brain, but this will require careful experiments, as one mistake could be fatal.

Claire and other experts believe that selectively modifying the DNA of living organisms will one day effectively treat neurological disorders from Parkinson's disease to dementia. CRISPR has unlocked new cancer treatments, treated different kinds of anemia, been trialed for sickle cell disease, and turned pigs into organ donors. CRISPR has also been used to make new fruits, to change a flower's color, and to eradicate disease-carrying mosquitos. CRISPR for certain forms of Parkinson's disease could become a reality in six to ten years.

Albert Einstein worried that his work could fuel a nuclear revolution. Similarly, Jennifer Doudna and Emmanuelle Charpentier, the Nobel laureates behind the CRISPR technology, have publicly worried about the ethics of gene editing. Treating human disease seems reasonable; however, permanently changing someone's genetic makeup requires an important dialogue about the consequences of using genetic scissors.[20,25–27]

Claire and her graduate student Sally Salomonsson recently reviewed the ways that CRISPR gene therapies could be rethought, built for good, and used as pathways to treat neurological disease.[11] How would it work? A potential treatment would be loaded with "CRISPR gene-editing cargo." The packaging would need to facilitate efficient and safe delivery, in this case to the brain. For CRISPR therapy to be successful, the delivery method and package would need to be as precise as the gene-editing cargo. Once in the brain, the cargo for CRISPR editing, the CRISPR scissors, would travel to a specific site in the genome. How would it know where to go? It would be accompanied by a courier, known as a guide RNA. In tandem with the guide RNA, it would make a cut in a prespecified double-stranded DNA gene target.

Though the CRISPR technique has been successful in sickle cell disease and beta thalassemia, it must be rigorously tested and monitored to be sure that inadvertent insertions or deletions in a similar-looking target sequence do not occur. Off-target or unintended editing can result in disastrous consequences, such as the future formation of a tumor. Scientists have maintained that the targets must be verified in the laboratory by a minimum of two different methods and that the delivery box should self-destruct or be designed to be easily broken down by the body.

Claire explains that many recent advances in gene editing have been game changers, making the process more efficient. Base editing can be employed when a single mutation in a gene, called a point mutation, is found to be causative for a disease. Alternatively, base editing can change gene expression and improve symptoms of a particular disease. Another, newer technique is to use premanufactured templates to create precise deletions in the genome. This templated CRISPR has the potential to inactivate a single member of a gene pair by carrying a dominant or a gain-of-function variant. This change results in an altered gene product gaining a new molecular function or pattern of expression. Templated CRISPR can correct a point mutation or replace a part of the gene that is defective. Finally, a templated CRISPR strategy can be used to treat a disease by upregulating or souping up another gene.[11]

Claire believes that Parkinson's is an ideal disease for targeting by CRISPR. She also believes we could use CRISPR to answer critical questions such as whether alpha-synuclein overexpression plays a role in the development of Parkinson's disease or whether enhancing the normal function of alpha-synuclein could be a treatment. She also believes that the technology could be applied to study the mysterious "spreading" of Parkinson's protein (alpha-synuclein) throughout the brain.

How will we test new therapies like CRISPR? It will be important to know when and when not to apply CRISPR. In Parkinson's gene mutations that lead to a loss of cell function like *GBA* or *PRKN* (another rare gene that can cause Parkinson's), these therapies may, for example, be better suited for gene therapy rather than for CRISPR. We will need to rethink and to develop a clear and safe path forward for this technology if we are to apply it to Parkinson's disease.

RESTARTING COMBINATION THERAPIES

When the chemist Jerome Horwitz first synthesized the compound AZT (zidovudine) in the 1960s, his hopes were in the clouds. He sought to derail the runaway genetic material that was occupying the insides of malignant cancer cells. The project was a failure—or so it seemed. Thirty years later, on October 26, 1990, the Food and Drug Administration (FDA) approved AZT—but not for cancer. Overnight, AZT became the transformative hope for a new disease, HIV/AIDS.[28–30] Horwitz's "failed" drug would pave the road for a new generation of therapies, and it emerged from an unexpected place.

AZT was initially a small breakthrough for HIV, because it was not that effective when used alone. The HIV virus was smarter than the drug and could mutate and move past it. The fortunes for this drug changed quickly with the introduction of several more HIV drugs to the market. The "aha" moment was when doctors combined the drugs into a highly active antiretroviral therapy (HAART).[31,32] HAART was effective against HIV because it targeted the virus in many ways. Each of the HAART drugs included in the cocktail targeted HIV in different stages of its life cycle. The combination of drugs made it difficult for the HIV virus to adapt and gave the body's immune system the upper hand. Overnight, HIV was transformed from a death sentence into a chronic, livable condition. People like Magic Johnson, the beloved basketball star diagnosed over thirty years ago, are still alive and thriving because of combination therapy. Recognizing the gains from the use of combination therapy in HIV will be important as we build combination therapies for Parkinson's disease.

Combination therapies have also been successful in treating cancer. Up until the 1960s, cancer survivors were an endangered species. Emil Freireich, a curmudgeon at the National Cancer Institute, was the least likely person to improve the situation. A pioneer of chemotherapy, he was a "pain in the ass" to work with, and he was even more annoying to be in the same room with. Author Malcolm Gladwell described him as "possessing both the sense of urgency for those dying of leukemia and the disagreeableness necessary to disrupt conventional thought." However, the oncologist was relentless in his pursuits and was still working at age ninety-three, when he succumbed to complications related to a Covid-19 infection. Emil sought to combine four chemotherapy drugs into one powerful concoction. This approach would create a highly charged torpedo that could be aimed at cancer cells. It was somewhat nonspecific, and it was designed to destroy as many cells as possible without killing the patient. Surprisingly, this blunt-force approach, which was far from the typical one drug, one-target approach, worked. The survival rate for leukemia following introduction of the concoction jumped from 30% to 90%.[33-36] HIV and cancer provide a fundamental lesson: there is power in recognizing the gains from combination therapy.

As in the case of chemotherapy and cancer, multiple studies comparing patients who lived pre- and postlevodopa have revealed that the introduction of the simple combination therapy carbidopa-levodopa increased life expectancy.[37-44] Disappointingly, fifty years after this success, no more progress on life expectancy or disease modification has been made.

Why use combination therapies for Parkinson's disease? The answer is simple: it has worked. It has worked in Parkinson's disease, and it has worked in cancer, HIV, and other diseases. What if we could activate cells to resist degenerating or dying? We could deliver a titanic blow to Parkinson's disease.

Regrettably, the early successful model of a combination therapy for Parkinson's (carbidopa plus levodopa) was not followed by development of other combinations to treat the symptoms or to slow Parkinson's disease progression. Carbidopa was necessary to get more dopamine to the brain and to reduce nausea and other side effects. Though we have welcomed more than a dozen symptomatic therapies since levodopa (and later its combination with carbidopa) was introduced, we desperately need something that will slow disease progression. The Parkinson's Plan will need to restart combination therapies.

Combining two approaches can lead to summation of their benefits $(1 + 1 = 2)$. Combination therapies in tuberculosis, leprosy, HIV, and cancer have all led to more than the sum of their parts; they have led to actual synergy $(1 + 1 = 3)$. Yet, since the most famous combination therapy of all time, Sinemet, the field has not pivoted to embrace combination therapies for disease modification. If we build on top of the carbidopa-levodopa success in Parkinson's, as well as the triumphs in HIV and cancer, we can, as Winston Churchill famously said, "Come back from our recent setbacks." Of course we will need better drug therapies to drive the combinations, and we anticipate that this will become a reality in a ten-plus-year frontier.

RAISING NANOMEDICINE

When Raag Airan worked in the laboratory of Karl Deisselroth, one of the fathers of optogenetics, his mentor tried to convince him to go into psychiatry. Raag believed, however, that radiology was his perfect fit. It was the place where technology could drive the next generation of modern medicine. There Raag could begin to figure out how to uncage drugs in order to impact lives.[45-48]

Drug uncaging has the potential to reduce Parkinson's disease symptoms, pain, and more.[49-54] Uncaging is when you load up an inactive or caged form of a drug and send it into the body, where it can be activated, or "uncaged." Raag has been drawn to the precise control over timing and location of drug activations, which he believes have the potential, perhaps in a ten-plus-year frontier, to reduce side effects and make a dent in unmet needs for Parkinson's disease.

The term *nanomedicine* is being used more and more in modern medicine, but what does it mean? It derives from the Greek word *nanos*, meaning "dwarf," and the Latin word *medicina*, which means "healing." How small is a nano? It is one-billionth of a meter. A gold nanoparticle, sometimes used in medicine, is about one-thousandth the width of a human hair. The beauty of using a nanoparticle as a treatment is that a nanoparticle has a large surface area relative to its volume. This property allows injected nanoparticles to interact in new biological environments. In Parkinson's, the interest in a nanoparticle to deliver drugs or modulate circuits is considerable.

The cliché that big things come in small packages perfectly suits nanoparticles. Nanoparticles are so small that they can evade the immune system and circulate for longer periods in the bloodstream than an unencapsulated drug. This makes them more attractive than many other therapies. Not only can the particles reach the target more efficiently, but scientists have also designed sustained-release versions, which is particularly enticing in a chronic disease like Parkinson's.

Studies using nanoparticle technology may form the foundation for novel Parkinson's disease therapies. Subsequent research efforts should raise the profile of nanomedicine and prioritize addressing the logistical and methodological challenges associated with translating these therapeutic approaches into clinical practice.

As we raise the profile for nanomedicine in the ten-year-plus frontier, there are many important questions facing the future of nanoparticles. Could nanoparticles be used to deliver antioxidant or anti-inflammatory therapies?

Could they be engineered to deliver gene therapies or to aid the scissors in CRISPR gene editing? Could we use nanoparticles to deliver the Miracle-Gro® (neurotrophic factors) to specific parts of the brain? One day scientists hope that we may be able to treat and simultaneously monitor Parkinson's, and it is possible nanoparticles will pave the road forward.

BEING READY

Science means "knowing." The word *science* derives from the Latin *scientia*. Science is greater than knowledge. Science is understanding. Science is not, however, serendipity. But when serendipity meets science, the benefits can be robust. To fully realize the frontiers in Parkinson's treatments, we need to be ready when opportunity strikes.

Christian Busch at New York University and the London School of Economics and Political Science credits serendipity with playing a "major role in the success of both individuals and organizations." Unfortunately, there remains a lack of conceptual clarity and structure, leading ultimately to a universal failure to operationalize, validate, and measure its actionability. Busch believes we should refocus on three domains to understand serendipity: agency, surprise, and value. All three must be present in order to differentiate serendipity from related concepts, such as "luck or targeted innovation." We should better appreciate the ideas in Busch's 2020 book, *The Serendipity Mindset: The Art and Science of Creating Good Luck*, as we progress toward the frontiers of Parkinson's therapies.[55]

What is the game plan for lab-based researchers seeking to better understand Parkinson's disease? First, ask a good question. Next, learn "why." Finally, conduct careful laboratory and then human-based experiments. Could we deviate from this tried-and-true scientific method to include serendipity? Could this be an opportunity?

When serendipity reveals itself in medicine, it usually manifests in one of three ways: (1) A drug administered for one purpose accidentally reveals an unexpected benefit or new indication, (2) Something of value is revealed when not sought, (3) The application of a flawed rationale tips the emergence of an unexpected finding. We have to be ready to receive all three forms if they reveal themselves.

In the 1960s, amantadine, a colorless crystalline solution, was commonly employed to prevent and treat flu. Nearly half of people in early flu studies benefited from amantadine, and virologists observed that the drug produced a "force field" around human cells. Amantadine rapidly received FDA approval in 1966 for its protection against infection with the Asian version of influenza. A decade later, it was also approved for use in influenza A. Amantadine as an antiviral treatment persisted for about forty years until a surplus of mutations in the flu virus rendered the pill ineffective. In 1969 serendipity revealed itself for the use of amantadine in Parkinson's disease, and the treatment remains in use today, after fifty-five years and counting— even longer than levodopa.[56]

In April 1968, a single woman with Parkinson's disease consumed amantadine for flu, and a remarkable story unfolded. Her Parkinson's symptoms improved. When she discontinued the drug, they immediately returned. Her doctor, a Harvard sailor and neurologist, Robert Schwab, was the perfect man for the moment.

Schwab was a "matchless storyteller, was never self-seeking, unpleasantly aggressive nor insecure."[57] Schwab made many "chance observations," but none were completely accidental. His observations were the product of awareness, recognition, and follow-through. What was Schwab's secret sauce? The doctor demonstrated that "a wise and clever individual, using simple techniques and striving for quantitation, can, by means of new insights and ideas in his clinical activities, open up unexplored areas of research and practice." In Parkinson's disease, beyond amantadine, he also pioneered the use of intravenous apomorphine, which tickles dopamine receptors and rapidly reverses Parkinson's disease. Schwab recognized this benefit "long before L-DOPA was considered," and it wasn't until 2004 that the world caught up to him when the FDA approved apomorphine hydrochloride injections.

Though the pharmaceutical company Smith, Kline & French owned the rights to the drug amantadine, they agreed to allow Robert Schwab to test it on ten people. Seven of these initial persons with Parkinson's improved. Within just months, Schwab conducted a formal clinical trial replicating his previous findings. He even went so far as to create a protocol to characterize tricky and ambiguous cases for which he employed, without consent, the use of a placebo pill. Schwab concluded that about two-thirds of his Parkinson's disease patients improved when he prescribed them amantadine.[58-61]

Following the publication of his study, the major neurological society of the time, the American Neurological Association, lauded Schwab in its published *Transactions*, citing the critical importance of the "unexpected and fortuitous therapeutic effect of amantadine." The authors were commended for their serendipitous observation and follow-up efforts, which led to "another drug added to our armamentarium." Five short years following this single patient–driven serendipitous finding, amantadine was approved for use in Parkinson's disease by the FDA.

Amantadine today continues to be prescribed heavily for the treatment of tremor and other Parkinson's disease motor features; however, its greatest benefit emerged in a second serendipitous lightning strike. Concurrent with the introduction of amantadine, the advent of levodopa revolutionized treatment of Parkinson's in the late 1960s and early 1970s. However, after a few short years, long-term levodopa-related side effects emerged, including a strange dance-like behavior. Frustrated by this afterbirth, doctors realized that when they added amantadine to levodopa, the movements unexplainably lessened and, in some cases, ceased. Later, the dancing was given a name, dyskinesia.

Since the early descriptions of amantadine dampening dyskinesia, multiple multicenter, double-blind, randomized, placebo-controlled trials have confirmed its ability to suppress the emergence of "disco dyskinesia."[62-68] Today, over fifty years after its introduction for flu, amantadine remains the single-best medication for Parkinson's-related dyskinesia. The dual serendipity of the discovery of amantadine for use in the primary treatment of Parkinson's as well as to address levodopa-related side effects has left crucial breadcrumbs for scientists to follow as they seek targets and treatments.

Can we teach clinicians and researchers to search for or be ready for serendipity? The answer is yes. David Perell argues in his blogs that "serendipity is a state of mind, and thus it can be learned." Christian Busch puts it more bluntly, sharing that what is needed is "sensemaking, event-based discussion and theorizing."[55] Serendipity can be cultivated. We are beginning to appreciate the "how, why and when factors to leverage value from the unexpected." The exemplification of this point in Parkinson's disease can be summarized in the obituary for Robert Schwab, which said that "serendipity, for him, was an example of chance favoring the prepared mind."

REINVIGORATING A NEW GENERATION

Joe Jankovic was born in the western region of Czechoslovakia, a place today better known for producing hockey players than for churning out doctors. His father died of tuberculosis when he was two, and his mother was an Auschwitz survivor. Joe grew up a poor Jewish kid in Czechoslovakia and had close to a zero chance of being accepted to medical school, so he decided that he would focus on studying engineering and playing his piano.

In 1965, at the age of seventeen and hardly speaking any English, he was invited by his uncle for a one-week vacation to the United States. Once he escaped the grip of the Iron Curtain, he never looked back. He was adopted by a family in Phoenix, Arizona, and triumphantly returned to Czechoslovakia decades later, after the fall of the Berlin Wall. Upon his return he was a doctor, a professor of neurology, an author of over 1,000 papers, and a world-renowned expert in Parkinson's disease.

When you ask Joe where to spend money to "develop new therapies in Parkinson's disease," his answer is simple and direct. Grow the next generation of clinicians, clinician-scientists, and researchers. Create opportunities for them, like the opportunity that was created for him. Only about fifty Parkinson's specialists are trained per year in the United States. This is not enough. Unless we nurture and grow the next generation, our climb to beat Parkinson's will only grow steeper.

REINVESTING OUR DOLLARS

We have spent the better part of the last year interviewing people and asking them where we should put our chips down to develop new Parkinson's therapies. For us, it starts with making the funnel bigger and funding more research. Our red card campaign, which was part of our last book, *Ending Parkinson's Disease*, flooded the White House with thousands of postcards advocating for increasing the investment in Parkinson's research by a factor of ten. We need to double down on this objective. Concurrently, we will need to better appreciate and embrace failure. We need many more failures to reach the types of successes we aspire to achieve.

We pushed hard with many partners for the passage of the National Plan to End Parkinson's Act. When it became law in 2024, this was a huge recognition of the efforts, and a critical step toward gaining the attention and funding necessary, to move the Parkinson's disease research needle. The work is not done; it is just getting started.

We need to invest many more dollars into prevention-based research, since, shockingly, only a few cents of every dollar we spend now go in this direction. It doesn't make sense to fund only new treatments, especially if the best treatment is prevention. We should fund the education of more and younger investigators interested in unravelling the "why" of Parkinson's disease. Once we understand the why, the therapies will flow.

It is also clear that we need to fund the development of more tools and better delivery systems for our therapies, and we need to improve the development of mini-brains in the dish. These steps will push us forward faster. We should fund better care models, more navigators, and more practitioners. We will, in our quest, not forget the living.

One of our mentors, Mahlon DeLong, appreciated that his seminal hypothesis on the circuits responsible for Parkinson's disease would and should be refined and possibly one day replaced. We should all embrace this approach as we push for more science and attract more young people into the field. We should step up and ask why clinical trials are failing. We should follow the script of HIV and cancer and double down on combination therapies. We should grow what we are doing now, from biomarkers to drugs, from the microbiome to electricity, and from vaccines to immunotherapy. We should nurture "outside-the-box" therapies like repurposing old drugs, reaching for new drugs, regenerating circuits, rejuvenating stem cells, rethinking gene editing, raising nanomedicine, and realizing serendipity. We should be courageous, welcome what lies "beyond," and be ready to act when serendipity reveals itself.

CONCLUSION

10

THE PLAN

The Secretary of Health and Human Services . . .
shall carry out a national project to prevent
and cure Parkinson's, ameliorate its symptoms,
and slow or stop its progression.

—National Plan to End Parkinson's Act[1]

ON WORLD PARKINSON'S DAY IN APRIL 2023, CONGRESSWOMAN Jennifer Wexton disclosed that she had been diagnosed with the disease. "I want to bring about as much good from this diagnosis as I can."[2] Five months later she would reveal that her diagnosis had been changed to progressive supranuclear palsy (PSP)—"a kind of Parkinson's on steroids."[2]

Wexton, a former prosecutor and judge (**Figure 1**), entered Congress in 2018 motivated to fight childhood cancer after a young girl in her northern Virginia community died of a brain tumor.[2] While the cause of her parkinsonian disorder is uncertain, Wexton, a mother of two, used to live near a landfill. She is left wondering if the polluted site may have contributed to her PSP.

The condition has robbed Wexton of much of her mobility and speech but has strengthened her resolve. She was one of the sponsors of the

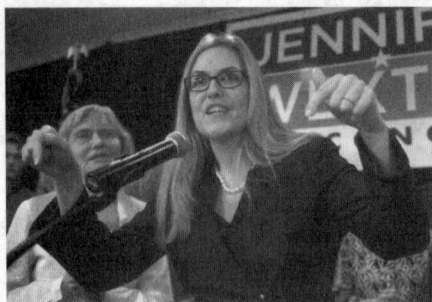

Figure 1. Jennifer Wexton after she was elected to Congress in 2018. Photo by Andrew Caballero-Reynolds/AFP via Getty Images.

Dr. Emmanuel Bilirakis and Honorable Jennifer Wexton National Plan to End Parkinson's Act, which passed the US House of Representatives 407–9.

Wexton, who remained an active legislator until her retirement in 2025, uses text-to-speech software to communicate. Three days after she gave a stirring speech at our Brain and Environment Symposium in Washington, DC, on May 20, 2024, the US Senate unanimously passed the bill, and President Joe Biden later signed it into law. Thanks to the act, the federal government will, for the first time, create a national plan to prevent and cure the disease.

In the preceding chapters, we have outlined the rationale for and introduced elements of our "PLAN." Here, we assemble those elements into a complete plan not just for the federal government but for all of us (**Figure 2**).

PREVENT

Chemicals in our food, water, and air are ubiquitous, and many are fueling the rise of Parkinson's. Most are ingested or inhaled, and the pathology of Parkinson's likely begins in the gut or the nose. The chemicals in question share a common characteristic: they damage the energy-producing parts of cells, which are critical to the health of nerves that make dopamine. While more work remains, epidemiological studies link these chemicals to Parkinson's in humans, and researchers have confirmed this relationship in laboratory animals.

In the Parkinson's 25, we detail steps individuals can take to reduce their risk of Parkinson's or, if they already have the disease, to possibly slow its progression. However, our environment largely reflects choices made by

The Parkinson's PLAN

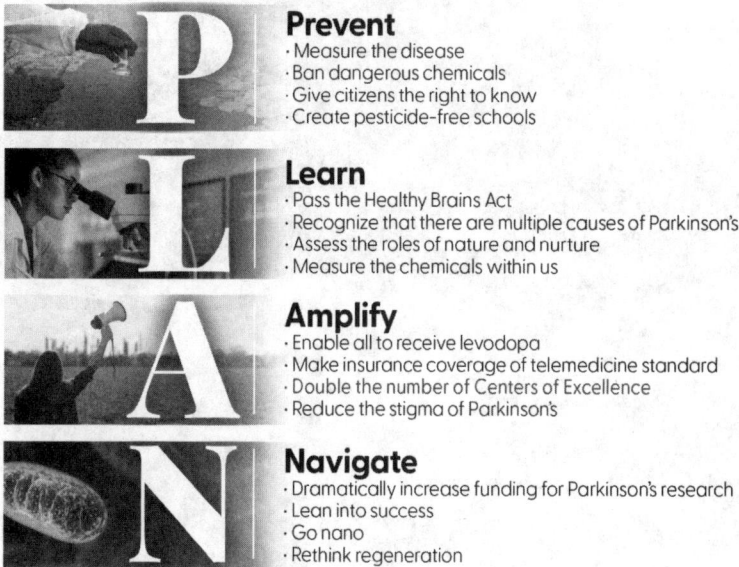

Prevent
· Measure the disease
· Ban dangerous chemicals
· Give citizens the right to know
· Create pesticide-free schools

Learn
· Pass the Healthy Brains Act
· Recognize that there are multiple causes of Parkinson's
· Assess the roles of nature and nurture
· Measure the chemicals within us

Amplify
· Enable all to receive levodopa
· Make insurance coverage of telemedicine standard
· Double the number of Centers of Excellence
· Reduce the stigma of Parkinson's

Navigate
· Dramatically increase funding for Parkinson's research
· Lean into success
· Go nano
· Rethink regeneration

Figure 2. Overview of the PLAN.

communities and nations, not individuals. To that end, here we introduce the Parkinson's Prevention Pyramid (**Figure 3**) to highlight actions individuals, communities, and nations can take to prevent the disease.

GLOBAL ACTION

1. Measure the Disease

What gets measured gets managed.[3] Right now, we fail to measure even the most basic aspects of Parkinson's: how many people have it and how many are developing it. Not surprisingly, the condition is out of control.

We don't know how many people actually have Parkinson's—not for the world, any country, any state or province, or any city. The values provided in this book are frequently based on models with multiple inputs, including reviews of medical records, claims data, or analyses from several studies. For

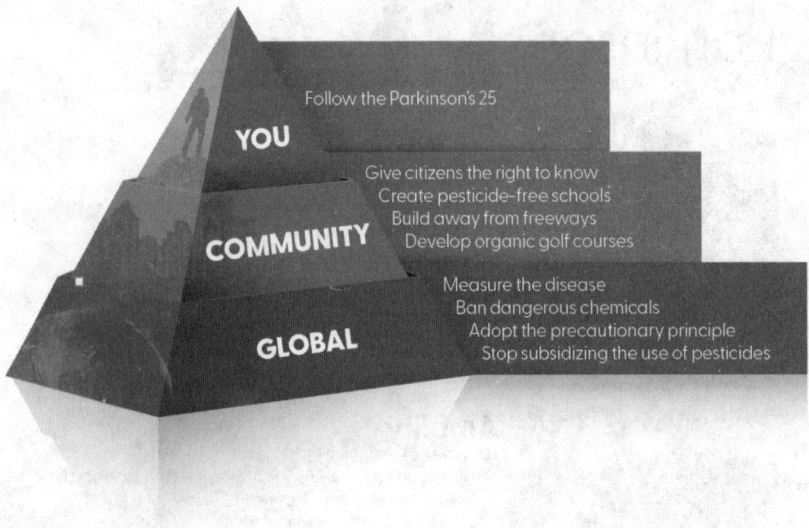

Figure 3. Parkinson's Prevention Pyramid.

example, one recent prevalence estimate for Parkinson's in the United States (930,000 people affected in 2020) relied on data from multiple studies.[4] The variability in the estimates generated from these investigations was high: 50% for women and twice that for men.[4]

In addition, no one knows how many Americans were newly diagnosed with Parkinson's in 2024. And researchers are even less certain how many are undiagnosed. The last time researchers checked in the United States was in 1978. They found that 42% of individuals identified with the disease in Copiah County, Mississippi, did not even know they had it.[5] Today, as Dr. Allison Willis, one of the field's most highly regarded epidemiologists, points out, the number may still be large. People with environmental exposures (like farmers) frequently suffer from other disabling conditions, have less access to care, and thus go uncounted.

The absence of data is not just a US problem. No country has such data. Even the Global Burden of Disease study, funded by the Bill & Melinda Gates Foundation, which provides the most detailed measures of disease burden, has not published estimates on the number of new cases (incidence) of Parkinson's. Only a handful of studies have examined trends in disease incidence. However, these studies are usually limited to a specific community, such as Rochester, Minnesota.[6,7] While these studies provide valuable data, they may not be generalizable, because the causes of Parkinson's in Rochester, for example, are likely different than those in Los Angeles or Dyersville, Iowa.

If we want to prevent and ultimately end Parkinson's, we must first measure it well, widely, and regularly.

2. Ban Dangerous Chemicals

For sixty years, paraquat and chlorpyrifos have been used to kill weeds and insects.[8] The health risks of both pesticides are well established, and multiple countries have long banned both substances. It is time for the United States to do the same. The Environmental Protection Agency (EPA) issued a rule effectively banning chlorpyrifos in 2021; however, two years later, a court of appeals set aside its rule and allowed for the continued use of chlorpyrifos on foods we eat.[8] These legal challenges, many by the pesticide's manufacturer, are not new. When the EPA announced its ban of DDT in 1972, major legal challenges were already underway.[8]

In December 2024, the EPA banned both trichloroethylene (TCE) and perchloroethylene (PCE). However, in January 2025, that action was delayed as part of a regulatory freeze.[9] TCE, first created in the 1800s, has caused cancer and probably contributed to Parkinson's for a century. PCE has likely done the same. The toxicity of TCE has been known for at least ninety years.[10] Companies promote safer alternatives for degreasing and dry cleaning;[11,12] it is time that we put them to the test in the United States and beyond.

3. Adopt the Precautionary Principle

In 1998, a group of thirty-five scientists, lawyers, environmentalists, and policy makers convened for a three-day conference in Racine, Wisconsin, on the shore of Lake Michigan. They were worried about toxic substances and the existing regulations that had "failed to protect adequately human health and the environment."[13,14] In place of reactionary regulations, they argued,

It is necessary to implement the Precautionary Principle: When an activity raises threats of harm to human health or the environment, precautionary measures should be taken even if some cause and effect relationships are not fully established scientifically.

In this context the proponent of an activity, rather than the public, should bear the burden of proof.[14,15]

As retired Master Sergeant Jerry Ensminger, whose daughter Janey died from leukemia at Camp Lejeune, said, "The benefit of the doubt should go to the people, not the chemical."[16] Such an approach would ensure that chemicals introduced into the environment are safe rather than requiring scientists, regulators, and policy makers to determine that a chemical is harmful after it is already on the market.

Before approving new medications, the US Food and Drug Administration (FDA) requires that a drug be safe and effective. The burden of demonstrating the safety and efficacy of a product thus falls on the company or sponsor, which stands to benefit if such evidence is generated. Such an approach has worked well for drugs since 1962. It is time to apply it to the chemical industry.

4. Stop Subsidizing the Use of Pesticides

The US federal government spends about $15 billion a year on farm subsidies.[17] Most of that goes to conventional farming, which uses pesticides.[18] In the United States, the two most subsidized crops are corn and soybeans,[19] and according to the US Geological Survey, paraquat is sprayed the most on those fields.[20] In essence, billions of taxpayer dollars are subsidizing the production of crops on fields that are sprayed with millions of pounds of paraquat.[19,20]

The Department of Agriculture does have a few programs to incentivize organic farming. However, the size of these programs is approximately 1% the size of the subsidies for farms using pesticides.[21] If we are going to subsidize farming, we should support programs that improve, rather than harm, the health of farmers, rural communities, and consumers.

COMMUNITY ACTION

5. Give Citizens the Right to Know

According to the *Guardian*, the manufacturer of paraquat adopted a "freedom to sell" campaign to protect sales of its blockbuster product.[22] If companies have a freedom to sell, then consumers should have the freedom to know.

One of the great travesties of Camp Lejeune is that even after the Marine Corps knew about the contamination, it refused to notify those who served there. According to one researcher, "From the time of detection in 1980 until a Congressional mandate in 2007, the Marine Corps made little to no effort to notify the affected veterans and their families of the potential for health problems, and failed to fully disclose the true extent of the contamination."[23] As a result, individuals were likely diagnosed with cancer at much later stages than they could have been. A great tragedy was made worse by the refusal to confront the truth.

The truth is also concealed from civilians. As discussed, many urban and suburban residents live or lived near a dry cleaner. Ray, one of the authors, was among them. During medical school, Ray and his young family lived in a high-rise apartment in Philadelphia that was located above a dry cleaner. Twenty-five years later, Ray called the dry cleaner and was relieved to find that the operation was just a storefront. The dry cleaning was done off-site. Others are not as fortunate.

From Hopewell Junction, New York, to Mountain View, California, residents have unknowingly lived on top of TCE-contaminated plumes for years.[24-27] In countless cases, people live, work, or study near a toxic site, oblivious to the risk. These sites are unmarked and often unfenced, and the dangers are invisible.

For years, Ray drove past *four* state Superfund sites less than ten minutes from his home, unaware that TCE and PCE were in the soil and groundwater. At one, a former metal printing and plating facility in suburban Pittsford, New York, the level of contamination may have been greater than that at Camp Lejeune.[28] And almost no one knew, likely for decades.

Today, many residents of Love Canal, New York, home of the country's first Superfund site, have little to no idea of its toxic past or any remaining contamination.[29]

This all must end. People who live, work, or study near a contaminated site should be notified regularly (e.g., annually) of their proximity to a Superfund or other toxic site, and the sites should be marked, so the public knows. In addition, organizations, including golf courses, schools, and towns, that release chemicals into our shared environment should have to report them. In the United States, such reporting is required of larger companies under the Emergency Planning and Community Right to Know Act. This effort could readily be expanded.[30,31] Citizens can then determine whether the release is warranted, test their homes and wells, and protect themselves and their families.

6. Create Pesticide-Free Schools

In 1998, Robina Suwol dropped off her son Nicholas, a kindergartner, at Sherman Oaks Elementary School in Los Angeles. As Nicholas was turning to kiss his mother good-bye, he encountered a cloud of weed killer sprayed by a man in a hazmat suit who had been treating the school's hedges. Nicholas said, "It tastes terrible," and began to wheeze. He asked his mom if this would happen again. His mom promised it wouldn't.[32–35]

Two years later, spurred by Suwol's activism, the California legislature passed the Healthy Schools Act. The law requires that all K-12 public schools and licensed child-care centers develop programs that minimize the use of chemicals and focus instead on weeding, removing dead plants, and employing traps. The bill bans the use of high-risk pesticides on schools and surrounding parks, and schools that use pesticides must notify parents annually.[36] The right-to-know law should serve as a model for schools nationally and beyond.[35]

7. Build Homes and Schools Away from Freeways

In California, air-quality officials recommend that homes be built at least five hundred feet from highways.[37] Yet over one million Southern Californians live within that distance. Another million live within 1,000 feet.[38] As reported in the *Los Angeles Times* in 2017, Mike Sanchez, his wife, and two young daughters live in housing that is just one hundred feet away from a freeway. He was reluctant to buy a house so close to traffic, but it was "one of the sacrifices [his family] made to get into a new home."[38,39]

At least the Sanchez family lives near only one freeway. Some live near two. Residents near a recent development at the intersection of the Hollywood (101) and Harbor (110) freeways prefer the convenient location but not the air pollution. One resident says that when she walks out on her fourth-floor balcony overlooking the freeway, her "feet turn black."[38] It is unlikely that the soot is just affecting her feet. Numerous studies from all over the world have found that living in areas with high levels of traffic-related air pollution is associated with an increased risk of Parkinson's, not to mention Alzheimer's.[40–46]

In the United States, sixty million people, one-fifth of the population, live near roads with high air pollution. Those with the least means to address this pollution are often among the most exposed. According to a recent study, "Racial/ethnic minorities and lower-income groups in the USA are at a higher risk of death from exposure to [particulate matter] than are other population/income groups."[47]

The problem is global. In Canada, 10 million people, almost a third of the population, live near polluted roads.[48] In New Delhi, India, 41% of the population is exposed to traffic-related air pollution. In Beijing, it is 66%. European cities are even worse. In Paris, the proportion is 67%, and in Barcelona, it's an astounding 96%.[49]

Schools are also at risk. As we saw in Mexico City, air pollution plants the seeds of Parkinson's at a very young age. We should protect children who may be especially vulnerable because of their size, development, greater activity, and higher breathing rates.[37,48] The particulate matter generated by cars does not stop at a school's doors but can make its way into the classroom.[37] If your child's school is located near a highway or in a polluted area, the EPA recommends installing roadside barriers (large walls) and planting vegetation, which together can reduce downwind pollution by up to 60%. In addition, closing windows and improving air-filtration systems can reduce exposure to particulate matter by 80% to 90%.[37] Regardless of the situation, schools can take measures to reduce childhood (and adult) exposure to air pollution and enable all to live longer, healthier lives.

8. Develop Organic Golf Courses

For many, golf is a wonderful sport. It occurs outdoors, fosters friendship and community, and requires physical activity. But golf should not contribute to Parkinson's disease for those who work, play, or live nearby. Organic golf courses, free of pesticides, are beginning to emerge, but according to a 2021 article in *Golf*, only one golf course is 100% organic—the Vineyard Golf Club in Martha's Vineyard.[50] Local residents required that it be so because they did not want to be exposed to chemicals or have toxicants pollute the island's only aquifer.[50]

Other golf courses, including Laurelwood in Eugene, Oregon, have been dramatically reducing their pesticide use. In the *Golf* article, author Olivia White, a Generation Z college golfer, concluded, "Perhaps the most important takeaway is that community voices matter; Vineyard Golf Club would have never been organic without pressure from the community. Golfers and non-golfers alike have the power to demand more from the courses they enjoy, knowing that their demands are realistic."[50]

LEARN

There are many unanswered questions about the origins of Parkinson's that we can address. We need to shift our scientific thinking "upstream" to the beginning of the disease rather than focusing on the end.

9. Pass the Healthy Brains Act

Congressman Gus Bilirakis and Congresswoman Jennifer Wexton recognize that we need to move upstream in our thinking, so in 2024, they introduced the Healthy Brains Act. The bill would create the first-ever program to study the relationship between environmental factors and all neurodegenerative diseases, including Parkinson's, PSP, and amyotrophic lateral sclerosis (ALS).

Research aimed at identifying the underlying causes of Parkinson's is woefully underfunded. Only two cents of every Parkinson's research dollar is devoted to preventing the disease (**Figure 4**).[51-55] Homes in Miami

Only 2 Cents
of every research dollar
goes to prevention

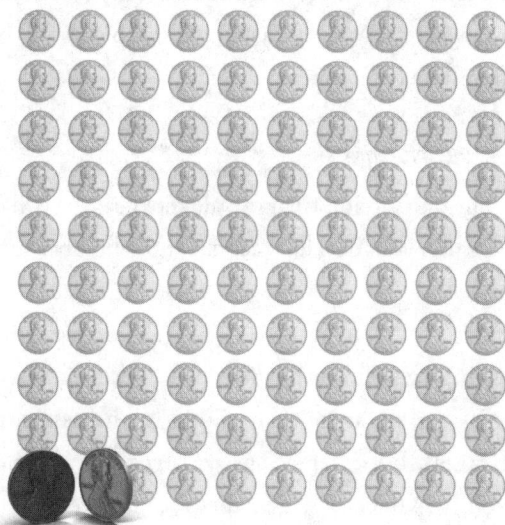

Figure 4. Proportion of Parkinson's research funding devoted to prevention.

sell for more money than the United States spends annually on preventing Parkinson's.[56,57]

In introducing the legislation, Congressman Bilirakis said, "We know that research is the key to developing a better understanding of diseases and holds the promise for the development of more effective treatments and potential cures." Congresswoman Wexton added, "We have a lot of work to do to understand how to prevent these diseases in the first place." The bipartisan bill sets aside $50 million to do just that.[58,59]

10. Recognize That There Are Multiple Causes of Parkinson's

We must appreciate that Parkinson's disease is actually Parkinson's *diseases*.[60] Like breast cancer, which can be due to chemicals, radiation, genetics, and other factors,[61] Parkinson's has many different causes.

We also now know that, for many, Parkinson's has its origins outside the brain. It is time that we study the entire bodies of affected individuals.[62] This can be done through imaging, as Dr. Per Borghammer and his colleagues in

Denmark do, or through pathological examination of bodies (and brains) after people have passed. There are likely clues in individuals' guts and noses, not to mention their hearts, skin, lungs, kidneys, and other organs that might be affected by chemicals like TCE. If we methodically assess the whole body and map changes over time, we can assemble the pieces of the Parkinson's puzzle and identify all its true origins.

11. Assess the Roles of Nature and Nurture

Smoking causes lung cancer, but only about 10% of smokers get it.[63] There must be other factors that determine who develops cancer and who does not. The same is true for Parkinson's.

Not every farmer who sprays paraquat, not every Marine drinking in TCE, and not everyone breathing in polluted air develops Parkinson's. We must learn why. As we have discussed, some of it is due to the exposure (dose, duration, route, and timing), but interactions with genes and other environmental factors and modifiers like stress and diet are important too. However, they are poorly understood.

Most genetic causes of Parkinson's alone are also insufficient to cause the disease. Some genetic causes—*LRRK2* mutations, for example—may have important interactions with TCE, while individuals carrying *GBA* mutations may be especially sensitive to the effects of pesticides.[64] Better understanding of these relationships will pave the way for more effective prevention and treatment strategies.

12. Measure the Chemicals Within Us

We know that chemicals contribute to Parkinson's. We now need to measure them in humans. We test adults for cholesterol to prevent heart disease and children for lead to avoid intellectual disabilities. Both efforts have had tremendous health benefits. For example, compared to the 1970s, the level of lead in children's blood today is 90% lower.[65] Bans on lead in gasoline and paint have made us all smarter.[66,67]

We should use that intelligence to expand testing for chemicals that are known to cause cancer and likely Parkinson's. At a minimum, we can start with those at greater risk, beginning with workers in high-risk occupations (e.g., farmers), those who live or have lived near contaminated sites (e.g., Camp Lejeune; Newport Beach, California), and those with the disease. Testing could also include clusters, as in Hebron, New York, or even graduates of the US Air Force Academy like Jana Reed and Sara Whittingham.

In Italy in the 1990s, researchers tested the blood of the general population for common environmental pollutants, including TCE and PCE. They discovered these chemicals in about three-quarters of the population.[68] What would the results be today? In Italy? The United States? China? We should find out.

In addition to measuring these toxic chemicals in our bodies, we should carefully evaluate their effects in laboratory animals and use alternatives like mini-brains in a dish. Doing so will help us learn why these toxicants likely lead to Parkinson's and what therapies could slow or arrest the damage that they cause.

AMPLIFY

Nearly twelve million people are now living with Parkinson's globally. Many more are undiagnosed. Together, the majority of these individuals go without adequate care or treatment.[69] Almost all need more help and support, and they need it now. We must increase resources and amplify the voices of those affected—patients, caregivers, and families—to reduce everyone's burden.

13. Enable All to Receive Levodopa

Fifty years after the introduction of levodopa, many countries around the world lack access to the highly effective medication.[70] According to the World Health Organization (WHO), only 37 of 110 countries globally have access to levodopa in clinics.[71] And where available, it is often unaffordable.[72,73] In low-income nations, it is not available at all.[71] We have failed to deliver a simple, safe, effective, low-cost tablet to millions of people with a treatable disease.

This lack of access must end. Those with HIV receive far more expensive, complex medications for their condition. We should enable those with Parkinson's to receive appropriate treatment for theirs.

How do we get levodopa to underserved populations?[71] We can learn from HIV/AIDS and buoy generic drug manufacturing and begin the process of contracting with UNICEF and other agencies to produce generic versions of the medicine. If cheap manufacturing can be accomplished within a country, availability and affordability will follow.

We need to borrow a page from the Clinton Foundation's Medicines, Technologies and Research program, which works with generic drug makers to guarantee the purchase of a minimum volume of medications. This approach has been a game changer for providing a steady drug supply for other chronic diseases.[74-78]

We also need to partner with the WHO[71] to achieve prequalification of newer and potentially more effective pharmaceutical products. We will need to pay particular attention to performance and labeling of drugs and to provide assurances to countries that the medications meet internationally accepted requirements for human use.

Finally, we need to invest in building logistics to procure, deploy, track, and distribute Parkinson's medications throughout lower-income nations. We will need a global fund capable of buying drugs from multiple countries, and we need to put in place tracking measures to judge both success and failure. In the interim, we should invest in programs that promote a growing supply of dopamine through planting and processing the dopamine-rich plant *Mucuna pruriens*, as this may be sustainable in some regions of the world.[71,79]

14. Make Insurance Coverage of Telemedicine Standard

Telemedicine for Parkinson's only became a widespread reality during the Covid-19 pandemic. However, in the United States, the provision was a time-limited teaser. Following the publication of *Ending Parkinson's Disease*, we launched a "Give a Dime for Parkinson's Disease" campaign that sent 30,000 postcards to the White House calling for the coverage to be made permanent. However, it is still temporary, and many benefits are slated to expire in early 2025.

We must make telemedicine an option for all as it can help reach those who are most underserved or most disabled.[80,81] No one should be left behind because of who they are or where they live.

15. Double the Number of Centers of Excellence

We have too few hubs of Parkinson's care. Currently, there are only a few dozen Centers of Excellence worldwide, and the US Department of Veterans Affairs has only six Parkinson's Disease Research, Education and Clinical Centers. We propose that for every 10,000 persons with Parkinson's, a Center of Excellence be available. To meet this need in the United States alone would require increasing the number of centers to about 100 and a commensurate rise in public and private funding.

As Dr. Allison Willis has demonstrated, better care results in better outcomes. Individuals with Parkinson's who see a neurologist are about 20% less likely to fracture a hip, to be placed in a skilled nursing facility, or to die prematurely compared to those who do not.[82] Yet 40% of Americans do not see a neurologist of any kind within four years of diagnosis.

In Europe, the first right endorsed by the European Parkinson's Disease Association Charter is care from a doctor with a special interest in Parkinson's, but many do not receive such care.[69] China has an estimated 1.4 million to 3.6 million people with Parkinson's;[83,84] however, the country only has 150 Parkinson's specialists.[85] Caring for the growing Parkinson's population will require new centers and models that embrace technology.[69]

16. Reduce the Stigma of Parkinson's

The stigma associated with Parkinson's is tremendous and often unaddressed. People with Parkinson's and their families, friends, and caregivers are all impacted. Research has helped us appreciate the deleterious short- and long-term effects of social isolation, emotional distress, and decreased self-esteem associated with Parkinson's disease.[60,86,87]

Dr. Indu Subramanian at the University of California, Los Angeles, has proposed a path forward that raises awareness, promotes inclusion, provides family support, fosters open communication, and deploys antistigma campaigns.[88–94] Thanks to the awareness generated by Muhammad Ali, Michael J. Fox, Brian Grant, Davis Phinney, and many others, the burden of Parkinson's has been reduced for many.

However, the stigma of Parkinson's persists. Self-described "reckless optimist" Omotola Thomas, a native of Nigeria with degrees in system engineering and project management, was diagnosed with Parkinson's in 2016 at age thirty-five. Omotola's wait for her diagnosis took years and spanned countries. After her diagnosis, she founded Parkinson's Africa to increase access to care and to confront the stigma that remains in many African communities, where cultural misconceptions pose serious challenges.[95] For example, in some Kenyan villages, people believe that individuals with Parkinson's are under a spell, possessed by demons, or suffering for the wrongs of family members. Consequently, many do not seek, much less receive, care.[96,97]

To help reduce stigma, media can be a powerful tool. Michael J. Fox has done this through his own career. The star actor Harrison Ford recently portrayed a wise, funny therapist with Parkinson's in the comedy series *Shrinking*.[98] Filmmakers have produced the moving documentary *Shaking Hands with the Devil* to help reduce the stigma of the disease in Africa.[99] Much more is needed. Parkinson's presents enough challenges as it is. Stigma need not be another.

NAVIGATE

The road to better treatments for Parkinson's will require a new direction. We must, as we did for HIV/AIDS and cancer, move toward combination therapies. We must develop more practical biomarkers that can monitor progression and assess the effectiveness of new therapies. We must think outside the box by using genes and "omics" technologies to uncover new drugs and targets for regenerative medicine. We must also advance gene editing, nanomedicine, neuromodulation, and neuroimmune approaches including vaccines. Finally, we need to incorporate artificial intelligence to catapult us toward identifying individual Parkinson's-specific fingerprints.

17. Dramatically Increase Funding for Parkinson's Research

Every six minutes we delay developing a new therapy, another diagnosis of Parkinson's is made. The current National Institutes of Health (NIH) research funding of $251 million a year will not move the needle and is a fraction of what we invest in HIV/AIDS (**Figure 5**).[55] Even after adding the support from the US Department of Defense ($16 million)[100] and

	Prevalence	Incidence	Funding
HIV/AIDS	**1.2 million** people living with HIV	**32,000** new infections/year	**$3.29 billion**
Parkinson's disease	**1.2 million** people living with PD	**90,000** new cases/year	**$251 million**

Figure 5. Comparison of NIH funding for HIV/AIDS and Parkinson's disease, 2022.

other federal sources (e.g., the Department of Veterans Affairs), the needle is stuck.[101] This amount of investment is simply insufficient.

If we want to succeed, we propose an Operation Warp Speed for Parkinson's. We need to increase funding tenfold and reach $3 billion in federal support annually. As a starting point, this money could be allocated equally to each part of the PLAN—prevent, learn, amplify, and navigate (**Figure 6**).

This level of expenditure has had immeasurable benefits for preventing and treating HIV. Millions of us have never been infected, and millions receive appropriate treatment for HIV because of that investment. With wise investment, the same can be realized for Parkinson's.

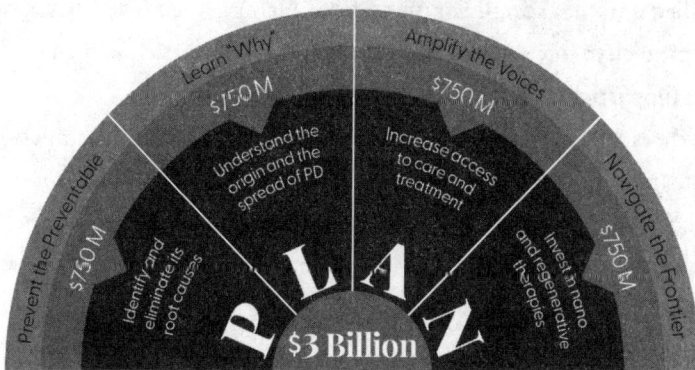

Funding the **PLAN**

Learn "Why" $750 M — Understand the origin and the spread of PD

Amplify the Voices $750 M — Increase access to care and treatment

Prevent the Preventable $750 M — Identify and eliminate its root causes

Navigate the Frontier $750 M — Invest in nano and regenerative therapies

$3 Billion

Figure 6. Proposed allocation of increased federal funding for Parkinson's disease.

18. Lean into Success

The oil tycoon John D. Rockefeller famously said, "Don't be afraid to give up the good to go for the great." Both levodopa and deep brain stimulation can be helpful treatments, yet both can be improved. Over time, larger and more frequent doses of levodopa are often required, leading to more side effects, including excessive dance-like movements called dyskinesia. Pumps are on the horizon that deliver a more constant dose of levodopa under the skin, much like insulin pumps for diabetes. Improving access to these types of innovative approaches could reduce symptoms and improve quality of life.[102]

Similarly, deep brain stimulation can turn back the clock for some individuals, but it too is far from a panacea. The wires and the stimulating device that deliver the electrical current to the brain will soon sense brain waves and adjust the stimulation to improve symptoms. The stimulating device will soon also become a sensing one, a powerful combination that will enhance function for many.

19. Go Nano

For Parkinson's research, we should think large but not forget to invest in the very small. Nanomedicine holds immense promise for both diagnosis and treatment. Nanomaterials will improve our diagnostic imaging, and nanosensors will detect biomarkers in the blood and other body fluids. Nanomedicine will improve drug delivery, reduce side effects, and enhance our ability to target specific brain regions. Nanomedicine will penetrate the brain's protective force field, called the blood-brain barrier, and enable delivery of nanoparticles, genes, and proteins.

The therapeutic potential is large. To reduce harmful inflammation, we can load nanoparticles with anti-inflammatory drugs. To rescue a brain damaged by a chemical, we can deliver nanoparticles to restore function of the energy-producing mitochondria. To fix damaged parts of the brain, we can deploy nanorobots, and to prevent the spread of misfolded proteins, we can utilize nanovaccines.

Nanomedicine opens the door to the previously unimaginable.

20. Rethink Regeneration

For many individuals, the most disabling features of Parkinson's are not the tremor or slowness of movements. Instead, "nonmotor" features, including thinking difficulties and mood disorders, are the greatest source of disability. Current treatments are not satisfying. New approaches are needed. Cell transplants and regenerative medicine will be an option to improve memory, thinking, and learning.

The new target may be an area of the brain (the basal forebrain) that does not use the chemical dopamine. It uses another chemical messenger called acetylcholine. Acetylcholine is critical for cognitive processes like memory, attention, and learning. Transplantation of acetylcholine-producing cells into brains of those with Parkinson's could improve memory and cognitive function. Similarly, approaches using gene therapy, CRISPR gene editing, and other technologies should be embraced and funded.

AMBITIOUS PLAN, AMBITIOUS GOALS

In 2014, the Joint United Nations Programme on HIV/AIDS (UNAIDS) set an ambitious target to help end the AIDS epidemic. It aimed to move beyond incremental progress with a goal that was "nothing less than the end of the AIDS epidemic by 2030."[103] To do so, UNAIDS established 90-90-90 targets for 2020 that would diagnose 90% of people living with HIV, provide appropriate treatment to 90% of these individuals, and suppress levels of the virus in 90% of those receiving treatment.[104]

While no country has yet met these goals, many are close,[105] and the global campaign against HIV has been highly successful. In the United States, HIV was a top-fifteen cause of disability in 1990. Today, it is not even in the top fifty.[106] Life expectancy in sub-Saharan Africa, which dropped in many nations in the early 2000s, is now at an all-time high.[107,108] Deaths due to HIV/AIDS have halved in the last decade, and the number of new infections is lower than at any point since 1990.[108,109]

Can we do the same for Parkinson's? As we have outlined here, we can. In **Figure 7**, we present 0-10-100 targets to prevent and reduce suffering due to Parkinson's by 2035.

2035 Parkinson's Goals

0·10·100

0% rise in new cases of Parkinson's	10x increase in research funding and percentage devoted to prevention	100% access to levodopa

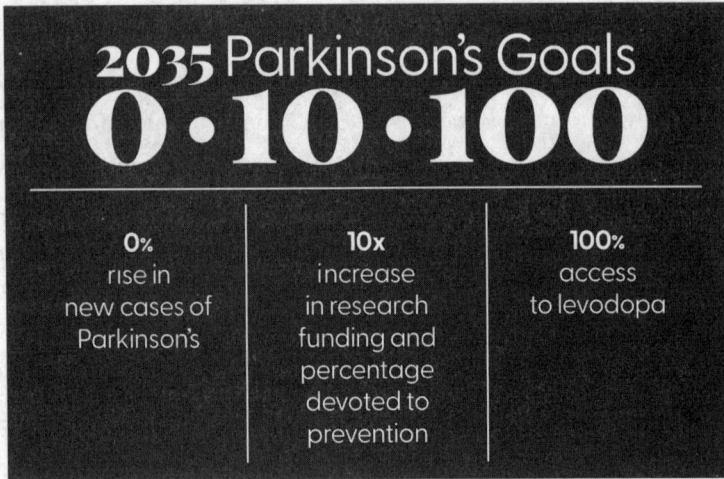

Figure 7. 0-10-100 Parkinson's goals for 2035.

Goal 1: 0% Rise in New Cases of Parkinson's

In the next decade, we can stop the rise of Parkinson's in both the United States and globally. The Rotterdam Study in the Netherlands offers hope for a world where Parkinson's is increasingly rare. The study, conducted in a port city in the south of Holland, found, after adjusting for age, a remarkable 60% decline in the number of new cases of Parkinson's between 1990 and 2000.[7] No other study, to our knowledge, has found such a remarkable decline. While the findings require replication and additional investigation, the decline followed substantial (75% to 90%) reductions in levels of pesticides in fat, quick prohibition of the use of paraquat, an early ban on and low levels of TCE in the environment, and large decreases in multiple air pollutants.[110]

As countries and entire continents clean their food, water, and air, we should begin to see the fall of Parkinson's. We may be seeing these first signs in Europe, although they are far from definitive. European nations were among the first to ban DDT, and the 2001 Stockholm Convention accelerated the elimination of other pesticides (called organochlorines) that dissolve in fat and are implicated in Parkinson's.[111] In 2013, the European Union severely restricted the use of TCE.[112] Air quality in Europe is dramatically better than it was in the past. Some air pollutants in Europe are down 80% or more from their peak in the 1980s.[113]

These reductions in three major classes of toxicants may be bearing fruit. After adjusting for age, Europe has the slowest rate of increase in the number of affected individuals, and in a few countries (e.g., France, Italy, and the Netherlands), the number may falling.[84,114]

While Parkinson's is poised to fall in some parts of the world, it is rising rapidly in those where chemicals are spreading. The country with the fastest increasing rise is China, where the prevalence of Parkinson's (again adjusted for age) more than doubled between 1990 and 2016.[114] During this period, China's use of pesticides doubled.[115,116] China also accounts for half the world's market of TCE, and its use is increasing.[117-119] Finally, as many know, China's air quality is among the world's worst.[120]

However, China is improving its environment. It has banned paraquat. China, by far the world's largest consumer of pesticides,[121] has also implemented policies to reduce their use and to decrease water and soil pollution.[122] Since peaking in 2015, pesticide use is now decreasing.[116] In response to its polluted skies, China in 2013 launched an antipollution campaign, and its skies are 50% cleaner.[123] It now has the world's fastest-improving air quality.[123]

Despite this progress, challenges remain. Historically, most countries in Africa have had limited use of pesticides and industrial chemicals and consequently have had clean air.[124-126] Unfortunately, that is changing. Over the past thirty years, pesticide use has nearly tripled in Africa.[119] Many of the chemicals being employed, including ones related to DDT, have been banned in other countries.[127] This rise is especially concerning as roughly 60% of the African population is engaged in agricultural production.[128] Without better safeguards (including personal protective equipment), many Africans could be developing Parkinson's in record numbers in the decades and generations to come.

Africa is not the only region with cause for concern. Per capita pesticide use in Central and South America is greater than any other region in the world.[129] Many of these pesticides are linked to Parkinson's.[129] Air pollution in the Middle East is mushrooming.[130] The United States has been unable or unwilling to ban some of the world's most toxic pesticides.

After adjusting for aging, a 0% rise in new cases for Parkinson's can happen in the next decade, but we must first eliminate, reduce, and mitigate its causes.

Goal 2: 10-Fold Increase in Research Funding and in the Percentage Devoted to Prevention

A dramatic increase in NIH funding has precedent. In 2011, Republican Senator Susan Collins and Democratic Senator Edward Markey cosponsored the National Alzheimer's Project Act, which is now law.[131] Following its passage, the Department of Health and Human Services set out an ambitious goal to "prevent and effectively treat Alzheimer's disease by 2025." In 2016, NIH funding for Alzheimer's research increased 56% to nearly $1 billion. By 2024, it was $3.6 billion, seven times what it was just nine years earlier.[55,132]

However, more money alone will not be enough. Dr. Edward de Bono, the Maltese physician who originated the term *lateral thinking*, said, "You cannot look in a new direction by looking harder in the same direction."[133] A new direction is needed. We need to learn "why," and that begins by identifying the environmental causes of Parkinson's. For decades, these causes have been underinvestigated by academics and obscured by industry.[22,62] Two pennies of every research dollar will not answer why the disease is spreading; two dimes might.

Goal 3: 100% Access to Levodopa

Just as we are seeking to provide everyone with HIV with appropriate treatment, we should do the same for Parkinson's. The WHO has called for increasing access to levodopa.[71] It is time to heed that call. Globally, we are making progress toward treating infectious diseases, and access to medications is part of the solution.[134,135] It is time that we apply those lessons to chronic conditions like Parkinson's disease.

THE ECONOMICS OF PREVENTION

The Parkinson's Plan will also have immense economic benefits. Part of the rationale for increasing NIH funding for Alzheimer's research was financial. The economic burden of Alzheimer's in the United States alone exceeds $300 billion.[136,137] The cost to Medicare (the health insurance program for Americans over sixty-five) is $155 billion.[136] Against this backdrop, investing $3.6 billion to prevent and treat the disease makes sense.

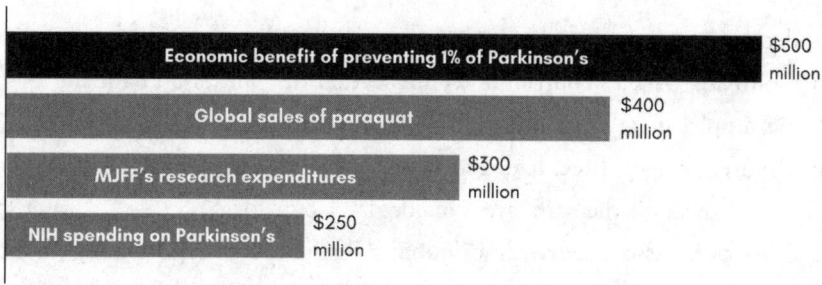

Figure 8. The economic benefits of preventing Parkinson's. MJFF = Michael J. Fox Foundation.

The benefits of preventing Parkinson's are similarly immense. The US disease burden has ballooned to over $50 billion.[138] Half is borne by Medicare due to additional health care costs. The other half is from the loss of income for affected individuals due to missed work, disability, and caregiving. Preventing just 1% of Parkinson's in the United States alone would have a value of $500 million per year. This is far more than the NIH or the Michael J. Fox Foundation spends on Parkinson's research annually (**Figure 8**).[139–141]

This level of prevention is readily achievable. For example, if paraquat is accountable for just 1% of Parkinson's, a ban would have enormous economic benefits. The $500 million savings would be more than the *Guardian's* estimate of paraquat's $400 million global *sales*.[22] Paraquat's economic burden in terms of Parkinson's—most of it paid for by taxpayers—likely far exceeds the company's sales of a weed killer.

Similar arguments could be made for TCE and PCE, which together likely contribute to a substantial proportion of Parkinson's in the United States and globally.[142] In essence, our immense public and private expenditures for Parkinson's are helping subsidize the true economic costs of these toxic chemicals. When these subsidies end, so too will the suffering.

COMMON CAUSE

Pesticides, TCE, PCE, and air pollution don't just contribute to Parkinson's. They can lead to miscarriages, congenital abnormalities, asthma, cancer, and countless other medical conditions. Pesticides—many of which are nerve toxins—likely contribute to intellectual disabilities and autism.[143,144] For example, increasing levels of chlorpyrifos are associated with lower IQ in children at ages three, five, and seven.[145-147] Pesticides, which can also be absorbed through the skin, are a major risk factor for ALS.[148-150] TCE also appears to be associated with a doubling of the risk of ALS among Camp Lejeune veterans.[151] Brain cancer has been reported in both media and scientific reports of likely TCE contamination.[118,152-154] Finally, air pollution is a major risk factor for Alzheimer's disease.[155]

The shared roots provide an opportunity to foster collaboration across disease foundations and organizations, which are often organized in silos and operate independently of one another. Dr. Bruce Lanphear, a physician scientist at Simon Fraser University in Vancouver, British Columbia, who has studied the impact of toxic chemicals on children, sees a new way forward. In reviewing this book, he wrote to Ray and said, "We are all competing for limited resources to support our causes, yet we share a larger goal: eliminating toxic chemicals that contribute to one-fourth of all diseases worldwide. You may be fighting for Parkinson's, another group for breast cancer, and another for autism. What would happen if we advocated for our own specific causes *and* highlighted the common environmental hazards driving all these diseases?"

A GIFT

Brain diseases are now the world's leading source of disability.[155] Parkinson's is among the fastest growing. This is the challenge of our time, and time is not on our side.

To address this challenge, we have detailed a plan that we can implement as individuals, in our communities, through our organizations, and with our political representatives to prevent and treat this terrible disease. If we do so, by 2035 we can create a world where Parkinson's is no longer rising but receding. By then, we can identify, understand, reduce, and eliminate many of its root causes. And finally, for the first time, we can provide access to treatment for all those in need.

Recent generations have given us a world largely free of polio, one where drinking and driving is socially unacceptable, and where HIV is both preventable and treatable. These are gifts. We have an obligation to receive gifts, and we have a duty to reciprocate.[156] Through our collective efforts, let future generations say that we answered the call, developed a plan, executed it, and created a world free of Parkinson's.

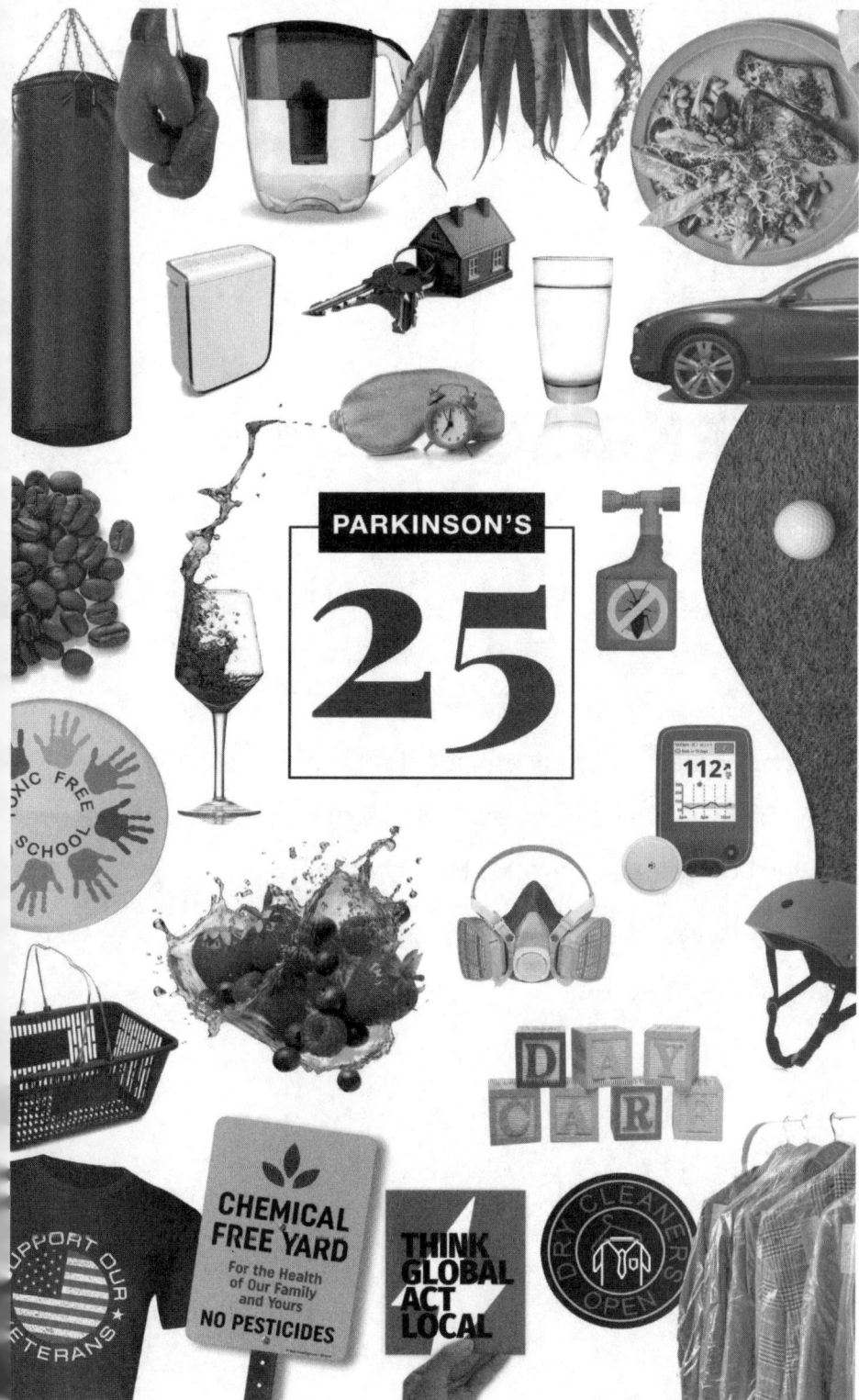

PARKINSON'S

25

TOXIC FREE SCHOOL

112

SUPPORT OUR VETERANS

CHEMICAL FREE YARD
For the Health
of Our Family
and Yours
NO PESTICIDES

THINK GLOBAL ACT LOCAL

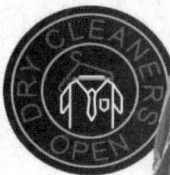

DRY CLEANERS OPEN

DAY CARE?

THE
PARKINSON'S 25

Here are 25 actions to lower your risk of Parkinson's. For those with the disease, some may even slow progression. Most apply to all of us regardless of age, sex, disability, or geography. These recommendations may be especially important for those with a family history of Parkinson's, those at genetic risk, or those who have been exposed to toxic chemicals.

Let's all live longer, healthier lives and say good-bye to Parkinson's disease.

1 Wash your produce, even your organic ones

Pesticides have contaminated our food supply. Remnants of pesticides are found in 20% of common foods. Organic produce, dairy products, and meat can reduce exposure but can still have unsafe residues of pesticides. So wash your produce at least with water and consider simple vegetable washes, vinegar, or salt solutions, too.

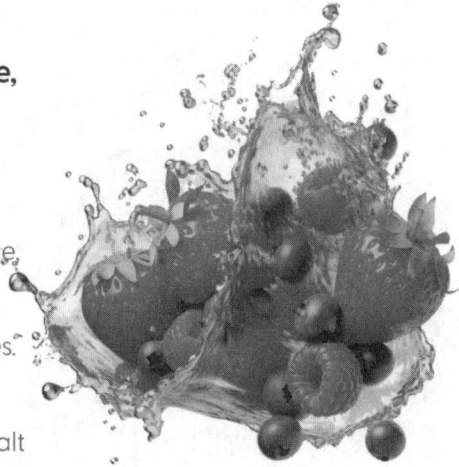

Change your diet

2

Individuals who eat a Mediterranean diet – high in fruits and vegetables and low in animal products – may lower their risk of Parkinson's. Such a diet may also be beneficial for those who already have the disease. The reasons for the benefit are not certain and may include reduced exposure to pesticides, which can concentrate in meat and dairy as they make their way up the food chain.

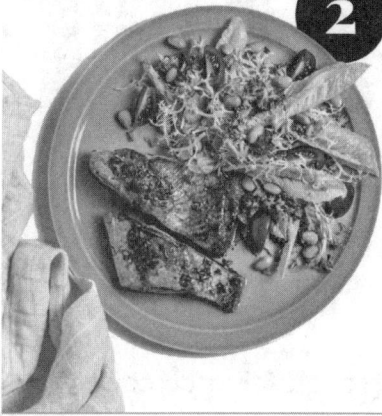

Make sure your grocery store is safe

3

Perchloroethylene (PCE), the dry cleaning chemical, can readily spread beyond the walls of a dry cleaner. In Germany, PCE, which dissolves in fat, has been found in dairy products in supermarkets near dry cleaners. Germany now prohibits supermarkets from being located close to dry cleaners. You may want to steer away from them as well.

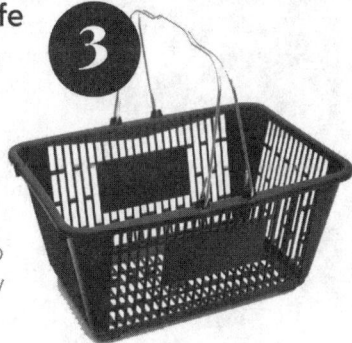

4
Enjoy wine without pesticides

Like produce, organic wines are not immune to pesticide contamination, but they have lower levels and thus reduced health risks. In addition, organic vineyards are likely safer for those who work there and for those who live nearby. Organic choices in what we eat and drink can improve the health of consumers, farmers, and communities.

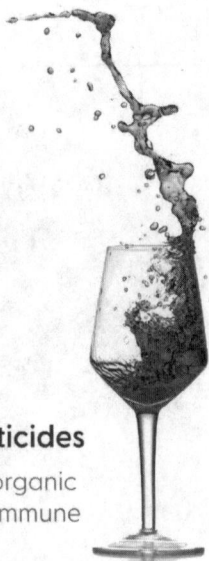

5
Avoid, or at least manage, diabetes

Diabetes is associated with a higher future risk of Parkinson's and may lead to a faster rate of progression. While it is unlikely a root cause of the disease, diabetes is probably an important modifier of risk and progression. So avoid diabetes by eating a healthy diet and staying active, and if you already have it, control your blood sugar levels.

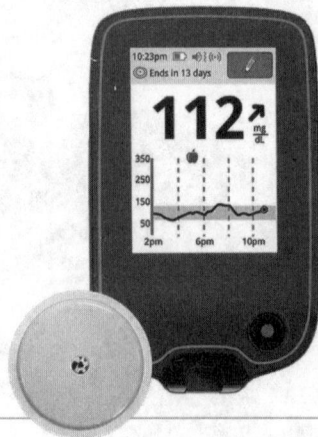

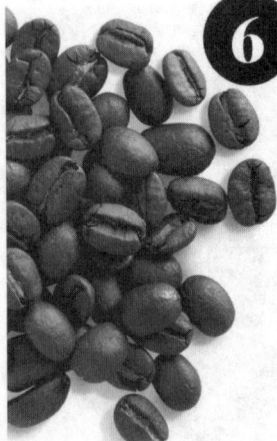

10:23pm Ends in 13 days

112 mg dL

350
250
150
50
2pm 6pm 10pm

6
Have a cup of caffeinated coffee

Caffeine consumption is associated with a decreased risk of Parkinson's. Caffeine may protect the dopamine-producing nerve cells from the damage that results from exposure to environmental toxicants. The benefits appear to be present regardless of your beverage of choice (e.g., coffee or tea) but are not present with decaffeinated beverages. Of course, caffeine has its own health risks, such as anxiety and headache. But you now have another reason to enjoy your morning cup of coffee.

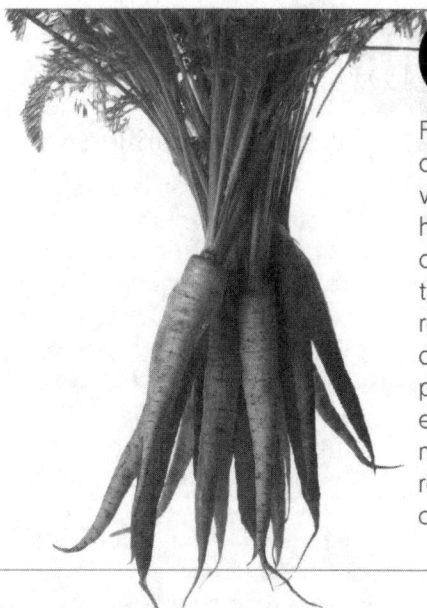

7 Farm safely

Farming is the world's most common job. Farmers who work with certain pesticides have a higher risk of Parkinson's. Farmers can lower their risk by decreasing the amount of pesticides used, reducing their frequency of administration, and using lower-risk pesticides. Personal protective equipment, including gloves, masks, and goggles, can also help reduce exposure and lower the risk of Parkinson's.

Check your well

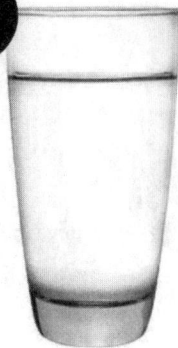

Up to 1 in 8 Americans have a private well. Unlike municipal or "city" water, these wells are not regulated by the Safe Drinking Water Act. They are infrequently tested and prone to contamination from pesticides and industrial chemicals. If you have one, test it regularly for pesticides and chemicals like trichloroethylene (TCE) in addition to the usual bacteria. Testing for these chemicals is often not done. The EPA provides a list of laboratories that are certified to test water, and mail-in options are available.

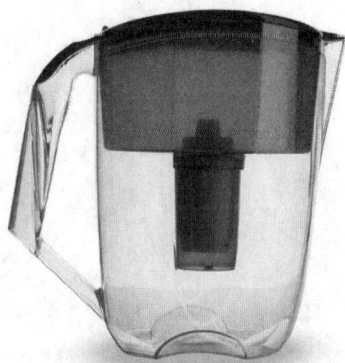

9 Use a water filter

A simple carbon water filter, widely available in supermarkets, can reduce exposure to pesticides, TCE, and other chemicals that may be in your water. These carbon filters can be installed for the whole house at the "point of entry" or at the point of use, such as faucets or even a water pitcher.

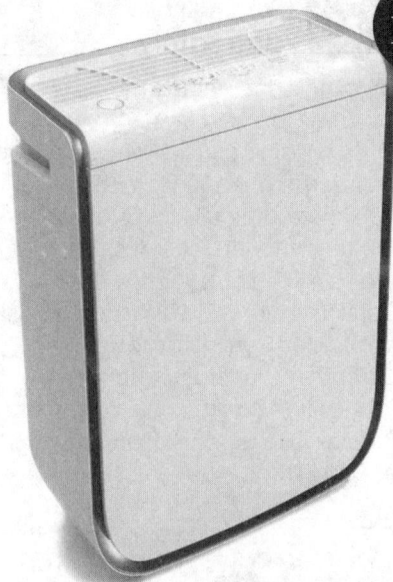

Consider air purifiers

Air purifiers are an easy and effective way to lower your risk of disease from indoor air pollution. Air purifiers do range in cost (as low as $10 to as high as $1000), require periodic cleaning and filter changes, and may need to be installed in multiple places depending on the size of the home, school, or work place. Be sure to use air purifiers with carbon filters designed to remove "volatile organic chemicals," like TCE.

Don't poison yourself

Sometimes the remedy is worse than the disease. Insects, including fleas, ants, and moths, can be unwanted guests. Unfortunately, some common pesticides can increase the risk of Parkinson's. For example, the pesticide permethrin, found in flea collars, ant sprays, moth balls, and outdoor apparel, can reduce dopamine-producing nerve cells in laboratory animals. Consider safer alternatives and, if necessary, minimize exposure by wearing a mask, increasing ventilation, and avoiding spraying near children.

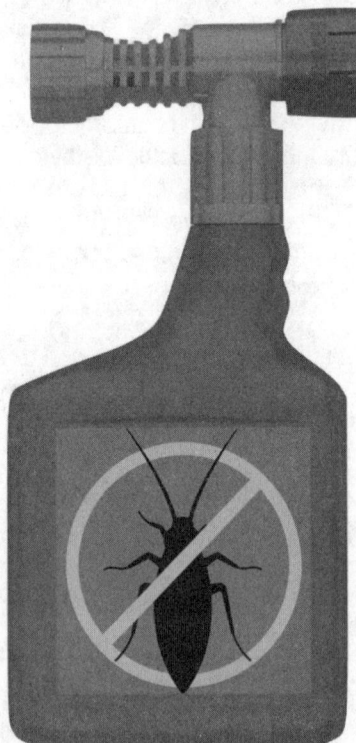

12 Choose your home carefully

Seventy million Americans live within three miles of a Superfund site. Most are unmarked, unfenced, and largely invisible. The EPA has a database where you can search for these sites, but less contaminated ones may be harder to find. If you live near a TCE- or PCE-contaminated site, you can test (usually through an environmental firm) your indoor air. If either chemical is present, a mitigation system, like the ones used for radon, can pump air from below your foundation to above your roof so you and your family can breathe easy.

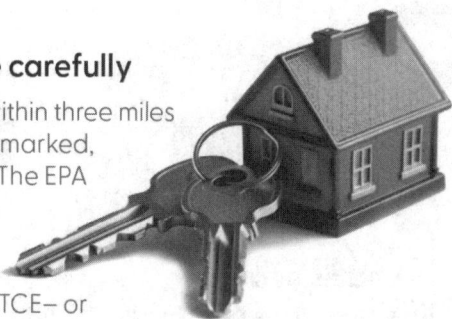

13 Dry-clean cautiously

Dry-cleaned clothes release dangerous chemicals like TCE and PCE into your car or home. To limit exposure, first, consider minimizing your dry cleaning. Second, find a dry cleaner that does not use PCE (also called "perc"). Third, if your dry cleaner does use PCE, "air" out your clothes before taking them inside the home. Take off the plastic bag and let the clothes breathe, so you don't have to breathe in the chemicals.

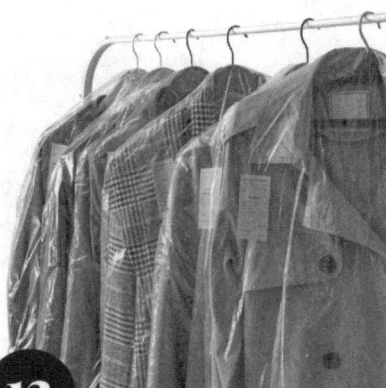

14 Check the ground floor

Before moving into a high rise, check what is on the ground floor. Because if there is a dry cleaner, the air inside may not be safe. If there is one, ask if dry cleaning is done on site and whether they use PCE (commonly known as "perc"). If they do, test your indoor air.

15

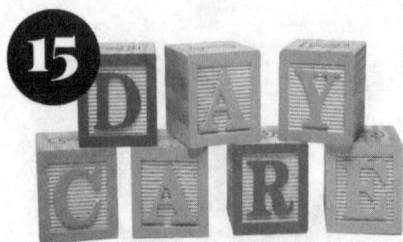

See what is near your child's day care center

Dry cleaners can also contaminate soil and groundwater, and these volatile chemicals can enter nearby homes, schools, and child care centers. Some day care centers are located near dry cleaners (for example, in strip malls). If so, you may want to ask if they have tested their indoor air or consider one that is not located near a dry cleaner.

16 Roll up your windows in traffic

Traffic-related air pollution, like that found on congested highways, is associated with an increased risk of Parkinson's and Alzheimer's. Next time you find yourself stuck in traffic or traveling through a tunnel full of cars, roll up your windows, and circulate the air within your car to avoid bringing toxic fumes inside.

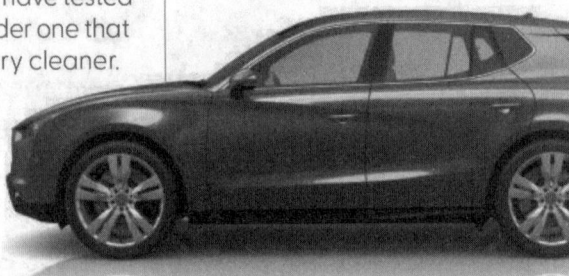

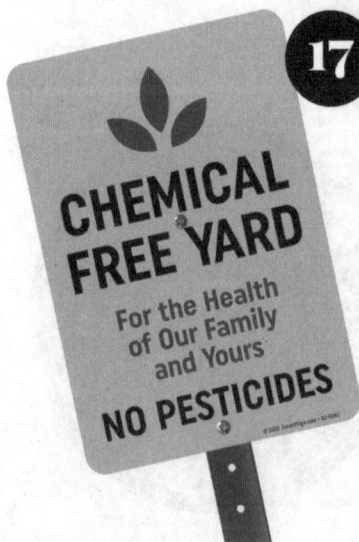

17 Garden with care

Plants, like chrysanthemum ("mums"), do not like to be eaten by insects, so many produce their own pesticides. Some of these natural pesticides are linked to Parkinson's. Amateur gardeners who spend an average of 160 days with weed killers in their yard, for example, have a 70% increased risk of Parkinson's. Gardeners should wear gloves, and if you work extensively with plants, you may want to adopt other protections, such as a mask or working in a well-ventilated space.

18 Be mindful of the greens

Those who live near or work on golf courses may have a higher risk of Parkinson's. What are golfers to do? Ask your favorite course or club what pesticides they use and when they spray. Encourage them to use less. Have them consider safer alternatives. In the interim, avoid playing on courses just after they have been sprayed. And don't lick your golf ball. Swallowing pesticides is not healthy either.

19 Look around your child's school

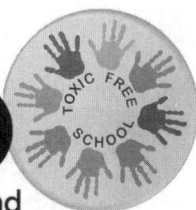

Over 4,000 U.S. elementary schools are located within 200 feet of crop fields. In Iowa, 90% of public school districts have buildings within 2,000 feet of a farm field. Also check out the playground and soccer field, where pesticides, often dangerous ones, are commonly used. Parents can ask their school leaders about what pesticides are used on their kids' playgrounds and fields, and sports teams at all levels can reduce their use of toxic pesticides.

20 Use personal protective equipment

Personal protective equipment (PPE) can protect against the toxic effects of chemicals. PPE, like long sleeves, pants, goggles, and respirators, can protect farmers, landscapers, pesticide applicators, and those who work with industrial chemicals like TCE and PCE. If you are an employer, protect your employees by providing them the appropriate PPE for the work required. If you are a worker, use them. It may save you and your family a lot of personal suffering and financial hardship in the future.

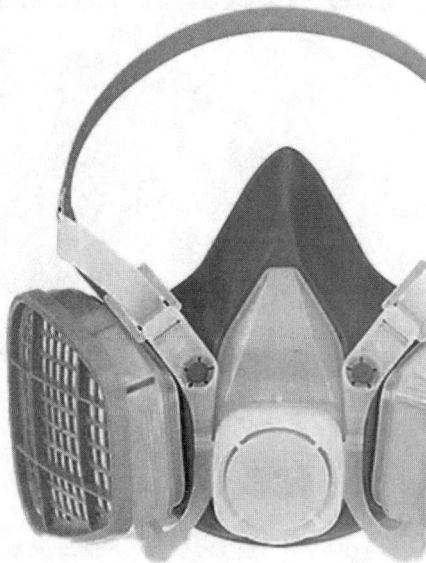

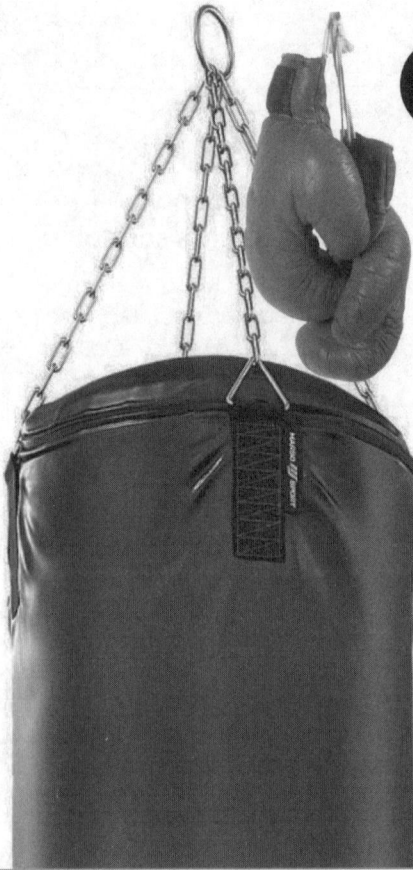

21

Exercise

In his best-selling book *Outlive*, Dr. Peter Attia wrote, "I now tell patients that exercise is, full stop and hands down, the best tool we have in the neurodegeneration prevention tool kit." Vigorous exercise can lower the risk of developing Parkinson's, and moving every day is also beneficial for those who already have the disease. In a recent study, aerobic exercise (stationary bike at least three times per week) reduced brain atrophy and stabilized disease progression.

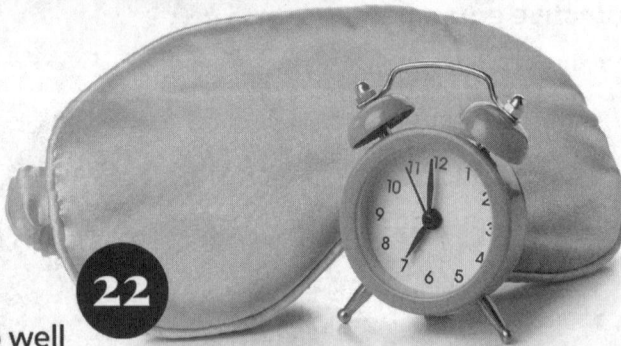

22

Sleep well

Improving sleep is important to maintaining brain health and may be important for preventing neurodegenerative diseases. Sleep is restorative and has been shown to clear toxins from the brain, including the Parkinson's-related protein called alpha-synuclein. When you sleep poorly, these proteins and other waste products accumulate. Improving sleep may help flush these toxins and minimize brain inflammation.

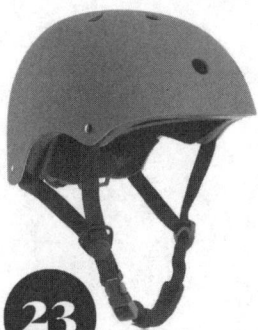

23
Avoid head trauma

Head trauma increases the risk of Parkinson's and may amplify the risk of pesticide exposure. So what to do? First, wear seat belts. Second, exercise caution with sports with a high risk of head injury, such as football, especially in children. Modifications (for example, no heading in soccer) may make sports safer and more enjoyable. Third, wear a helmet when you bike, skate, or ski.

24
Act locally

Much of our local environment is under our control. We can reduce pesticide use in our communities by speaking with mayors, town supervisors, and members of city council. Simple measures, such as reducing or eliminating use of pesticides in schools, parks, medians, and sports fields, are readily achievable. Doing so can improve health and save money.

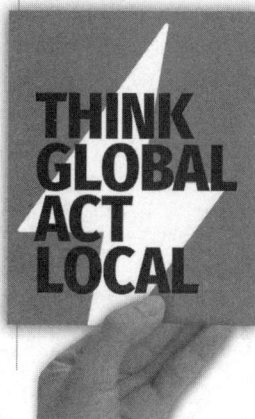

THINK GLOBAL ACT LOCAL

25
Support our veterans

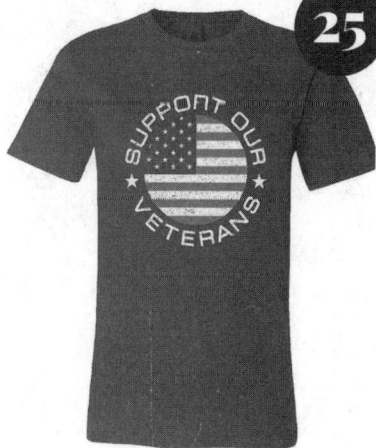

Veterans make up 6% of the US population but 10% of individuals with Parkinson's. Veterans are at increased risk for at least three reasons – exposure to certain pesticides, TCE, and head trauma. Some of these exposures are amenable to prevention efforts by reducing use of toxic chemicals, cleaning up or remediating polluted sites, and providing better equipment.

Resources

The following pages contain **resources** and **organizations** that provide more information on

Preventing the preventable
Learning why
Amplifying the voices of those affected
Navigating new frontiers of treatments

The list is not comprehensive but just serves as a starting point

Contact Us

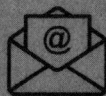

PDplan.org   info@PDplan.org

Children

HealthyChildren.org
healthychildren.org

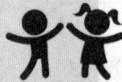

Healthy Schools Act,
California Department of
Pesticide Regulation
cdpr.ca.gov

Moms Across America
momsacrossamerica.com

Protect America's Children
from Toxic Pesticides Act
congress.gov/bill/118th-
congress/senate-bill/269

Toxic Chemicals

Agency for Toxic Substances
and Disease Registry
atsdr.cdc.gov

Beyond Pesticides
beyondpesticides.org

Pesticide Action &
Agroecology Network
panna.org

US Environmental Protection
Agency Superfund Sites
epa.gov/superfund

The Environment

Earthjustice
earthjustice.org

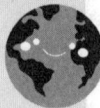

Environmental Working
Group
ewg.org

Facts and Stats

Global Burden of Disease Study
healthdata.org/research-
analysis/gbd

Our World in Data
ourworldindata.org

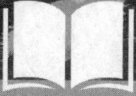

Books

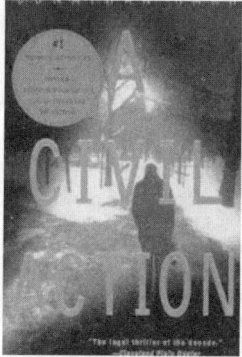

A CIVIL ACTION

"The legal thriller of the decade." —Cleveland Plain Dealer

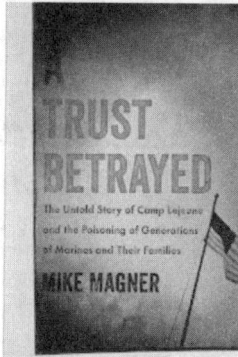

A TRUST BETRAYED

The Untold Story of Camp Lejeune and the Poisoning of Generations of Marines and Their Families

MIKE MAGNER

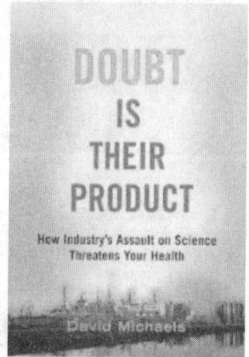

DOUBT IS THEIR PRODUCT

How Industry's Assault on Science Threatens Your Health

David Michaels

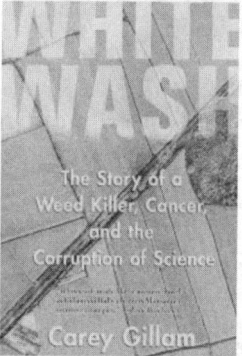

WHITE WASH

The Story of a Weed Killer, Cancer, and the Corruption of Science

Carey Gillam

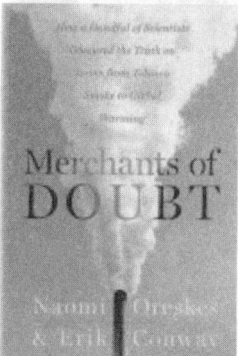

Merchants of DOUBT

Naomi Oreskes & Erik Conway

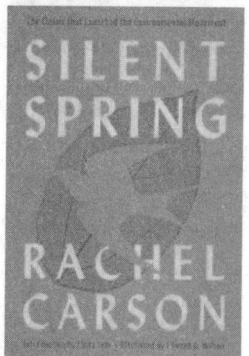

SILENT SPRING

RACHEL CARSON

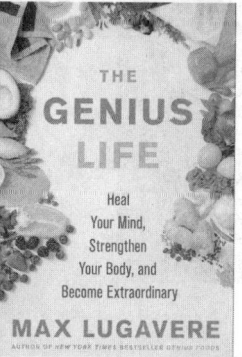

THE GENIUS LIFE

Heal Your Mind, Strengthen Your Body, and Become Extraordinary

MAX LUGAVERE
AUTHOR OF NEW YORK TIMES BESTSELLER GENIUS FOODS

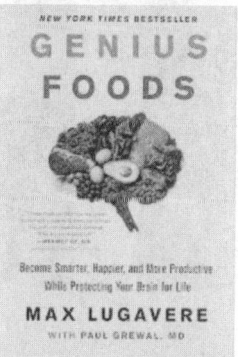

NEW YORK TIMES BESTSELLER

GENIUS FOODS

Become Smarter, Happier, and More Productive While Protecting Your Brain for Life

MAX LUGAVERE
WITH PAUL GREWAL, MD

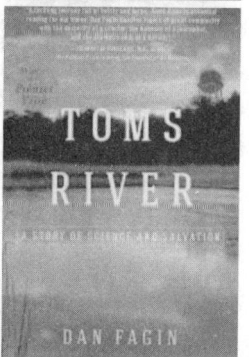

TOMS RIVER

A STORY OF SCIENCE AND SALVATION

DAN FAGIN

info@PDplan.org

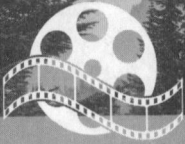

Movies

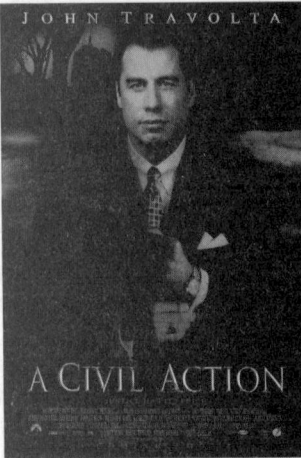

JOHN TRAVOLTA

A CIVIL ACTION

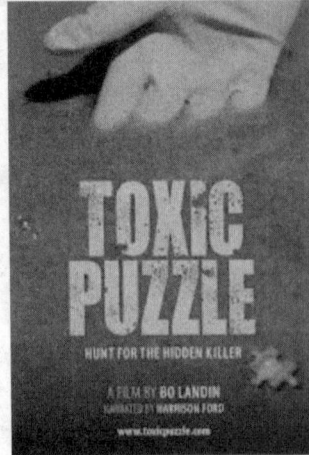

TOXiC PUZZLE

HUNT FOR THE HIDDEN KILLER

A FILM BY BO LANDIN
NARRATED BY HARRISON FORD

www.toxicpuzzle.com

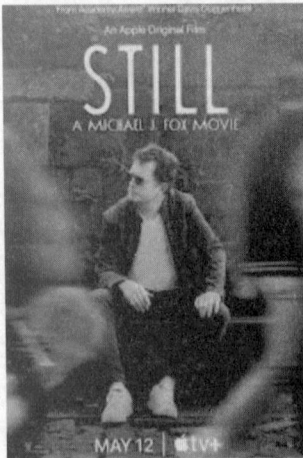

An Apple Original Film

STILL

A MICHAEL J. FOX MOVIE

MAY 12 | tv+

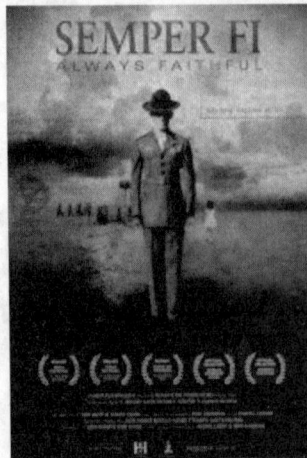

SEMPER FI
ALWAYS FAITHFUL

Aligning Science Across Parkinson's
parkinsonsroadmap.org

HEALTHY BRAINS Act
congress.gov/bill/118th-
congress/house-bill/9233

National Institute of Neurological
Disorders and Stroke
ninds.nih.gov/health-
information/disorders/parkinsons-
disease

National Institute of Environmental
Health Sciences
niehs.nih.gov

Parkinson's Secrets
parkinsonsecrets.com

Science of Parkinson's
scienceofparkinsons.com

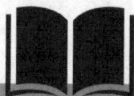

Books

A PRESCRIPTION
for ACTION

ENDING

PARKINSON'S

DISEASE

Ray Dorsey, MD · Todd Sherer, PhD
Michael S. Okun, MD
Bastiaan R. Bloem, MD, PhD

JON PALFREMAN

BRAIN
STORMS

THE RACE TO UNLOCK
THE MYSTERIES OF
PARKINSON'S
DISEASE

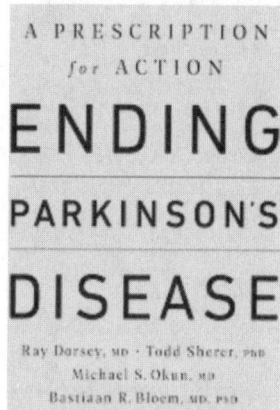

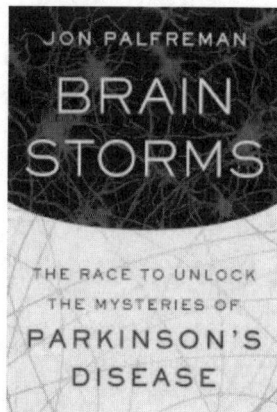

info@PDplan.org

Organizations

Movies

Dance for PD
danceforparkinsons.org

InMotion
beinmotion.org

International Parkinson and Movement
Disorder Society
movementdisorders.org

Mediflix
mediflix.com/topics/parkinsons-disease

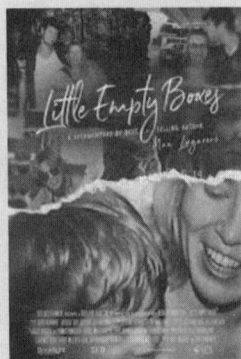

Parkinson's Foundation
parkinson.org/resources-support

Parkinsonz by Sara Whittingham
parkinsonz.org

PD Avengers
pdavengers.com

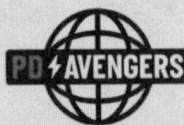

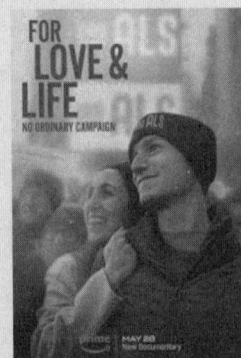

Rock Steady Boxing
rocksteadyboxing.org

World Parkinson Coalition
worldpdcoalition.org

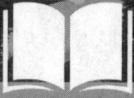

Books

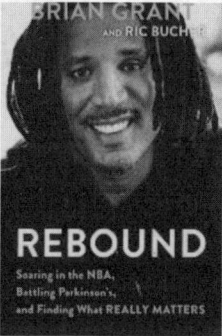

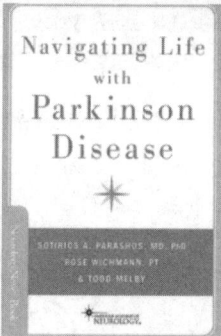

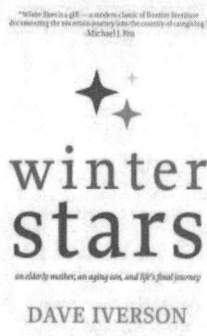

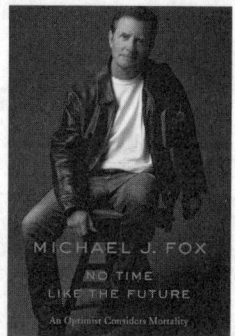

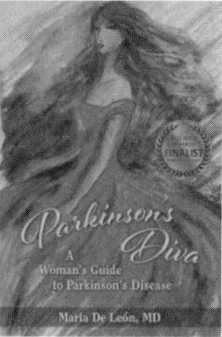

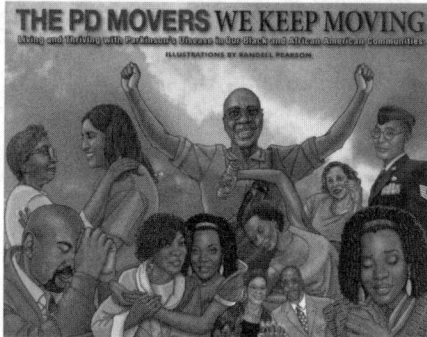

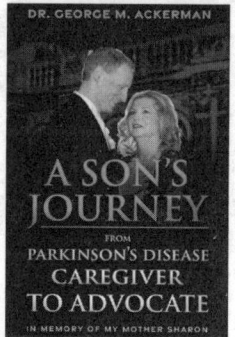

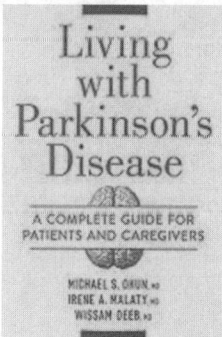

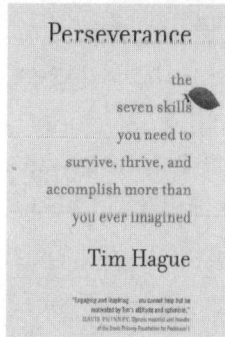

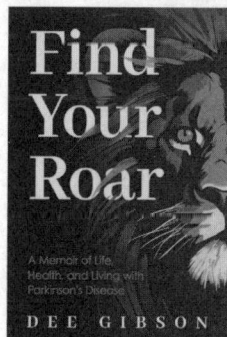

info@PDplan.org

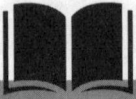

Books

Alberto Espay · Benjamin Stecher

BRAIN
FABLES

THE HIDDEN HISTORY OF
NEURODEGENERATIVE DISEASES
AND A BLUEPRINT TO CONQUER THEM

TRANSLATED INTO 20+ LANGUAGES
The Most Read Parkinson's Disease Treatment Book In The World

PARKINSON'S
TREATMENT

10 Secrets to a Happier Life

ENGLISH EDITION

Michael S. Okun, M.D.

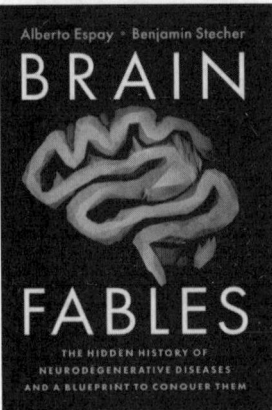

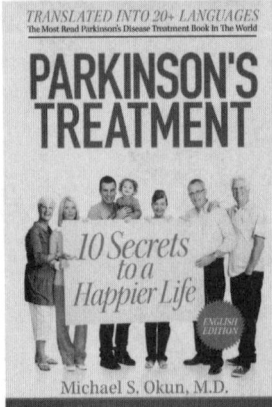

Organizations

American Parkinson's Disease Association
Center for Advanced Research
apdaparkinson.org

ClinicalTrials.gov
clinicaltrials.gov

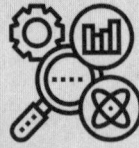

NIH RePORT
report.nih.gov

parkinsons Wellness project
parkinsonswellnessproject.org

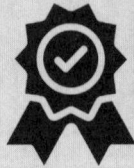

Parkinson's Foundation Global Care Network
parkinson.org/living-with-parkinsons/finding-
care/global-care-network

US Department of Veterans Affairs, Parkinson's
Disease Research, Education and Clinical Centers
parkinsons.va.gov

ORGANIZATIONS

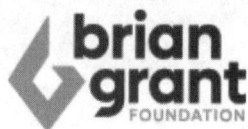

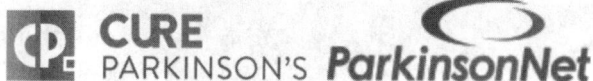

Brian Grant Foundation
briangrant.org

Davis Phinney Foundation
davisphinneyfoundation.org

International Parkinson and
Movement Disorder Society
movementdisorders.org

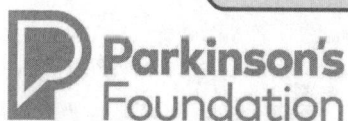

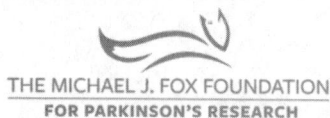

Parkinson's Foundation
parkinson.org

ParkinsonNet
parkinsonnet.com

PD Avengers
pdavengers.com

The Michael J. Fox Foundation
michaeljfox.org

The Cure Parkinson's Trust
cureparkinsons.org.uk

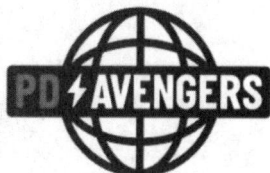

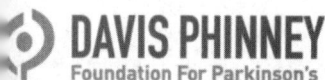

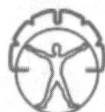

info@PDplan.org

PHONE HELPLINES

American Parkinson's Disease Association

Availability: Monday-Friday 9am to 5pm EST

Services:
- Answers questions about symptoms, medications, and resources
- Refers patients to local APDA chapters, support groups, and movement disorder specialists
- Offers educational materials for patients, caregivers, and healthcare professionals
- Facilitates access to programs like exercise classes and wellness initiatives

1-800-223-2732

Michael J. Fox Foundation Parkinson's Support

Email: ask@michaeljfox.com

Services:
- Provides information on clinical trials and research
- Offers guidance on navigating Parkinson's resources and support options
- Connects patients with local and national Parkinson's resources, including those on emerging therapies and patient advocacy

1-800-708-7644

PDplan.org

PHONE HELPLINES

Parkinson's UK Helpline (for people in the UK)

Languages: English and translation services available for non-English speakers

Availability: Monday–Friday 9am to 6pm (Wednesdays until 7pm), and Saturday 10am to 2pm

Services:
- Provides support and advice for people living with Parkinson's, their caregivers, and families
- Offers information on treatments
- Refers to support groups all across the UK
- Provides legal advice, including employment and benefits

0-808-800-0303

Parkinson's Foundation Helpline

Availability: Monday–Friday 9am to 7pm EST

Languages: English and Spanish

Services:
- Answers questions about symptoms, medications, and treatment options
- Provides referrals to local resources including doctors and support groups
- Offers emotional support and guidance for patients and caregivers
- Helps navigate health insurance and Social Security disability benefits
- Provides information on clinical trials

1-800-473-4636

info@PDplan.org

Veterans Affairs (VA) Parkinson's Disease Helpline (US)

Phone: The VA provides direct support through their Parkinson's Disease Research, Education, and Clinical Centers (PADRECCs). Veterans can access general information by contacting the general health care helpline at 1-877-222-8387.

Services:
- Assistance with Parkinson's care for veterans
- Information on specialized services available at the VA, including clinical trials and treatments

1-800-708-7644

REGIONAL ORGANIZATIONS

Australia

Parkinson's Australia
parkinsons.org.au

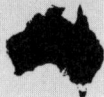

Shake It Up Australia Foundation
shakeitup.org.au

Asia

Parkinson's Disease and
Movement Disorder Society
(India)
parkinsonssocietyindia.com

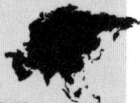

Europe

European Parkinson's Disease
Association
epda.eu.com

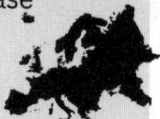

Dutch Parkinson's Disease Association
parkinson-vereniging.nl

Parkinson Federación Española (Spain)
esparkinson.es/

Parkinson's Society Nova Scotia
parkinsonsocietynovascotia.com

Parkinson's UK
parkinson.org.uk

Pan America

American Parkinson Disease
Association
apdaparkinson.org

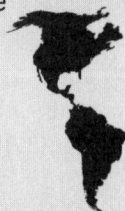

Associação Brasil Parkinson
parkinson.org.br/

Fundación Parkinson de Colombia
parkinsoncolombia.org/

Parkinson Canada
parkinson.ca

Africa

Parkinson's Africa
parkinsonsafrica.org

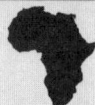

Parkinson's Disease South Africa
parkinsonsza.org/

More

Movement Disorders > For Patients
movementdisorders.org/For-
Patients.htm

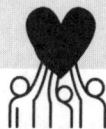

info@PDplan.org

DISCLOSURES

We are both neurologists and researchers who rely on and are thankful for the generous support of funders for our work. In addition, we have worked with companies and organizations that are engaged in Parkinson's disease advocacy, care, education, or research. These relationships undoubtedly influence our perspectives. For transparency, we disclose our relationships since 2022 here.

Ray has served as a consultant to Abbvie, Biohaven, BioSensics, Cerevance, DConsult2, Genentech, HanAll BioPharma, Health & Wellness Partners, HMP Education, Included Health, Karger, Mediflix, MedRhythms, Mitsubishi Tanabe Pharma, Novartis, Sanofi, Seelos Therapeutics, and Vivosense. He has received grant or research support from Averitas Pharma, Biogen, Burroughs Wellcome Fund, Department of Defense, Michael J. Fox Foundation, National Institutes of Health (NIH), PhotoPharmics, Roche, and the Thomas Golisano Foundation. Ray also has ownership interests in Included Health, Mediflix, SemCap, and Synapticure.

Michael serves as the medical advisor at the Parkinson's Foundation and has received research grants from the NIH, Parkinson's Foundation, Michael J. Fox Foundation, Parkinson Alliance, Smallwood Foundation, Tourette Association of America, and University of Florida Foundation. Michael's research is supported by NIH grants (R01NS131342, R01NR014852, R01NS096008, UH3NS119844, U01NS119562, UH3NS095553,

R42NS132614). He is also multiprincipal investigator of the NIH R25NS108939 Training Grant. Michael has received royalties for publications from Hachette Book Group, Demos, Manson, Amazon, Smashwords, Books4Patients, Perseus, Robert Rose, Oxford, Elsevier, and Cambridge. Michael is an associate editor for the *New England Journal of Medicine Journal Watch Neurology* and *JAMA Neurology*. He has participated in educational activities on movement disorders sponsored by WebMD/Medscape, RMEI Medical Education, American Academy of Neurology, Movement Disorders Society, Mediflix, and Vanderbilt University. He has also been a site principal investigator and/or coinvestigator for several NIH-, foundation-, and industry-sponsored trials but has not received honoraria. Research projects at the University of Florida Fixel Institute, where he works, receive device and drug donations.

EXPERTS INTERVIEWED

To help identify new treatment approaches for Parkinson's disease, Michael formally and informally interviewed many of the world's leading experts, whom we thank here:

Charles Adler, MD, PhD, Mayo Clinic, United States
Raag Airan, MD, PhD, Stanford University, United States
Roger Barker, MBBS, PhD, University of Cambridge, United Kingdom
Per Borghammer, MD, PhD, DMSc, Aarhus University, Denmark
Dawn Bowers, PhD, University of Florida, United States
Ed Boyden, PhD, MIT, United States
Claire Clelland, MD, PhD, University of California, San Francisco, United States
William Dauer, MD, University of Texas Southwestern, United States
Ted Dawson, MD, PhD, Johns Hopkins University, United States
Mahlon DeLong, MD, Emory University, United States (deceased)
Alberto Espay, MD, University of Cincinnati, United States
Stewart Factor, DO, Emory University, United States
Kelly Foote, MD, University of Florida, United States
Thomas Gasser, MD, PhD, University of Tübingen, Germany
Aryn Gittis, PhD, Carnegie Mellon University, United States
Mark Hallett, MD, National Institutes of Health, United States
Christopher Hess, MD, University of Florida, United States
Andrew Horne, MBCHB, PhD, University of Edinburgh, United Kingdom
Joseph Jankovic, MD, Baylor College of Medicine, United States

Hyder (Buz) Jinnah, MD, PhD, Emory University, United States

Lorraine Kalia, MD, PhD, University of Toronto, Canada

Christine Klein, MD, University of Lübeck, Germany

Jeffrey Kordower, PhD, Arizona State University, United States

Anthony Lang, MD, University of Toronto, Canada

Matthew Lavoie, PhD, University of Florida, United States

Irene Malaty, MD, University of Florida, United States

Helen Mayberg, MD, Mount Sinai, United States

Svjetlana Miocinovic, MD, PhD, Emory University, United States

Jill Ostrem, MD, University of California, San Francisco, United States

Greg Pontone, MD, University of Florida, United States

Adolfo Ramirez-Zamora, MD, University of Florida, United States

Timothy Sampson, PhD, Emory University, United States

Andrew Siderowf, MD, MSCE, University of Pennsylvania, United States

Ellen Sidransky, MD, National Institutes of Health, United States

Andrew Singleton, PhD, National Institutes of Health, United States

David Vaillancourt, PhD, University of Florida, United States

Jerrold Vitek, MD, PhD, University of Minnesota, United States

Thomas Wichmann, MD, PhD, Emory University, United States

ACKNOWLEDGMENTS

THE PARKINSON'S PLAN IS PART OF A JOURNEY TO HELP PREVENT, treat, and end this terrible disease. That journey has been enabled by many whom we thank here.

We first thank Congressman Gus Bilirakis and Congresswoman Jennifer Wexton for their moving foreword and incredible dedication to addressing the Parkinson's pandemic. They know parkinsonian disorders intimately and have been courageous, tireless, and fearless advocates and an inspiration to us both. The passage of the Dr. Emmanuel Bilirakis and Honorable Jennifer Wexton National Plan to End Parkinson's Act was a watershed moment in the fight against this terrible disease. We are thankful to its lead sponsors, including Congressman Paul Tonko, Senators Shelley Moore Capito and Chris Murphy, and their incredible staffs. We are also appreciative of the work of Ted Thompson, the former senior vice president of public policy at the Michael J. Fox Foundation; John Lehr, CEO of the Parkinson's Foundation; and the many Parkinson's foundations and advocates who helped push for passage of this bill.

Books need stories, and this one is filled with the frequently moving accounts of many amazing individuals. We thank Drs. Jana Reed and Sara Whittingham for allowing us to share the story of Parkinson's through their lived experiences. We are in awe of their service and inspired by their actions. Among the many who contributed their experiences are Peter Spencer, Stein Nilsen, Tim Greenamyre, Steve Phillips, Carey Gillam, Matt Mortellaro, Sarah Teale, George Flint, Brian Grant, Jerry Ensminger, Samuel Goldman, Amy Lindberg, Melody Howarth, Adeline Cassin, Briana De Miranda, Dan Kinel, Patti Burnett, Dave Toth, Catherine Keligan, Harrison Avisto, Mike

Nathanson, Brittany Krzyzanowski, Karl Robb, Per Borghammer, Jacob Horsager, Alastair Noyce, John Duda, Katie Carpenter, Bobbie Lindsay, the "Songbirds," Rick Johnson, Dan McDonald, Sirwan Darweesh, Bastiaan Bloem, Nathan Slewett, Sarah Johnston, Jim Jones, Indu Subramanian, Sol De Jesus, Guo Hu, Jake Taylor, Sally Johnston, Darla King, Diane Waxman, Jennifer Wexton, Allison Willis, Omotola Thomas, the dozens of experts whom we interviewed for this book who are listed on the preceding pages, and many others.

We also want to thank our friends and colleagues who generously reviewed different sections of the manuscript—and in a few cases the entire book. They helped ensure that our stories were true, our science accurate, and our writing clear. They include Jana Reed, Sara Whittingham, Larry Gifford, Soania Mathur, Brian Cook, Matt Mortellaro, Tim Greenamyre, Sarah Teale, Carey Gillam, Steve Phillips, Peter Spencer, Beate Ritz, Brian Grant, Katrina Kahl, Amy Lindberg, Melody Howarth, Jerry Ensminger, Samuel Goldman, Adeline Cassin, Kevin Hylton, Dan Kinel, Patti Burnett, Dave Toth, Briana De Miranda, Mike Nathanson, Stein Nilsen, Catherine Keligan, Harrison Avisto, Brittany Krzyzanowski, Per Borghammer, Ralph Jozefowicz, Katie Carpenter, Bobbie Lindsay, John Duda, Alastair Noyce, Allison Willis, Mark Zupan, Christopher Carlsten, Karen Berger, Norm Yung, Bruce Lanphear, Thomas Dorsey, Zena Shuber, Mike Rajkovic, Donna Rajkovic, Shen-Yang Lim, Lauren Fixel, and Omotola Thomas.

We dedicated this book to the PD Avengers, which formed after our first book, *Ending Parkinson's Disease*. We are inspired by the actions of this global community, led by Larry Gifford, Soania Mathur, and Tim Hague Sr. The end of any pandemic, from polio to HIV, has at its heart individuals who not only bear the burden of the disease but reduce it for others. They refuse to allow future generations to suffer the consequences that they have had to endure.

We thank Dr. Todd Sherer from the Michael J. Fox Foundation and Dr. Bastiaan Bloem from Radboud University, who cowrote *Ending Parkinson's Disease* with us and continue to be our partners in our efforts to end this debilitating and deadly disease. We also want to acknowledge the incredible work of Dr. Caroline Tanner, a neurologist and epidemiologist at the University of California, San Francisco. Her research over the past forty years fills the pages of this book. More than any other, she has detailed the environmental roots of Parkinson's in our food, water, and air. If we follow her work, we will prevent and end Parkinson's.

Authors like us need help, and we received plenty of it. Sarrah Hussain and Kathryn Murphy managed countless drafts, provided invaluable feedback, created compelling visuals, and handled hundreds of references. Reenie Marcello is the world's best and kindest assistant. Monica Piraino from Brand & Butter designed many of the beautiful figures in the book and has been an endless source of creativity. Katie Adams, who has worked as a senior editor for some of New York's top publishing houses, edited the entire book and provided amazing guidance and suggestions to improve it. Don Fehr at the Trident Media Group has provided us with great advice and guidance, including having us return to the wonderful Colleen Lawrie and PublicAffairs. Colleen has had unwavering faith in two academic neurologists. She is kind, patient, and insightful and a great editor. We thank her and the outstanding PublicAffairs team, including Brian Distelberg, Jennifer Kelland, Michelle Welsh-Horst, Jenny Lee, Jessica Breen, Alcimary Pena, Angela Messina, Alex Cullina, and many others, for helping bring *The Parkinson's Plan* to all of you. We also thank the team at Dey., including Rimjhim Dey, Andrew DeSio, and Jessica Zagacki, for helping us reach new audiences for this book in our effort to prevent and treat this disease.

The work that we do is supported by some generous individuals who share our vision for creating a world without Parkinson's. Among these individuals who look at the world differently are Nomi Bergman, Tom Golisano, Joann Stang, the Edmond J. Safra Foundation, John Lehr, John Kozyak, Steve Figueroa, Margaret Friend, Tara Hearns, Melissa Himes, Lisa Warren, Chuck Jacobson, Doug Jackson, Sabra Willis, Rick and Michelle Staab (Tyler's Hope), Anne and John Curtis, Jim and Sharen Green, Sally Muller (Smallwood Foundation), the Fixel Family, Robert Dein, John Gabriel, Karen Wilder Scott (BJ and Eve Wilder Family Foundation), Jack and Ron Belz, Judith Barrett, Jeff Fitzsimmons, Becky and Bob Allen, David

Rembert, Jenny and Eric Scott, John and Patty Noel, Rich Blaser, Griffin Greene, Michelle Streitmater, Will Markel, Bob Anderson, Jeff Smith, John and Susan McCallan, the Bosshardt family, and the Criser family.

Finally, and most importantly, we thank our wonderful wives, Zena and Leslie. They not only help us to do what we do but also put up with our endless discussions on the topic. Their ceaseless encouragement propels us forward, and we hope that we can match their support in their passions to improve the world.

REFERENCES

Graphics were created using Canva.com, BioRender.com, and other tools.

Introduction

1. Smith D. Doctor with Parkinson's finishes grueling 140.6-mile triathlon: "You can be active again." *USA Today*. November 5, 2023. https://www.usatoday.com/story/news/health/2023/11/05/ohio-doctor-parkinsons-ironman/71420547007.

2. Parkinson J. An essay on the shaking palsy. 1817. *Journal of Neuropsychiatry and Clinical Neurosciences*. Spring 2002;14(2):223–236; discussion 222. doi:10.1176/jnp.14.2.223.

3. Goodwin VA, Richards SH, Taylor RS, Taylor AH, Campbell JL. The effectiveness of exercise interventions for people with Parkinson's disease: a systematic review and meta-analysis. *Movement Disorders*. 2008;23(5):631–640. doi:10.1002/mds.21922.

4. O'Brien K, Vasquez I. Michael J. Fox says Parkinson's disease "sucks" but he has "a great life": "I have no regrets." *People*. March 14, 2023. https://people.com/health/michael-j-fox-parkinsons-disease-sucks-but-has-great-life-no-regrets.

5. Braak H, Rüb U, Gai WP, Del Tredici K. Idiopathic Parkinson's disease: possible routes by which vulnerable neuronal types may be subject to neuroinvasion by an unknown pathogen. *Journal of Neural Transmission*. May 2003;110(5):517–536. doi:10.1007/s00702-002-0808-2.

6. Borghammer P, Van Den Berge N. Brain-first versus gut-first Parkinson's disease: a hypothesis. *Journal of Parkinson's Disease*. 2019;9(s2):S281–S295. doi:10.3233/jpd-191721.

7. Bogers JS, Bloem BR, Den Heijer JM. The etiology of Parkinson's disease: new perspectives from gene-environment interactions. *Journal of Parkinson's Disease*. 2023;13(8):1281–1288. doi:10.3233/jpd-230250.

8. Deng H, Wang P, Jankovic J. The genetics of Parkinson disease. *Ageing Research Reviews*. March 1, 2018;42:72–85. doi:10.1016/j.arr.2017.12.007.

9. Sellbach AN, Boyle RS, Silburn PA, Mellick GD. Parkinson's disease and family history. *Parkinsonism & Related Disorders*. October 1, 2006;12(7):399–409. doi:10.1016/j.parkreldis.2006.03.002.

10. Cook L, Verbrugge J, Schwantes-An T-H, et al. Parkinson's disease variant detection and disclosure: PD GENEration, a North American study. *Brain*. August 1, 2024;147(8):2668–2679. doi:10.1093/brain/awae142.

11. Feigin VL, Nichols E, Alam T, et al. Global, regional, and national burden of neurological disorders, 1990–2016: a systematic analysis for the Global Burden of Disease Study 2016. *The Lancet Neurology*. May 1, 2019;18(5):459–480. doi:10.1016/S1474-4422(18)30499-X.

271

12. Steinmetz JD, Seeher KM, Schiess N, et al. Global, regional, and national burden of disorders affecting the nervous system, 1990–2021: a systematic analysis for the Global Burden of Disease Study 2021. *The Lancet Neurology.* 2024;23(4):344–381. doi:10.1016/S1474-4422(24)00038-3.

13. Global, regional, and national burden of neurological disorders during 1990–2015: a systematic analysis for the Global Burden of Disease Study 2015. *The Lancet Neurology.* November 2017;16(11):877–897. doi:10.1016/s1474-4422(17)30299-5.

14. Willis AW, Roberts E, Beck JC, et al. Incidence of Parkinson disease in North America. *npj Parkinson's Disease.* December 15, 2022;8(1):170. doi:10.1038/s41531-022-00410-y.

15. García Ruiz PJ. Prehistoria de la enfermedad de Parkinson [Prehistory of Parkinson's disease]. *Neurologia.* December 2004;19(10):735–737.

16. Ovallath S, Deepa P. The history of parkinsonism: descriptions in ancient Indian medical literature. *Movement Disorders.* May 2013;28(5):566–568. doi:10.1002/mds.25420.

17. Zhang Z-X, Dong Z-H, Román GC. Early descriptions of Parkinson disease in ancient China. *Archives of Neurology.* 2006;63(5):782–784. doi:10.1001/archneur.63.5.782.

18. Ritchie H, Roser M. Air pollution. Our World in Data. October 2017, last revised February 2024. https://ourworldindata.org/air-pollution.

19. Ritchie H, Roser M, Rosado P. Pesticides. Our World in Data. 2022. https://ourworldindata.org/pesticides.

20. Dorsey ER, Elbaz A, Nichols E, et al. Global, regional, and national burden of Parkinson's disease, 1990–2016: a systematic analysis for the Global Burden of Disease Study 2016. *The Lancet Neurology.* 2018;17(11):939–953. doi:10.1016/S1474-4422(18)30295-3.

21. PD Avengers. https://www.pdavengers.com. Accessed August 8, 2024.

22. Schiess N, Cataldi R, Okun MS, et al. Six action steps to address global disparities in Parkinson disease: a World Health Organization priority. *JAMA Neurology.* September 1, 2022;79(9):929–936. doi:10.1001/jamaneurol.2022.1783.

23. EPA proposes ban on all consumer and many commercial uses of perchloroethylene to protect public health. US EPA. June 8, 2023. https://www.epa.gov/newsreleases/epa-proposes-ban-all-consumer-and-many-commercial-uses-of-perchloroethylene-protect.

24. EPA finds trichloroethylene poses an unreasonable risk to human health. US EPA. January 9, 2023. https://www.epa.gov/chemicals-under-tsca/epa-finds-trichloroethylene-poses-unreasonable-risk-human-health.

25. James I. Arizona awaits EPA decision on adding toxic Phoenix site to Superfund list. AZCentral. May 14, 2020. https://www.azcentral.com/story/news/local/arizona-environment/2020/05/14/cleanup-phoenix-toxic-water-epa-superfund-west-van-buren/3080970001.

26. Dorsey ER, Constantinescu R, Thompson JP, et al. Projected number of people with Parkinson disease in the most populous nations, 2005 through 2030. *Neurology.* January 30, 2007;68(5):384–386. doi:10.1212/01.wnl.0000247740.47667.03.

27. USAFA Association of Graduates. Harnessing swarms. *Checkpoints* 2023;52(3). https://issuu.com/usafaaog/docs/checkpoints_december_2023-finalonline.

28. Mench C. An Air Force veteran and doctor with Parkinson's disease shares her journey running an Ironman triathlon. *Men's Journal.* October 16, 2023. https://www.mensjournal.com/news/air-force-veteran-parkinsons-disease-ironman-triathlon.

Chapter 1: Pesticides in Our Food, Farms, and Fields

1. Monmaney T. This obscure malady. *New Yorker.* October 21, 1990.

2. Reid LA. Origin of Guam's Indigenous people. https://www.guampedia.com/origin-of-guams-indigenous-people. Accessed September 17, 2024.

3. Hirano A, Kurland LT, Krooth RS, Lessell S. Parkinsonism-dementia complex, an endemic disease on the island of Guam: I. clinical features. *Brain*. 1961;84(4):642–661. doi:10.1093/brain/84.4.642.

4. Morris HR, Steele JC, Crook R, et al. Genome-wide analysis of the parkinsonism-dementia complex of Guam. *Archives of Neurology*. 2004;61(12):1889–1897. doi:10.1001/archneur.61.12.1889.

5. Spencer PS. Cycad toxins driving the ALS-parkinsonism-dementia complex. Virtual World Congress on Controversies in Neurology. *Video Journal of Neurology*. October 19, 2020.

6. Cox PA, Sacks OW. Cycad neurotoxins, consumption of flying foxes, and ALS-PDC disease in Guam. *Neurology*. 2002;58(6):956–959. doi:10.1212/WNL.58.6.956.

7. Chamorro people. Wikipedia. https://en.wikipedia.org/wiki/Chamorro_people. Accessed August 5, 2024.

8. The Chamorro: caught in the middle. National Park Service. https://npshistory.com/publications/wapa/npswapa/extContent/wapa/guides/outbreak/sec5.htm. Accessed August 5, 2024.

9. Iwamoto N. Caught between the sun and stars: the Chamorro experience during the Second World War. *Hohonu*. 2020;18:11–18. https://hilo.hawaii.edu/campuscenter/hohonu/volumes/documents/CaughtBetweentheSunandStarsTheChamorroExperienceDuringtheSecondWorldWar.pdf.

10. Taitano GE. CHamorus: a people divided. Guampedia. https://www.guampedia.com/chamorros-a-people-divided.

11. Spencer PS, Nunn PB, Hugon J, et al. Guam amyotrophic lateral sclerosis–parkinsonism–dementia linked to a plant excitant neurotoxin. *Science*. 1987;237(4814):517–522. doi:10.1126/science.3603037.

12. Cox PA, Banack SA, Murch SJ. Biomagnification of cyanobacterial neurotoxins and neurodegenerative disease among the Chamorro people of Guam. *Proceedings of the National Academy of Sciences of the United States of America*. November 11, 2003;100(23):13380–13383. doi:10.1073/pnas.2235808100.

13. Arnst C. Guam's flying fox bat: a deadly delicacy? *BusinessWeek*. December 1, 2003. https://www.bloomberg.com/news/articles/2003-12-01/guams-flying-fox-bat-a-deadly-delicacy.

14. Carrera JB. Neurologist: neurodegenerative disease may end on Guam. *Guam Daily Post*. February 12, 2012. https://www.postguam.com/news/local/neurologist-neurodegenerative-disease-may-end-on-guam/article_ec3cca5b-a500-5c0f-8d24-db65272e1b3c.html.

15. Spencer PS, Palmer VS, Kisby GE. Seeking environmental causes of neurodegenerative disease and envisioning primary prevention. *NeuroToxicology*. September 1, 2016;56:269–283. doi:10.1016/j.neuro.2016.03.017.

16. Goldwyn, E. The poison that waits. Goldwyn Associates. Vimeo. August 28, 2008. https://shorturl.at/Yg5NG.

17. Smith RJ. Hawaiian milk contamination creates alarm. *Science*. 1982;217(4555):137–140. doi:10.1126/science.7089547.

18. Hong S, Hwang J, Kim JY, Shin KS, Kang SJ. Heptachlor induced nigral dopaminergic neuronal loss and parkinsonism-like movement deficits in mice. *Experimental & Molecular Medicine*. February 28, 2014;46(2):e80. doi:10.1038/emm.2014.12.

19. Park M, Ross GW, Petrovitch H, et al. Consumption of milk and calcium in midlife and the future risk of Parkinson disease. *Neurology*. 2005;64(6):1047–1051. doi:10.1212/01.WNL.0000154532.98495.BF.

20. Abbott RD, Ross GW, Petrovitch H, et al. Midlife milk consumption and substantia nigra neuron density at death. *Neurology.* February 9, 2016;86(6):512–519. doi:10.1212/wnl.0000000000002254.

21. Contaminated milk problem in Hawaii nears end. *New York Times.* May 23, 1982. https://www.nytimes.com/1982/05/23/us/contaminated-milk-problem-in-hawaii-nears-end.html.

22. Wong MH, Leung AOW, Chan JKY, Choi MPK. A review on the usage of POP pesticides in China, with emphasis on DDT loadings in human milk. *Chemosphere.* August 1, 2005;60(6):740–752. doi:10.1016/j.chemosphere.2005.04.028.

23. Tanner CM, Ottman R, Goldman SM, et al. Parkinson disease in twins: an etiologic study. *JAMA.* 1999;281(4):341–346. doi:10-1001/pubs.JAMA-ISSN-0098-7484-281-4-joc81035.

24. Bond C, Buhl K, Stone D. Pyrethrins general fact sheet. National Pesticide Information Center, Oregon State University Extension Services. November 2014. http://npic.orst.edu/factsheets/pyrethrins.html.

25. Public health statement for pyrethrins and pyrethroids. Agency for Toxic Substances and Disease Registry (ATSDR). 2014. https://wwwn.cdc.gov/TSP/PHS/PHS.aspx?phsid=785&toxid=153.

26. Costa LG. Chapter 9—The neurotoxicity of organochlorine and pyrethroid pesticides. In: Lotti M, Bleecker ML, eds. *Handbook of Clinical Neurology.* Elsevier; 2015:135–148.

27. Ascherio A, Chen H, Weisskopf MG, et al. Pesticide exposure and risk for Parkinson's disease. *Annals of Neurology.* 2006;60(2):197–203. doi:10.1002/ana.20904.

28. Tanner CM, Kamel F, Ross GW, et al. Rotenone, paraquat, and Parkinson's disease. *Environmental Health Perspectives.* 2011;119(6):866–872. doi:10.1289/ehp.1002839.

29. Van Maele-Fabry G, Hoet P, Vilain F, Lison D. Occupational exposure to pesticides and Parkinson's disease: a systematic review and meta-analysis of cohort studies. *Environment International.* October 1, 2012;46:30–43. doi:10.1016/j.envint.2012.05.004.

30. Polaka S, Raji S, Singh A, Katare P, Tekade RK. Chapter 26—Connecting link between pesticides and Parkinson's disease. In: Tekade RK, ed. *Public Health and Toxicology Issues in Drug Research.* Academic Press; 2024:735–754.

31. Cabras P, Caboni P, Cabras M, Angioni A, Russo M. Rotenone residues on olives and in olive oil. *Journal of Agricultural and Food Chemistry.* 2002;50(9):2576–2580.

32. Gupta RC, Miller Mukherjee IR, Malik JK, Doss RB, Dettbarn W-D, Milatovic D. Chapter 26—Insecticides. In: Gupta RC, ed. *Biomarkers in Toxicology (Second Edition).* Academic Press; 2019:455–475.

33. Padamsey Z, Rochefort NL. Paying the brain's energy bill. *Current Opinion in Neurobiology.* February 1, 2023;78:102668. doi:10.1016/j.conb.2022.102668.

34. Watts ME, Pocock R, Claudianos C. Brain energy and oxygen metabolism: emerging role in normal function and disease. *Frontiers in Molecular Neuroscience.* 2018;11:216. doi:10.3389/fnmol.2018.00216.

35. Mamelak M. Parkinson's disease, the dopaminergic neuron and gammahydroxybutyrate. *Neurology and Therapy.* June 2018;7(1):5–11. doi:10.1007/s40120-018-0091-2.

36. Bolam JP, Pissadaki EK. Living on the edge with too many mouths to feed: why dopamine neurons die. *Movement Disorders.* October 2012;27(12):1478–1483. doi:10.1002/mds.25135.

37. Haddad D, Nakamura K. Understanding the susceptibility of dopamine neurons to mitochondrial stressors in Parkinson's disease. *FEBS Letters.* December 21, 2015;589(24 Pt A):3702–3713. doi:10.1016/j.febslet.2015.10.021.

38. Betarbet R, Sherer TB, MacKenzie G, Garcia-Osuna M, Panov AV, Greenamyre JT. Chronic systemic pesticide exposure reproduces features of Parkinson's disease. *Nature Neuroscience.* December 1, 2000;3(12):1301–1306. doi:10.1038/81834.

39. Wadman M. Twist of fate. *Science.* May 4, 2023. https://www.science.org/content/article /twist-fate-what-happens-when-top-parkinson-s-researcher-gets-disease.

40. Landrigan PJ, Powell KE, James LM, Taylor PR. Paraquat and marijuana: epidemiologic risk assessment. *American Journal of Public Health.* 1983;73(7):784–788.

41. Goodman E. Marijuana outrage. *Washington Post.* April 22, 1978. https://www .washingtonpost.com/archive/politics/1978/04/22/marijuana-outrage/5f62df59-4990-4351-99ef -c9e20de3679a.

42. Kornbluth J. Poisonous fallout from the war on marijuana. *New York Times.* November 19, 1978. https://www.nytimes.com/1978/11/19/archives/poisonous-fallout-from-the-war -on-marijuana-paraquat.html.

43. London J. Paraquat pot: the true story of how the US government tried to kill weed smokers with a toxic chemical in the 1980s. *Thought.is.* 2010. https://thought.is/paraquat-pot.

44. Project NWQ-A. Estimated annual agricultural pesticide use. https://water.usgs.gov /nawqa/pnsp/usage/maps/show_map.php?year=2018&map=PARAQUAT&hilo=L. Accessed September 1, 2024.

45. Gillam C, Uteuova A. Secret files suggest chemical giant feared weedkiller's link to Parkinson's disease. *The Guardian.* October 20, 2022. https://www.theguardian.com/us-news /2022/oct/20/syngenta-weedkiller-pesticide-parkinsons-disease-paraquat-documents.

46. Chen F, Ye Y, Jin B, Yi B, Wei Q, Liao L. Homicidal paraquat poisoning. *Journal of Forensic Sciences.* May 2019;64(3):941–945. doi:10.1111/1556-4029.13945.

47. Wells G, Horwitz J, Seetharaman D. Facebook knows Instagram is toxic for teen girls, company documents show. *Wall Street Journal.* September 14, 2021. https://www.wsj.com /articles/facebook-knows-instagram-is-toxic-for-teen-girls-company-documents-show-1163 1620739.

48. Myung W, Lee GH, Won HH, et al. Paraquat prohibition and change in the suicide rate and methods in South Korea. *PLOS One.* 2015;10(6):e0128980. doi:10.1371/journal .pone.0128980.

49. Costello S, Cockburn M, Bronstein J, Zhang X, Ritz B. Parkinson's disease and residential exposure to maneb and paraquat from agricultural applications in the central valley of California. *American Journal of Epidemiology.* April 15, 2009;169(8):919–926. doi:10.1093/aje /kwp006.

50. Brooks AI, Chadwick CA, Gelbard HA, Cory-Slechta DA, Federoff HJ. Paraquat elicited neurobehavioral syndrome caused by dopaminergic neuron loss. *Brain Research.* March 27, 1999;823(1):1–10. doi:10.1016/S0006-8993(98)01192-5.

51. Castello PR, Drechsel DA, Patel M. Mitochondria are a major source of paraquat-induced reactive oxygen species production in the brain. *Journal of Biological Chemistry.* 2007;282(19):14186–14193. doi:10.1074/jbc.M700827200.

52. Dinis-Oliveira RJ, Remião F, Carmo H, et al. Paraquat exposure as an etiological factor of Parkinson's disease. *NeuroToxicology.* December 1, 2006;27(6):1110–1122. doi:10.1016 /j.neuro.2006.05.012.

53. Arsac JN, Sedru M, Dartiguelongue M, et al. Chronic exposure to paraquat induces alpha-synuclein pathogenic modifications in *drosophila.* *International Journal of Molecular Sciences.* October 27, 2021;22(21): 11613. doi:10.3390/ijms222111613.

54. Cicchetti F, Lapointe N, Roberge-Tremblay A, et al. Systemic exposure to paraquat and maneb models early Parkinson's disease in young adult rats. *Neurobiology of Disease.* November 1, 2005;20(2):360–371. doi:10.1016/j.nbd.2005.03.018.

55. Dwyer Z, Rudyk C, Farmer K, et al. Characterizing the protracted neurobiological and neuroanatomical effects of paraquat in a murine model of Parkinson's disease. *Neurobiology of Aging.* April 1, 2021;100:11–21. doi:10.1016/j.neurobiolaging.2020.11.013.

56. Tangamornsuksan W, Lohitnavy O, Sruamsiri R, et al. Paraquat exposure and Parkinson's disease: A systematic review and meta-analysis. *Archives of Environmental & Occupational Health.* September 3, 2019;74(5):225–238. doi:10.1080/19338244.2018.1492894.

57. Kumar A, Leinisch F, Kadiiska MB, Corbett J, Mason RP. Formation and implications of alpha-synuclein radical in maneb- and paraquat-induced models of Parkinson's disease. *Molecular Neurobiology.* July 1, 2016;53(5):2983–2994. doi:10.1007/s12035-015-9179-1.

58. Dorsey ER, Ray A. Paraquat, Parkinson's disease, and agnotology. *Movement Disorders.* June 1, 2023;38(6):949–952. doi:10.1002/mds.29371.

59. Barbeau A, Roy M, Bernier G, Campanella G, Paris S. Ecogenetics of Parkinson's disease: prevalence and environmental aspects in rural areas. *Canadian Journal of Neurological Sciences / Journal canadien des sciences neurologiques.* 1987;14(1):36–41. doi:10.1017/S0317167100026147.

60. Michaels D. *Doubt Is Their Product: How Industry's Assault on Science Threatens Your Health.* Oxford University Press; 2008.

61. Markowitz G, Rosner D. *Deceit and Denial: The Deadly Politics of Industrial Pollution.* University of California Press; 2013.

62. Haffajee RL, Mello MM. Drug companies' liability for the opioid epidemic. *New England Journal of Medicine.* December 14, 2017;377(24):2301–2305. doi:10.1056/NEJMp1710756.

63. Schiebinger LP, Robert N. *Agnotology: The Making and Unmaking of Ignorance.* Stanford University Press; 2008.

64. Paraquat. Syngenta Global. https://www.syngenta.com/en/paraquat-in-the-media#parkinsons-disease. Accessed September 1, 2024.

65. Proctor RN. The history of the discovery of the cigarette–lung cancer link: evidentiary traditions, corporate denial, global toll. *Tobacco Control.* 2012;21(2):87–91.

66. Doll R, Hill AB. The mortality of doctors in relation to their smoking habits: a preliminary report. 1954. *BMJ.* June 26, 2004;328(7455):1529–1533; discussion 1533. doi:10.1136/bmj.328.7455.1529.

67. Hill AB. The environment and disease: association or causation? *Proceedings of the Royal Society of Medicine.* May 1, 1965;58(5):295–300. doi:10.1177/003591576505800503.

68. Bates C, Rowell A. Tobacco explained . . . the truth about the tobacco industry . . . in its own words. Paper WHO$_4$. Tobacco Control: Reports on Industry Activity. eScholarship. 1999. https://escholarship.org/content/qt9fp6566b/qt9fp6566b_noSplash_cf5479bcb22b38bca6c5db7a3ffb9dfe.pdf.

69. Lawsuit challenges EPA approval of deadly pesticide for 15 more years. Center for Biological Diversity. September 24, 2021. https://biologicaldiversity.org/w/news/press-releases/lawsuit-challenges-epa-approval-of-deadly-pesticide-for-15-more-years-2021-09-24.

70. Desk N. Lab tests on French wines find pesticide residue in every bottle. Food Safety News. September 30, 2013. https://www.foodsafetynews.com/2013/09/lab-tests-on-french-wines-find-pesticide-residue-in-every-bottle.

71. Ruitenberg R. French wine test finds pesticides in each of 92 bottles analyzed. Bloomberg. September 25, 2013. https://www.bloomberg.com/news/articles/2013-09-25/french-wine-test-finds-pesticides-in-each-of-92-bottles-analyzed.

72. Mustacich S. Study raises concerns over pesticide residues in French wines. *Wine Spectator.* September 26, 2013. https://www.winespectator.com/articles/study-raises-concerns-over-pesticide-residues-in-french-wines-48962.

73. Anson J. French study finds pesticide residues in 90% of wines. Decanter. February 19, 2013. https://www.decanter.com/wine-news/french-study-finds-pesticide-residues-in-90-of-wines-21199.

74. Pesticides in French wine. *New York Times.* January 3, 2014. https://www.nytimes.com/2014/01/03/opinion/pesticides-in-french-wine.html.

75. Organic farmer faces jail time for refusing to spray pesticide. Beyond Pesticides. February 26, 2014. https://beyondpesticides.org/dailynewsblog/2014/02/organic-farmer-faces-jail-time-for-refusing-to-spray-pesticide.

76. Baltazar MT, Dinis-Oliveira RJ, de Lourdes Bastos M, Tsatsakis AM, Duarte JA, Carvalho F. Pesticides exposure as etiological factors of Parkinson's disease and other neurodegenerative diseases—a mechanistic approach. *Toxicology Letters.* October 15, 2014;230(2):85–103. doi:10.1016/j.toxlet.2014.01.039.

77. Bao W, Liu B, Simonsen DW, Lehmler H-J. Association between exposure to pyrethroid insecticides and risk of all-cause and cause-specific mortality in the general US adult population. *JAMA Internal Medicine.* 2020;180(3):367–374. doi:10.1001/jamainternmed.2019.6019.

78. Hansen MRH, Jørs E, Lander F, et al. Neurological deficits after long-term pyrethroid exposure. *Environmental Health Insights.* 2017;11:1178630217700628. doi:10.1177/1178630217700628.

79. Sciolino E. In France, pesticides get in way of natural wines. *New York Times.* March 2, 2015. https://www.nytimes.com/2015/03/04/dining/in-france-pesticides-get-in-way-of-natural-wines.html.

80. Kab S, Spinosi J, Chaperon L, et al. Agricultural activities and the incidence of Parkinson's disease in the general French population. *European Journal of Epidemiology.* March 1, 2017;32(3):203–216. doi:10.1007/s10654-017-0229-z.

81. Baldi I, Cantagrel A, Lebailly P, et al. Association between Parkinson's disease and exposure to pesticides in southwestern France. *Neuroepidemiology.* 2003;22(5):305–310. doi:10.1159/000071194.

82. Yitshak Sade M, Zlotnik Y, Kloog I, Novack V, Peretz C, Ifergane G. Parkinson's disease prevalence and proximity to agricultural cultivated fields. *Parkinson's Disease.* 2015;2015:576564. doi:10.1155/2015/576564.

83. Pesticides. National Onion Association. https://www.onions-usa.org/onion-advocacy/pesticides. Accessed June 6, 2024.

84. Chlorpyrifos general fact sheet. National Pesticide Information Center. 2009. https://npic.orst.edu/factsheets/chlorpgen.html.

85. Rauh VA. Polluting developing brains—EPA failure on chlorpyrifos. *New England Journal of Medicine.* 2018;378(13):1171–1174. doi:10.1056/NEJMp1716809.

86. Deveci HA, Karapehlivan M. Chlorpyrifos-induced parkinsonian model in mice: behavior, histopathology and biochemistry. *Pesticide Biochemistry and Physiology.* January 1, 2018;144:36–41. doi:10.1016/j.pestbp.2017.11.002.

87. Freire C, Koifman S. Pesticide exposure and Parkinson's disease: epidemiological evidence of association. *NeuroToxicology.* October 1, 2012;33(5):947–971. doi:10.1016/j.neuro.2012.05.011.

88. Gorell JM, Johnson CC, Rybicki BA, Peterson EL, Richardson RJ. The risk of Parkinson's disease with exposure to pesticides, farming, well water, and rural living. *Neurology.* May 1998;50(5):1346–1350. doi:10.1212/wnl.50.5.1346.

89. Dhananjayan V, Ravichandran B. Occupational health risk of farmers exposed to pesticides in agricultural activities. *Current Opinion in Environmental Science & Health.* August 1, 2018;4:31–37. doi:10.1016/j.coesh.2018.07.005.

90. Spencer J. Kale, watermelon and even some organic foods pose high pesticide risk, analysis finds. *The Guardian.* April 18, 2024. https://www.theguardian.com/environment/2024/apr/18/fruits-vegetables-pesticide-consumer-reports.

91. Lardieri A. Cancer-causing ingredient in weedkiller found in Cheerios. *US News.* June 12, 2019. https://www.usnews.com/news/health-news/articles/2019-06-12/cancer-causing-ingredient-in-roundup-weedkiller-found-in-cheerios-nature-valley-products.

92. Picchi A. Cheerios, Nature Valley cereals contain Roundup ingredient, study finds. *CBS News*. June 13, 2019. https://www.cbsnews.com/news/glyphosate-breakfast-cereal-still -contains-roundup-ingredient-study-finds.

93. Gibson K. Pesticide linked to reproductive issues found in Cheerios, Quaker Oats and other oat-based foods. *CBS News*. February 20, 2024. https://www.cbsnews.com/news /cheerios-quaker-oats-infertility-chemicals-in-cereal-ewg.

94. Temkin AM, Evans S, Spyropoulos DD, Naidenko OV. A pilot study of chlormequat in food and urine from adults in the United States from 2017 to 2023. *Journal of Exposure Science & Environmental Epidemiology*. March 1, 2024;34(2):317–321. doi:10.1038/s41370-024 -00643-4.

95. Carson R. *Silent Spring* [1962]. Houghton Mifflin; 2009.

96. McKeith I, Mintzer J, Aarsland D, et al. Dementia with Lewy bodies. *The Lancet Neurology*. January 2004;3(1):19–28. doi:10.1016/s1474-4422(03)00619-7.

97. What is Lewy body dementia? Causes, symptoms, and treatments. National Institute on Aging. https://www.nia.nih.gov/health/lewy-body-dementia/what-lewy-body-dementia -causes-symptoms-and-treatments. Accessed June 6, 2024.

98. Lawson T. From the archives: Robin Williams talks growing up in Bloomfield Hills. *Entertainment*. August 13, 2014. https://www.hometownlife.com/story/entertainment/2014 /08/13/from-the-archives-robin-williams-talks-growing-up-in-bloomfield-hills/13990981.

99. Society BH. Stonycroft (Theodore F. MacManus) 1920–1960. https://www.bloomfield historicalsociety.org/53-stoneycroft-1920-1960. Accessed June 6, 2024.

100. Kosaka K, Oyanagi S, Matsushita M, Hori A, Iwase S. Presenile dementia with Alzheimer-, Pick- and Lewy-body changes. *Acta Neuropathologica*. September 1, 1976;36(3):221–233. doi:10.1007/BF00685366.

101. Kosaka K, Yoshimura M, Ikeda K, Budka H. Diffuse type of Lewy body disease: progressive dementia with abundant cortical Lewy bodies and senile changes of varying degree—a new disease? *Clinical Neuropathology*. September–October 1984;3(5):185–192.

102. Katayama N, Baba YG, Kusumoto Y, Tanaka K. A review of post-war changes in rice farming and biodiversity in Japan. *Agricultural Systems*. January 1, 2015;132:73–84. doi:10.1016/j. agsy.2014.09.001.

103. Watanabe H, Inao K, Vu SH, et al. Chapter 8—Pesticide exposure assessment in rice paddy areas: a Japanese perspective. In: Capri E, Karpouzas D, eds. *Pesticide Risk Assessment in Rice Paddies*. Elsevier; 2008:167–214.

104. Parada H, Jr., Wolff MS, Engel LS, et al. Organochlorine insecticides DDT and chlordane in relation to survival following breast cancer. *International Journal of Cancer*. February 1, 2016;138(3):565–575. doi:10.1002/ijc.29806.

105. Loganathan BG, Tanabe S, Hidaka Y, Kawano M, Hidaka H, Tatsukawa R. Temporal trends of persistent organochlorine residues in human adipose tissue from Japan, 1928–1985. *Environmental Pollution*. January 1, 1993;81(1):31–39. doi:10.1016/0269-7491(93)90025-J.

106. Toteja GS, Mukherjee A, Diwakar S, Singh P, Saxena BN. Residues of DDT and HCH pesticides in rice samples from different geographical regions of India: a multicentre study. *Food Additives & Contaminants*. October 2003;20(10):933–939. doi:10.1080/02652030310001 600939.

107. Eskenazi B, Chevrier J, Rosas LG, et al. The Pine River statement: human health consequences of DDT use. *Environmental Health Perspectives*. September 2009;117(9):1359–1367. doi:10.1289/ehp.11748.

108. Hatcher JM, Delea KC, Richardson JR, Pennell KD, Miller GW. Disruption of dopamine transport by DDT and its metabolites. *NeuroToxicology*. July 2008;29(4):682–690. doi:10.1016/j.neuro.2008.04.010.

109. Dardiotis E, Aloizou AM, Sakalakis E, et al. Organochlorine pesticide levels in Greek patients with Parkinson's disease. *Toxicology Reports.* 2020;7:596–601. doi:10.1016/j.toxrep.2020.03.011.

110. Kumar A, Calne SM, Schulzer M, et al. Clustering of Parkinson disease: shared cause or coincidence? *Archives of Neurology.* 2004;61(7):1057–1060. doi:10.1001/archneur.61.7.1057.

Chapter 2: Toxic Water

1. Grant B, Bucher, R. *Rebound: Soaring in the NBA, Battling Parkinson's, and Finding What Really Matters.* Triumph Books; 2022.

2. Summary of the water contamination situation at Camp Lejeune. Agency for Toxic Substances and Disease Registry (ATSDR). 2017. https://www.atsdr.cdc.gov/sites/lejeune/water modeling_summary.html.

3. Testimony of Richard Clapp, DSc, MPH, Committee on Science and Technology, Sub-committee on Investigations and Oversight. House Science, Space, and Technology Committee. September 16, 2012. https://republicans-science.house.gov/_cache /files/b/b/bbb9e53f-5d99-43e6-8376-07e3c2c92fb5/D8C64807420098F83F1234D BE1B35CE4.091610-clapp.pdf.

4. Dorsey ER, Bloem BR. Parkinson's disease is predominantly an environmental disease. *Journal of Parkinson's Disease.* 2024;14(3):451–465. doi:10.3233/JPD-230357.

5. Ceballos DM, Fellows KM, Evans AE, Janulewicz PA, Lee EG, Whittaker SG. Perchloroethylene and dry cleaning: it's time to move the industry to safer alternatives. *Frontiers in Public Health.* 2021;9:638082. doi:10.3389/fpubh.2021.638082.

6. IARC Working Group on the Evaluation of Carcinogenic Risks to Humans. *Trichloroethylene, Tetrachloroethylene, and Some Other Chlorinated Agents.* IARC Monographs on the Evaluation of Carcinogenic Risks to Humans 106. International Agency for Research on Cancer; 2014.

7. Dorsey ER, Zafar M, Lettenberger SE, et al. Trichloroethylene: an invisible cause of Parkinson's disease? *Journal of Parkinson's Disease.* 2023;13(2):203–218. doi:10.3233/JPD-225047.

8. Harr J. *A Civil Action.* Vintage; 2011.

9. Fagin D. *Toms River: A Story of Science and Salvation.* Bantam; 2013.

10. Cutler JJ, Parker GS, Rosen S, Prenney B, Healey R, Caldwell GG. Childhood leukemia in Woburn, Massachusetts. *Public Health Reports.* March–April 1986;101(2):201–205.

11. Schecter A, McFadden C, Chan M. Their babies died when Camp Lejeune's water was poisoned. But justice has been hard to find. September 18, 2023. *NBC News.* https://www.nbcnews .com/news/us-news/camp-lejeune-lawsuits-victims-miscarriage-difficult-fight-rcna97801.

12. Camp Lejeune: contamination and compensation, looking back, moving forward. Committee on Science and Technology, House of Representatives. November 2, 2010. https:// democrats-science.house.gov/hearings/camp-lejeune-contamination-and-compensation -looking-back-moving-forward.

13. Trichloroethylene (TCE). National Cancer Institute. https://www.cancer.gov /about-cancer/causes-prevention/risk/substances/trichloroethylene. Accessed August 6, 2024.

14. Trichloroethylene. National Toxicology Program. National Institute of Environmental Health Sciences. https://ntp.niehs.nih.gov/sites/default/files/ntp/roc/content/profiles/trichloro ethylene.pdf. Accessed September 1, 2024.

15. Tetrachloroethylene (perchloroethylene). EPA. April 1992. https://www.epa.gov/sites /default/files/2016-09/documents/tetrachloroethylene.pdf.

16. Clark J. Exclusive: the investigation into water contamination at Camp Lejeune may reopen soon. *Task & Purpose.* May 12, 2017. https://taskandpurpose.com/news/camp-lejeune -water-contamination-investigation-cdc.

17. Goldman SM, Quinlan PJ, Ross GW, et al. Solvent exposures and Parkinson disease risk in twins. *Annals of Neurology.* June 2012;71(6):776–784. doi:10.1002/ana.22629.

18. About the Brian Grant Foundation. Brian Grant Foundation. https://briangrant.org /about. Accessed September 1, 2024.

19. Correa D. NBA Star Brian Grant living on time with Parkinson's. *Brain & Life.* June 23, 2022. https://www.brainandlife.org/podcast/nba-star-brian-grant-living-with -parkinsons-disease.

20. Welcome to Naval Medical Center Camp Lejeune. Lejeune NMCCL. https://camp-lejeune .tricare.mil/About-Us. Accessed September 1, 2024.

21. Goldman SM, Weaver FM, Stroupe KT, et al. Risk of Parkinson disease among service members at Marine Corps Base Camp Lejeune. *JAMA Neurology.* 2023;80(7):673–681. doi:10.1001/jamaneurol.2023.1168.

22. Barringer F. E.P.A. charts risks of a ubiquitous chemical. *New York Times.* September 30, 2011. https://archive.nytimes.com/green.blogs.nytimes.com/2011/09/30/e-p-a-quantifies -trichloroethylene-risks.

23. Amarelo M. Notorious cancer-causing solvent TCE taints tap water for 14 million Americans. EWG. July 24, 2018. https://www.ewg.org/news-insights/news-release/notorious-cancer -causing-solvent-tce-taints-tap-water-14-million.

24. Superfund site: Love Canal, Niagara Falls, NY, cleanup activities. EPA. https://cumulis .epa.gov/supercpad/SiteProfiles/index.cfm?fuseaction=second.cleanup&id=0201290. Accessed September 1, 2024.

25. Ephron J. *Poisoned Ground: The Tragedy at Love Canal.* American Experience; 2024.

26. Love Canal—public health time bomb. New York State Department of Health. September 1978. https://www.health.ny.gov/environmental/investigations/love_canal/lctimbmb.htm.

27. What is Superfund? EPA. https://www.epa.gov/superfund/what-superfund. Accessed September 1, 2024.

28. Alves B. Number of hazardous waste sites in the United States as of June 2024, by state. Statista. September 9, 2024. https://www.statista.com/statistics/1147665/number-of -hazardous-waste-sites-in-the-united-states.

29. Population surrounding 1,857 Superfund remedial sites. EPA. Updated September 2020. https://www.epa.gov/sites/default/files/2015-09/documents/webpopulationrsuperfund sites9.28.15.pdf.

30. Superfund site: Shenandoah Road Groundwater Contamination, East Fishkill, NY, announcements and key topics. EPA. https://cumulis.epa.gov/supercpad/cursites/csitinfo .cfm?id=0204269. Accesed September 1, 2024.

31. Water Resources Mission Area. Domestic (private) supply wells. US Geological Survey. March 1, 2019. https://www.usgs.gov/mission-areas/water-resources/science /domestic-private-supply-wells.

32. Rajput A, Uitti RJ, Stern W, Laverty W. Early onset Parkinson's disease in Saskatchewan— environmental considerations for etiology. *Canadian Journal of Neurological Sciences.* 1986;13(4):312–316.

33. Gatto NM, Cockburn M, Bronstein J, Manthripragada AD, Ritz B. Well-water consumption and Parkinson's disease in rural California. *Environmental Health Perspectives.* 2009;117(12):1912–1918.

34. Jiménez-Jiménez FJ, Mateo D, Giménez-Roldán S. Exposure to well water and pesticides in Parkinson's disease: a case-control study in the Madrid area. *Movement Disorders.* 1992;7(2):149–152. doi:10.1002/mds.870070209.

35. Overview of the Safe Drinking Water Act. EPA. Updated January 23, 2025. https://www .epa.gov/sdwa/overview-safe-drinking-water-act.

36. Dorsey R, Sherer T, Okun MS, Bloem BR. *Ending Parkinson's Disease: A Prescription for Action*. Hachette UK; 2020.

37. Superfund site: Hopewell Precision, Hopewell Junction, cleanup activities. EPA. Updated August 9, 2024. https://cumulis.epa.gov/supercpad/SiteProfiles/index.cfm?fuseaction=second .cleanup&id=0201588.

38. Wickes Manufacturing TCE Plume. Michigan Department of Environment, Great Lakes, and Energy. January 2020. https://www.michigan.gov/egle/about/organization /remediation-and-redevelopment/wickes-manufacturing-tce-plume-2.

39. Axelson B. 20 most toxic places in upstate New York on the EPA's hazard list. NYup .com January 12, 2017. https://www.newyorkupstate.com/news/2017/01/most_toxic_places_in _upstate_new_york_superfund_priorities.html.

40. Scott CS, Chiu WA. Trichloroethylene cancer epidemiology: a consideration of select issues. *Environmental Health Perspectives*. September 2006;114(9):1471–1478. doi:10.1289/ ehp.8949.

41. Hazardous Waste Cleanup: 1033 Kings Highway, LLC in Saugerties, New York. EPA. Updated June 7, 2024. https://www.epa.gov/hwcorrectiveactioncleanups/hazardous-waste -cleanup-1033-kings-highway-llc-saugerties-new-york.

42. Watson JD, Crick FHC. Molecular structure of nucleic acids: a structure for deoxyribose nucleic acid. *Nature*. April 1, 1953;171(4356):737–738. doi:10.1038/171737a0.

43. McGovern L, Miller G, Hughes-Cromwick P. The relative contribution of multiple deter- minants to health. *Health Affairs Health Policy Brief*. 2014;10(10.1377).

44. Schroeder SA. We can do better—improving the health of the American people. *New England Journal of Medicine*. 2007;357(12):1221–1228. doi:10.1056/NEJMsa073350.

45. Polymeropoulos MH, Lavedan C, Leroy E, et al. Mutation in the alpha-synuclein gene identified in families with Parkinson's disease. *Science*. June 27, 1997;276(5321):2045–2047. doi:10.1126/science.276.5321.2045.

46. Cook L, Verbrugge J, Schwantes-An T-H, et al. Parkinson's disease variant detection and disclosure: PD GENEration, a North American study. *Brain*. August 1, 2024;147(8):2668–2679. doi:10.1093/brain/awae142.

47. Bloem BR, Okun MS, Klein C. Parkinson's disease. *The Lancet*. June 12, 2021;397(10291):2284–2303.

48. Borsche M, Pereira SL, Klein C, Grünewald A. Mitochondria and Parkinson's disease: clinical, molecular, and translational aspects. *Journal of Parkinson's Disease*. 2021;11(1):45–60. doi:10.3233/jpd-201981.

49. Moon HE, Paek SH. Mitochondrial dysfunction in Parkinson's disease. *Experimental Neurobiology*. June 2015;24(2):103–116. doi:10.5607/en.2015.24.2.103.

50. Narayan S, Sinsheimer JS, Paul KC, et al. Genetic variability in ABCB1, occupational pes- ticide exposure, and Parkinson's disease. *Environmental Research*. November 1, 2015;143:98–106. doi:10.1016/j.envres.2015.08.022.

51. van Dongen J, Slagboom PE, Draisma HH, Martin NG, Boomsma DI. The continuing value of twin studies in the omics era. *Nature Reviews Genetics*. September 2012;13(9):640–653. doi:10.1038/nrg3243.

52. Foltynie T, Sawcer S, Brayne C, Barker R. The genetic basis of Parkinson's disease. *Journal of Neurology, Neurosurgery, and Psychiatry*. 2002;73(4):363–370.

53. Tanner CM, Ottman R, Goldman SM, et al. Parkinson disease in twins: an etiologic study. *JAMA*. 1999;281(4):341–346. doi:10-1001/pubs.JAMA-ISSN-0098-7484-281-4-joc81035.

54. Dorsey ER, De Miranda BR, Horsager J, Borghammer P. The body, the brain, the environ- ment, and Parkinson's disease. *Journal of Parkinson's Disease*. 2024;14(3):363–381. doi:10.3233/ JPD-240019.

55. Martinez TN, Greenamyre JT. Toxin models of mitochondrial dysfunction in Parkinson's disease. *Antioxidants & Redox Signaling.* May 1, 2012;16(9):920–934. doi:10.1089/ars.2011.4033.

56. Gash DM, Rutland K, Hudson NL, et al. Trichloroethylene: parkinsonism and complex 1 mitochondrial neurotoxicity. *Annals of Neurology.* February 1, 2008;63(2):184–192. doi:10.1002/ana.21288.

57. Simpson C, Vinikoor-Imler L, Nassan FL, et al. Prevalence of ten LRRK2 variants in Parkinson's disease: a comprehensive review. *Parkinsonism & Related Disorders.* May 1, 2022;98:103–113. doi:10.1016/j.parkreldis.2022.05.012.

58. De Miranda BR, Castro SL, Rocha EM, Bodle CR, Johnson KE, Greenamyre JT. The industrial solvent trichloroethylene induces LRRK2 kinase activity and dopaminergic neurodegeneration in a rat model of Parkinson's disease. *Neurobiology of Disease.* June 2021;153:105312. doi:10.1016/j.nbd.2021.105312.

59. How Minnesota passed the country's first ban on trichloroethylene. Minnesota Pollution Control Agency. September 1, 2023. https://www.pca.state.mn.us/news-and-stories/tce-ban-in-effect.

60. Clukey K. New York state bans cancer-linked solvent used as degreaser. *Bloomberg Law.* December 24, 2020. https://news.bloomberglaw.com/environment-and-energy/new-york-state-bans-cancer-linked-solvent-used-as-degreaser.

61. EPA proposes ban on all consumer and many commercial uses of perchloroethylene to protect public health. EPA. June 8, 2023. https://www.epa.gov/newsreleases/epa-proposes-ban-all-consumer-and-many-commercial-uses-perchloroethylene-protect.

62. Biden-Harris administration proposes ban on trichloroethylene to protect public from toxic chemical known to cause serious health risks. EPA. October 23, 2023. https://www.epa.gov/newsreleases/biden-harris-administration-proposes-ban-trichloroethylene-protect-public-toxic. Accessed September 20, 2024.

63. Casey M. EPA proposes ban on cancer-causing chemical that contaminated Woburn water. WBUR. October 24, 2023. https://www.wbur.org/news/2023/10/24/epa-ban-tce-trichloroethylene-cancer-chemical-woburn.

64. Trichloroethylene (TCE). EPA. https://19january2017snapshot.epa.gov/assessing-and-managing-chemicals-under-tsca/trichloroethylene-tce_.html. Accessed June 8, 2024.

Chapter 3: An Invisible Cause Inside Our Homes

1. Pauley J. Michael J. Fox on Parkinson's and how he finds "optimism is sustainable." *CBS News.* April 30, 2023. https://www.cbsnews.com/news/michael-j-fox-on-parkinsons-and-how-he-finds-optimism-is-sustainable.

2. Gerusky TM. The Pennsylvania radon story. *Journal of Environmental Health.* 1987;49(4):197–200.

3. Legget M. The story of how radon was discovered in homes. BrickKicker of Georgia. July 26, 2019. https://www.georgia.brickkicker.com/the-story-of-how-radon-was-discovered-in-homes.

4. The radioactive nuclear plant worker. Institute of Physics. https://spark.iop.org/radioactive-nuclear-plant-worker. Accessed September 1, 2024.

5. Radionuclide basics: radon. EPA. Updated on May 6, 2024. https://www.epa.gov/radiation/radionuclide-basics-radon.

6. Radon in homes, schools and buildings. EPA. Updated on January 24, 2024. https://www.epa.gov/radtown/radon-homes-schools-and-buildings.

7. Banks K. How much do radon mitigation systems cost in 2024? *Forbes.* Updated July 26, 2024. https://www.forbes.com/home-improvement/home/radon-mitigation-system-cost-guide.

8. What is EPA's action level for radon and what does it mean? EPA. Updated on December 2, 2024. https://www.epa.gov/radon/what-epas-action-level-radon-and-what-does-it-mean.

9. A citizen's guide to radon. EPA. May 2012. https://www.epa.gov/sites/default/files/2016-02/documents/2012_a_citizens_guide_to_radon.pdf.

10. Radon testing and home sales: a case study. 2021. American Lung Association. https://www.lung.org/getmedia/220ca207-5852-4591-8b96-8bb89945fddf/ALA-Radon-Montgomery-County-Case-Study-2021_Final-revised-08-16-21_1.pdf.

11. Yao M, Ding K, Tang X, et al. Analysis and monitoring of indoor radon concentrations of 37 kindergartens—Beijing municipality, China, 2023. *China CDC Weekly*. March 29, 2024;6(13):272–276. doi:10.46234/ccdcw2024.053.

12. Giraldo-Osorio A, Ruano-Ravina A, Varela-Lema L, Barros-Dios JM, Pérez-Ríos M. Residential radon in Central and South America: a systematic review. *International Journal of Environmental Research and Public Health*. June 24, 2020;17(12). doi:10.3390/ijerph17124550.

13. Esan DT, Obed RI, Afolabi OT, Sridhar MK, Olubodun BB, Ramos C. Radon risk perception and barriers for residential radon testing in southwestern Nigeria. *Oxford Handbook of Public Health Practice*. November 2020;1:100036. doi:10.1016/j.puhip.2020.100036.

14. Feres M, Feres MFN. Absence of evidence is not evidence of absence. *Journal of Applied Oral Science*. March 27, 2023;31:ed001. doi:10.1590/1678-7757-2023-ed001.

15. Dorsey ER, Bloem BR. Parkinson's disease is predominantly an environmental disease. *Journal of Parkinson's Disease*. 2024;14(3):451–465. doi:10.3233/JPD-230357.

16. PubMed search with key words "parkinsons + genetics," "parkinsons + environment," "parkinsons + pesticides," "parkinsons + solvents," and "parkinsons + air pollution." https://pubmed.ncbi.nlm.nih.gov. Accessed May 8, 2024.

17. De Miranda BR, Goldman SM, Miller GW, Greenamyre JT, Dorsey ER. Preventing Parkinson's disease: an environmental agenda. *Journal of Parkinson's Disease*. 2022;12(1):45–68. doi:10.3233/JPD-212922.

18. Dorsey ER, Kinel D, Pawlik ME, et al. Dry-cleaning chemicals and a cluster of Parkinson's disease and cancer: a retrospective investigation. *Movement Disorders*. March 1, 2024;39(3):606–613. doi:10.1002/mds.29723.

19. What is vapor intrusion? EPA. 2023. https://www.epa.gov/vaporintrusion/what-vapor-intrusion.

20. De Miranda BR, Castro SL, Rocha EM, Bodle CR, Johnson KE, Greenamyre JT. The industrial solvent trichloroethylene induces LRRK2 kinase activity and dopaminergic neurodegeneration in a rat model of Parkinson's disease. *Neurobiology of Disease*. June 2021;153:105312. doi:10.1016/j.nbd.2021.105312.

21. McHugh T, Loll P, Eklund B. Recent advances in vapor intrusion site investigations. *Journal of Environmental Management*. December 15, 2017;204(Pt 2):783–792. doi:10.1016/j.jenvman.2017.02.015.

22. Department of Environmental Conservation, New York State. Environmental Site Database Search. 2024. Accessed July 1, 2024. https://dec.ny.gov/environmental-protection/site-cleanup/database-search.

23. Tüchsen F, Jensen AA. Agricultural work and the risk of Parkinson's disease in Denmark, 1981–1993. *Scandinavian Journal of Work, Environment & Health*. 2000;26(4):359–362.

24. History. https://www.fordnbfacts.com/history. Accessed October 22, 2024.

25. MIM-72 chaparral. Wikipedia. https://en.wikipedia.org/wiki/MIM-72_Chaparral. Accessed July 16, 2024.

26. Santa Ana Regional Water Quality Control Board and Ford Motor Company. Community fact sheet no. 13. August 2024. https://static1.squarespace.com/static/65402603749fb25a78b16cf8/t/66c52e283c99eb57a5c7f719/1724198441332/FordNB_CFS-13_Final_2024_07_30.pdf.

27. FordNBFacts.com. https://www.fordnbfacts.com. Accessed July 16, 2024.

28. Weber J. Ford Aerospace treated for years like a stepchild. *Los Angeles Times*. January 14, 1990. https://www.latimes.com/archives/la-xpm-1990-01-14-fi-390-story.html.

29. Coyote Canyon. County of Orange Waste & Recycling. https://oclandfills.com/landfills/closed-landfill-sites/coyote-canyon. Accessed September 9, 2024.

30. Wallace D, Groth E, III, Kirrane E, Warren B, Halloran J. Upstairs, downstairs: perchloroethylene in the air in apartments above New York City dry cleaners. CUNY Digital History Archive. October 1995. https://cdha.cuny.edu/files/original/f7d262bbd5d0fb33c26eb32a38978515.pdf.

31. Dry cleaner regulation. New York State Department of Environmental Conservation. https://dec.ny.gov/environmental-protection/air-quality/controlling-pollution-from-facilities/dry-cleaner-regulation. Accessed July 17, 2024.

32. McDermott MJ, Mazor KA, Shost SJ, Narang RS, Aldous KM, Storm JE. Tetrachloroethylene (PCE, Perc) levels in residential dry cleaner buildings in diverse communities in New York City. *Environmental Health Perspectives*. October 1, 2005;113(10):1336–1343. doi:10.1289/ehp.7414.

33. Clukey K. New York state bans cancer-linked solvent used as degreaser. *Bloomberg Law*. December 24, 2020. https://news.bloomberglaw.com/environment-and-energy/new-york-state-bans-cancer-linked-solvent-used-as-degreaser.

34. Gass-Poore J. Toxic fumes detected at popular Brooklyn shuffleboard club for past 2 years. *Gothamist*. March 9, 2023. https://gothamist.com/news/toxic-fumes-detected-at-popular-brooklyn-shuffleboard-club-for-past-2-years.

35. Velsey K. What Superfund? *Curbed*. June 27, 2024. https://www.curbed.com/article/gowanus-toxic-vapors-pollution-superfund-luxury-real-estate.html.

36. Calder R. 100 blocks by toxic NYC canal being tested for cancerous vapors—residents demand answers. *New York Post*. June 15, 2024. https://nypost.com/2024/06/15/us-news/100-blocks-by-gowanus-canal-in-nyc-being-tested-for-toxic-vapors.

37. Population surrounding 1,857 Superfund remedial sites. EPA. Updated September 2020. https://www.epa.gov/sites/default/files/2015-09/documents/webpopulationrsuperfundsites9.28.15.pdf.

38. LaRocco PS, David M. The Grumman Plume: decades of deceit. *Newsday*. February 18, 2020. https://projects.newsday.com/long-island/plume-grumman-navy.

39. Trichloroethylene (TCE). EPA. Updated March 8, 2024. https://clu-in.org/contaminantfocus/default.focus/sec/Trichloroethylene_(TCE)/cat/Treatment_Technologies.

40. Toxicological review of tetrachloroethylene (perchloroethylene). EPA. February 2012. https://cfpub.epa.gov/ncea/iris/iris_documents/documents/toxreviews/0106tr.pdf.

41. Altmann L, Neuhann HF, Kramer U, Witten J, Jermann E. Neurobehavioral and neurophysiological outcome of chronic low-level tetrachloroethene exposure measured in neighborhoods of dry cleaning shops. *Environmental Research*. May 1, 1995;69(2):83–89. doi:10.1006/enrs.1995.1028.

42. McCord CP. Toxicity of trichloroethylene. *Journal of the American Medical Association*. 1932;99(5):409–409. doi:10.1001/jama.1932.02740570055030.

43. Huber F. Zur Klinik und Neuropathologie der Trichloräthylenvergiftung [Clinical aspects and neuropathology of trichloroethylene poisoning]. *Zeitschrift fur Unfallmedizin und Berufskrankheiten*. 1969;62(4):226–267.

44. Guehl D, Bezard E, Dovero S, Boraud T, Bioulac B, Gross C. Trichloroethylene and parkinsonism: a human and experimental observation. *European Journal of Neurology*. 1999;6(5):609–611. doi:10.1046/j.1468-1331.1999.650609.x.

45. Gash DM, Rutland K, Hudson NL, et al. Trichloroethylene: parkinsonism and complex 1 mitochondrial neurotoxicity. *Annals of Neurology*. February 1, 2008;63(2):184–192. doi:10.1002/ana.21288.

46. Barringer F. Exposed to solvent, worker faces hurdles. *New York Times*. January 25, 2009. https://www.nytimes.com/2009/01/25/us/25toxic.html.

47. Dorsey ER, Zafar M, Lettenberger SE, et al. Trichloroethylene: an invisible cause of Parkinson's disease? *Journal of Parkinson's Disease*. 2023;13(2):203–218. doi:10.3233/jpd-225047.

48. Adamson A, Ilieva N, Stone WJ, De Miranda BR. Low-dose inhalation exposure to trichloroethylene induces dopaminergic neurodegeneration in rodents. *Toxicological Sciences*. November 28, 2023;196(2):218–228. doi:10.1093/toxsci/kfad090.

49. Barringer F. E.P.A. charts risks of a ubiquitous chemical. *New York Times*. September 30, 2011. https://archive.nytimes.com/green.blogs.nytimes.com/2011/09/30/e-p-a-quantifies-trichloroethylene-risks.

50. Doherty R. History of TCE. In: Gilbert KM, Blossom SJ, eds. *Trichloroethylene: Toxicity and Health Risks*. Humana Press; 2014:1–14.

51. Reis J, Benbrick E, Bonneterre V, Spencer PS. Parkinson's disease and solvents: is there a causal link? *Revue neurologique*. December 2016;172(12):761–765. doi:10.1016/j.neurol.2016.09.012.

52. Superfund site: Travis Air Force Base, Travis AFB, CA, contaminant list. EPA. https://cumulis.epa.gov/supercpad/SiteProfiles/index.cfm?fuseaction=second.contams&id=0902767. Accessed September 24, 2024.

53. Preliminary final environmental impact statement. Defense Technical Information Center. December 2000. https://apps.dtic.mil/sti/tr/pdf/ADA389944.pdf.

54. Superfund site: Wright-Patterson Air Force Base, Dayton, OH, contaminant list. EPA. https://cumulis.epa.gov/supercpad/SiteProfiles/index.cfm?fuseaction=second.contams&id=0504939. Accessed September 25, 2024.

55. Wright-Patterson Air Force Base—a case study. Agency for Toxic Substances and Disease Registry, CDC. 2001. https://www.atsdr.cdc.gov/HAC/landfill/PDFs/Landfill_2001_appd.pdf.

56. Broder JM. Pollution "hot spots" taint water sources. *Los Angeles Times*. June 18, 1990. https://www.latimes.com/archives/la-xpm-1990-06-18-mn-176-story.html.

57. Broder JM. U.S. military leaves toxic trail overseas. *Los Angeles Times*. June 18, 1990. https://www.latimes.com/archives/la-xpm-1990-06-18-mn-96-story.html.

58. Superfund site: Moffett Field Naval Air Station, Dayton, CA, Superfund site information. EPA. https://cumulis.epa.gov/supercpad/cursites/ccontinfo.cfm?id=0902734. Accessed September 25, 2024.

59. DeBolt D. Toxic vapors found in NASA Ames buildings. *Mountain View Voice*. April 26, 2013. https://www.mv-voice.com/news/2013/04/26/toxic-vapors-found-in-nasa-ames-buildings.

60. Barajas M. Questions linger over Kelly AFB contamination even after property changes hands. *San Antonio Current*. October 11, 2011. https://www.sacurrent.com/news/questions-linger-over-kelly-afb-contamination-even-after-property-changes-hands-2241824.

61. Vartabedian R. Cancer stalks a "toxic triangle." *Los Angeles Times*. March 30, 2006. https://www.latimes.com/archives/la-xpm-2006-mar-30-na-toxic30-story.html.

62. Osan Air Base drinking water consumer confidence report 2018 (covering calendar year 2017). Osan Air Base. 2018. https://www.osan.af.mil/Portals/72/Osan%20AB%202018%20CCR.PDF.

63. Maldonado A. Cleaning up Shaw's water. Air Force Civil Engineer Center. March 15, 2019. https://www.nellis.af.mil/News/Article/1786436/cleaning-up-shaws-water.

64. Superfund site: Hill Air Force Base, Hill AFB, UT, contaminant list. EPA. https://cumulis.epa.gov/supercpad/SiteProfiles/index.cfm?fuseaction=second.contams&id=0800753. Accessed September 24, 2024.

65. Goldman SM, Quinlan PJ, Ross GW, et al. Solvent exposures and Parkinson disease risk in twins. *Annals of Neurology*. June 2012;71(6):776–784. doi:10.1002/ana.22629.

66. Goldman SM, Weaver FM, Stroupe KT, et al. Risk of Parkinson disease among service members at Marine Corps Base Camp Lejeune. *JAMA Neurology.* 2023;80(7):673–681. doi:10.1001/jamaneurol.2023.1168.

67. Bergeson LL, Hutton CN. EPA delays effective date of TCE risk management rule. Bergeson & Campbell, P.C. January 30, 2025. https://natlawreview.com/article/epa-delays -effective-date-tce-risk-management-rule.

68. Solvent cleaning with 3M™ Novec™ Engineered Fluids. 3M. October 2017. https:// multimedia.3m.com/mws/media/1479638O/solvent-cleaning-with-3mtm-novectm-engineered -fluids.pdf.

69. Frequently asked questions about TCE alternatives. MicroCare. https://www.micro care.com/en-US/Resources/Resource-Center/FAQs/Frequently-Asked-Questions-About-TCE-Alternatives. Accessed September 17, 2024.

70. IARC Working Group on the Evaluation of Carcinogenic Risks to Humans. *Trichloroethylene, Tetrachloroethylene, and Some Other Chlorinated Agents.* IARC Monographs on the Evaluation of Carcinogenic Risks to Humans 106. International Agency for Research on Cancer; 2014.

71. Lomas C. Green dry cleaner. DW.com. June 18, 2013. https://www.dw.com/en /france-forces-dry-cleaners-to-use-safer-chemicals/a-16888476.

72. Yang W, Hamilton JL, Kopil C, et al. Current and projected future economic burden of Parkinson's disease in the U.S. *npj Parkinson's Disease.* July 9, 2020;6(1):15. doi:10.1038/ s41531-020-0117-1.

73. Abbott B, Loftus P. Cancer is capsizing Americans' finances. "I Was Losing Everything." *Wall Street Journal.* May 28, 2024. https://www.wsj.com/health/healthcare/cancer -cost-patient-debt-dd7c540c.

Chapter 4: The Brain's Front Door

1. Associated Press. Mexico City cleans up its reputation for smog. *NBC News.* December 26, 2008. https://www.nbcnews.com/id/wbna28391130.

2. Calderón-Garcidueñas L, Franco-Lira M, Mora-Tiscareño A, Medina-Cortina H, Torres-Jardón R, Kavanaugh M. Early Alzheimer's and Parkinson's disease pathology in urban children: friend versus foe responses—it is time to face the evidence. *BioMed Research International.* 2013;2013:161687. doi:10.1155/2013/161687.

3. Calderón-Garcidueñas L, González-Maciel A, Reynoso-Robles R, et al. Alzheimer's disease and alpha-synuclein pathology in the olfactory bulbs of infants, children, teens and adults ≤40 years in Metropolitan Mexico City. APOE4 carriers at higher risk of suicide accelerate their olfactory bulb pathology. *Environmental Research.* 2018;166:348–362.

4. Calderón-Garcidueñas L, Solt AC, Henríquez-Roldán C, et al. Long-term air pollution exposure is associated with neuroinflammation, an altered innate immune response, disruption of the blood-brain barrier, ultrafine particulate deposition, and accumulation of amyloid β-42 and α-synuclein in children and young adults. *Toxicologic Pathology.* 2008;36(2):289–310.

5. Calderón-Garcidueñas L, Gónzalez-Maciel A, Reynoso-Robles R, et al. Hallmarks of Alzheimer disease are evolving relentlessly in Metropolitan Mexico City infants, children and young adults. APOE4 carriers have higher suicide risk and higher odds of reaching NFT stage V at ≤40 years of age. *Environmental Research.* 2018;164:475–487.

6. Dattani S, Rodes-Guirao L, Ritchie H, Ortiz-Ospina E, Roser M. Life expectancy. Our World in Data. 2023. https://ourworldindata.org/life-expectancy.

7. Dorsey ER, Bloem BR. Parkinson's disease is predominantly an environmental disease. *Journal of Parkinson's Disease.* 2024;14(3):451–465. doi:10.3233/jpd-230357.

8. Steinmetz JD, Seeher KM, Schiess N, et al. Global, regional, and national burden of disorders affecting the nervous system, 1990–2021: a systematic analysis for the Global

Burden of Disease Study 2021. *The Lancet Neurology.* 2024;23(4):344–381. doi:10.1016/S1474-4422(24)00038-3.

9. Proctor RN. The history of the discovery of the cigarette–lung cancer link: evidentiary traditions, corporate denial, global toll. *Tobacco Control.* 2012;21(2):87–91.

10. Society AC. What causes lung cancer? American Cancer Society. January 29, 2024. https://www.cancer.org/cancer/types/lung-cancer/causes-risks-prevention/what-causes.html.

11. Beach TG, White CL, Hladik CL, et al. Olfactory bulb α-synucleinopathy has high specificity and sensitivity for Lewy body disorders. *Acta Neuropathologica.* February 1, 2009;117(2):169–174. doi:10.1007/s00401-008-0450-7.

12. Doty RL. Olfactory dysfunction in Parkinson disease. *Nature Reviews Neurology.* June 1, 2012;8(6):329–339. doi:10.1038/nrneurol.2012.80.

13. Haehner A, Hummel T, Reichmann H. Olfactory loss in Parkinson's disease. *Parkinson's Disease.* 2011;2011:450939. doi:10.4061/2011/450939.

14. Air quality in Mexico City. IQAir. https://www.iqair.com/us/mexico/mexico-city. Accessed September 20, 2024.

15. Jacobs C, Kelly WJ. *Smogtown: The Lung-Burning History of Pollution in Los Angeles.* Abrams; 2008.

16. Marshall C. Stories of cities #29: Los Angeles and the "great American streetcar scandal." *The Guardian.* April 25, 2016. https://www.theguardian.com/cities/2016/apr/25/story-cities-los-angeles-great-american-streetcar-scandal.

17. Smedley T. *Clearing the Air: The Beginning and the End of Air Pollution.* Bloomsbury Publishing; 2019.

18. Chiland E. Did a conspiracy really destroy LA's huge streetcar system? *Curbed Los Angeles.* September 20, 2019. https://la.curbed.com/2017/9/20/16340038/los-angeles-streetcar-conspiracy-theory-general-motors.

19. Historical timeline of Los Angeles. Discover Los Angeles. October 22, 2024. https://www.discoverlosangeles.com/things-to-do/historical-timeline-of-los-angeles.

20. Ovallath S, Deepa P. The history of parkinsonism: descriptions in ancient Indian medical literature. *Movement Disorders.* May 2013;28(5):566–568. doi:10.1002/mds.25420.

21. Nieuwenhuijsen MJ, Basagaña X, Dadvand P, et al. Air pollution and human fertility rates. *Environment International.* 2014;70:9–14.

22. Vizcaíno MAC, González-Comadran M, Jacquemin B. Outdoor air pollution and human infertility: a systematic review. *Fertility and Sterility.* 2016;106(4):897–904.e1.

23. Lelieveld J, Pozzer A, Pöschl U, Fnais M, Haines A, Münzel T. Loss of life expectancy from air pollution compared to other risk factors: a worldwide perspective. *Cardiovascular Research.* 2020;116(11):1910–1917.

24. Particulate matter (PM) basics. EPA. Updated on June 20, 2024. https://www.epa.gov/pm-pollution/particulate-matter-pm-basics.

25. Kwon D, Paul KC, Yu Y, et al. Traffic-related air pollution and Parkinson's disease in central California. *Environmental Research.* January 1, 2024;240(Pt 1):117434. doi:10.1016/j.envres.2023.117434.

26. Shukman D. Pollution particles 'get into brain.' *BBC News.* September 5, 2016. https://www.bbc.com/news/science-environment-37276219.

27. History. California Air Resources Board. https://ww2.arb.ca.gov/about/history. Accessed October 22, 2024.

28. Malmin J. Buildings in Los Angeles Civic Center are barely visible in picture looking east at 1st and Olive Streets when smog was at its peak. *Los Angeles Times.* 1955. https://www.latimes.com/local/la-me-air-pollution-0428-pictures-photogallery.html.

29. Guerin E. LA explained: smog. *LAist*. October 3, 2018. https://laist.com/news /climate-environment/la-explained-smog.

30. Barboza T. Los Angeles suffers worst smog in almost 30 years. *Los Angeles Times*. September 10, 2020. https://www.latimes.com/california/story/2020-09-10/los-angeles-had-it -worst-smog-in-26-years-during-heat-wave.

31. Willis AW, Roberts E, Beck JC, et al. Incidence of Parkinson disease in North America. *npj Parkinson's Disease*. December 15, 2022;8(1):170. doi:10.1038/s41531-022-00410-y.

32. Ritz B, Lee P-C, Hansen J, et al. Traffic-related air pollution and Parkinson's disease in Denmark: a case-control study. *Environmental Health Perspectives*. 2016;124(3):351–356. doi:10.1289/ehp.1409313.

33. Ai B, Zhang J, Zhang S, et al. Causal association between long-term exposure to air pollution and incident Parkinson's disease. *Journal of Hazardous Materials*. May 5, 2024;469:133944. doi:10.1016/j.jhazmat.2024.133944.

34. Chen T-B, Liang C-S, Chang C-M, et al. Association between exposure to particulate matter and the incidence of Parkinson's disease: a nationwide cohort study in Taiwan. *Journal of Movement Disorders*. 2024;17(3):313.

35. Lee PC, Liu LL, Sun Y, et al. Traffic-related air pollution increased the risk of Parkinson's disease in Taiwan: a nationwide study. *Environment International*. November 2016;96:75–81. doi:10.1016/j.envint.2016.08.017.

36. Krzyzanowski B, Searles Nielsen S, Turner JR, Racette BA. Fine particulate matter and Parkinson disease risk among Medicare beneficiaries. *Neurology*. 2023;101(21):e2058–e2067.

37. Dewitt E, Ladyzhets B. Top 10 U.S. counties with the worst air pollution. Healthline. Last medically reviewed on March 15, 2021. https://www.healthline.com/health/allergic-asthma /air-pollution.

38. Parkinson J. An essay on the shaking palsy. 1817. *Journal of Neuropsychiatry and Clinical Neurosciences*. Spring 2002;14(2):223–236. doi:10.1176/jnp.14.2.223.

39. The 20th century mortality files, 1901–2000. Office for National Statistics. March 11, 2011. https://www.data.gov.uk/dataset/2548e46b-873e-4668-968c-25d6c155dd73/the-20th -century-mortality-files.

40. Gowers WR. *A Manual of Diseases of the Nervous System*. Vol. 2. P. Blakiston, Son & Company; 1898.

41. Duvoisin RC, Schweitzer MD. Paralysis agitans mortality in England and Wales, 1855–1962. *British Journal of Preventive & Social Medicine*. 1966;20(1):27.

42. Roser M, Ritchie H. Outdoor air pollution. Our World in Data. 2019. https://our worldindata.org/outdoor-air-pollution.

43. Dorsey ER, Elbaz A, Nichols E, et al. Global, regional, and national burden of Parkinson's disease, 1990–2016: a systematic analysis for the Global Burden of Disease Study 2016. *The Lancet Neurology*. 2018;17(11):939–953. doi:10.1016/S1474-4422(18)30295-3.

44. Air quality and pollution city ranking at IQAir. 2021. iqair.com.

45. IARC Working Group on the Evaluation of Carcinogenic Risks to Humans. 1.2 Sources of air pollutants. In: *Outdoor Air Pollution*. IARC Monographs on the Evaluation of Carcinogenic Risks to Humans No. 109. International Agency for Research on Cancer; 2016. https:// www.ncbi.nlm.nih.gov/books/NBK368029.

46. Vatican hid pope's Parkinson's disease. *UPI*. March 19, 2006. https://www.upi.com /Top_News/2006/03/19/Vatican-hid-popes-Parkinsons-disease/48511142806424.

47. Blakemore W. St. John Paul II. *Encyclopedia Britannica*. https://www.britannica.com /biography/Saint-John-Paul-II. Accessed September 14, 2021.

48. Health of Pope John Paul II. Wikipedia. August 15, 2021. https://en.wikipedia.org/wiki /Health_of_Pope_John_Paul_II.

49. Pagani S. Surgeon: pope suffers from Parkinson's. *ABC News.* January 4, 2001. https://abcnews.go.com/International/story?id=81777&page=1.

50. Parkinson's expert sees decline in pope. *ABC News.* May 24, 2001. https://abcnews.go.com/GMA/story?id=126945&page=1.

51. Pedagogy of suffering: John Paul II's victory. *Millennial.* May 21, 2014. https://millennialjournal.com/2014/05/21/pedagogy-of-suffering-john-paul-iis-victory.

52. Boudreaux R. Visibly shaking John Paul II unable to finish speech in Armenia / Effects of Parkinson's overcome the pope. *SFGate.* September 26, 2001. https://www.sfgate.com/news/article/visibly-shaky-john-paul-ii-unable-to-finish-2874970.php.

53. Cornwell J. *The Pope in Winter: The Dark Face of John Paul II's Papacy.* Penguin UK; 2005.

54. Wingfield B. Vatican details final days of Pope John Paul II. *New York Times.* September 18, 2005. https://www.nytimes.com/2005/09/18/international/europe/vatican-details-final-days-of-pope-john-paul-ii.html.

55. Tycner A. 20 interesting facts about John Paul II's life: a courageous leader who fought against communism. Victims of Communism Memorial Foundation. June 13, 2022. https://victimsofcommunism.org/publication/20-interesting-facts-about-john-paul-ii.

56. Gigacz S. Universal brotherhood and solidarity: Cardijn & JPII. *Cardijn Research.* May 27, 2020. https://cardijnresearch.org/universal-brotherhood-and-solidarity-cardijn-and-john-paul-ii.

57. Pope John Paul II. Wikipedia. https://en.wikipedia.org/wiki/Pope_John_Paul_II. Accessed September 20, 2024.

58. Motyka J, Czop M. Vertical changes of iron and manganese concentration in water from abandoned "Zakrzówek" limestone quarry near Cracow (South Poland). In: Rapantova N, Hrkal Z, eds. *Mine Water and the Environment: Proceedings of the 10th IMWA Congress 2008: 2–5 June, 2008, Karlovy Vary, Czech Republic.* VŠB—Technical University of Ostrava, Faculty of Mining and Geology; 2008;167–170.

59. Olanow CW. Manganese-induced parkinsonism and Parkinson's disease. *Annals of the New York Academy of Sciences.* 2004;1012(1):209–223. doi:10.1196/annals.1306.018.

60. Guilarte TR. Manganese and Parkinson's disease: a critical review and new findings. *Environmental Health Perspectives.* 2010;118(8):1071–1080.

61. Couper J. On the effects of black oxide of manganese when inhaled into the lungs. *British Annals of Medicine and Pharmacology.* 1837;1:41–42.

62. Racette BA, Searles Nielsen S, Criswell SR, et al. Dose-dependent progression of parkinsonism in manganese-exposed welders. *Neurology.* 2017;88(4):344–351.

63. Gorell JM, Johnson CC, Rybicki BA, et al. Occupational exposures to metals as risk factors for Parkinson's disease. *Neurology.* March 1997;48(3):650–658. doi:10.1212/wnl.48.3.650.

64. Tanner CM, Ross GW, Jewell SA, et al. Occupation and risk of parkinsonism: a multi-center case-control study. *Archives of Neurology.* September 2009;66(9):1106–1113. doi:10.1001/archneurol.2009.195.

65. Zakrzówek Park & Reservoir. In Your Pocket. https://www.inyourpocket.com/krakow/zakrzowek-park-reservoir_50421v. Accessed July 22, 2024.

66. Zakrzówek has re-opened. Kraków Expats Directory. June 1, 2023. https://krakowexpats.pl/news-from-krakow/zakrzowek-re-opens.

67. Tymczak P. Kraków szykuje się do otwarcia Zakrzówka. Tak ma funkcjonować nowe kąpielisko. Na baseny wejdzie ograniczona liczba osób ZDJĘCIA. *Gazeta Krakowska.* March 27, 2023. https://gazetakrakowska.pl/krakow-szykuje-sie-do-otwarcia-zakrzowka-tak-ma-funkcjonowac-nowe-kapielisko-na-baseny-wejdzie-ograniczona-liczba-osob-zdjecia/ar/c7-17407543.

68. Johnson R, Plummer L, Chan J, Wills A-M. Feasibility and tolerability randomized clinical trial of golf versus tai chi for people with moderate Parkinson's disease (1962). *Neurology.* 2021;96(15_supplement):1962.

69. Bliss RR, Church FC. Golf as a physical activity to potentially reduce the risk of falls in older adults with Parkinson's disease. *Sports.* 2021;9(6):72.

70. Parrish ML, Gardner RE. Is living downwind of a golf course a risk factor for parkinsonism? *Annals of Neurology.* 2012;72(6):984.

71. Toxic fairways: risking groundwater contamination from pesticides on Long Island golf courses. Beyond Pesticides. December 1995. https://www.beyondpesticides.org/assets/media /documents/documents/toxic-fairways-1995.pdf.

72. Uteuova A. "Botox for your lawn": the controversial use of pesticides on golf courses. *The Guardian.* August 6, 2022. https://www.theguardian.com/us-news/2022/aug/06/pesticides-golf -courses-health-problems.

73. de Graaf L, Boulanger M, Bureau M, et al. Occupational pesticide exposure, cancer and chronic neurological disorders: a systematic review of epidemiological studies in greenspace workers. *Environmental Research.* 2022;203:111822.

74. Braak H, Rüb U, Gai WP, Del Tredici K. Idiopathic Parkinson's disease: possible routes by which vulnerable neuronal types may be subject to neuroinvasion by an unknown pathogen. *Journal of Neural Transmission.* May 2003;110(5):517–536. doi:10.1007/s00702-002 -0808-2.

75. Borghammer P, Van Den Berge N. Brain-first versus gut-first Parkinson's disease: a hypothesis. *Journal of Parkinson's Disease.* 2019;9(s2):S281–S295. doi:10.3233/JPD-191721.

76. McKeith I, Mintzer J, Aarsland D, et al. Dementia with Lewy bodies. *The Lancet Neurology.* January 2004;3(1):19–28. doi:10.1016/s1474-4422(03)00619-7.

77. Lewy body dementia. National Institute on Aging. https://www.nia.nih.gov/health /lewy-body-dementia. Accessed October 22, 2024.

78. Weintraub D. What's in a name? The time has come to unify Parkinson's disease and dementia with Lewy bodies. *Movement Disorders.* November 2023;38(11):1977–1981. doi:10.1002/mds.29590.

79. Borghammer P, Okkels N, Weintraub D. Parkinson's disease and dementia with Lewy bodies: one and the same. *Journal of Parkinson's Disease.* 2024;14:383–397. doi:10.3233/ JPD-240002.

80. Dorsey ER, De Miranda BR, Horsager J, Borghammer P. The body, the brain, the environment, and Parkinson's disease. *Journal of Parkinson's Disease.* 2024;14(3):363–381. doi:10.3233/ JPD-240019.

81. Chen H, Wang K, Scheperjans F, Killinger B. Environmental triggers of Parkinson's disease—implications of the Braak and dual-hit hypotheses. *Neurobiology of Disease.* 2022;163:105601.

82. Why do a child's age and developmental stage affect physiological susceptibility to toxic substances? Agency for Toxic Substances and Disease Registry, CDC. https://www.atsdr.cdc.gov /csem/pediatric-environmental-health/child_age.html. Accessed August 13, 2023.

83. Adamson A, Ilieva N, Stone WJ, De Miranda BR. Low-dose inhalation exposure to trichloroethylene induces dopaminergic neurodegeneration in rodents. *Toxicological Sciences.* November 28, 2023;196(2):218–228. doi:10.1093/toxsci/kfad090.

84. Vilchez D, Saez I, Dillin A. The role of protein clearance mechanisms in organismal ageing and age-related diseases. *Nature Communications.* December 8, 2014;5(1):5659. doi:10.1038/ ncomms6659.

85. Knopman DS. The enigma of decreasing dementia incidence. *JAMA Network Open.* 2020;3(7):e2011199–e2011199. doi:10.1001/jamanetworkopen.2020.11199.

86. Wolters FJ, Chibnik LB, Waziry R, et al. Twenty-seven-year time trends in dementia incidence in Europe and the United States: the Alzheimer Cohorts Consortium. *Neurology.* August 4, 2020;95(5):e519–e531. doi:10.1212/wnl.0000000000010022.

87. Wang X, Younan D, Millstein J, et al. Association of improved air quality with lower dementia risk in older women. *Proceedings of the National Academy of Sciences of the United States of America.* January 11, 2022;119(2):e2107833119. doi:10.1073/pnas.2107833119.

Chapter 5: Learn Why

1. Tindle HA, Stevenson Duncan M, Greevy RA, et al. Lifetime smoking history and risk of lung cancer: results from the Framingham Heart Study. *Journal of the National Cancer Institute.* November 1, 2018;110(11):1201–1207. doi:10.1093/jnci/djy041.

2. Villeneuve PJ, Mao Y. Lifetime probability of developing lung cancer, by smoking status, Canada. *Canadian Journal of Public Health.* November–December 1994;85(6):385–388.

3. Ranger GS. Alexander the Great may have died from a perforated peptic ulcer. *Journal of Clinical Gastroenterology.* 1999;28(3):279–280.

4. Hunt PS. Surgical management of bleeding chronic peptic ulcer. A 10-year prospective study. *Annals of Surgery.* January 1984;199(1):44–50. doi:10.1097/00000658-198401000-00008.

5. Kraus M, Mendeloff G, Condon RE. Prognosis of gastric ulcer: twenty-five year followup. *Annals of Surgery.* October 1976;184(4):471–476. doi:10.1097/00000658-197610000-00010.

6. Pincock S. Nobel Prize winners Robin Warren and Barry Marshall. *The Lancet.* October 22–28, 2005;366(9495):1429. doi:10.1016/S0140-6736(05)67587-3.

7. Marshall B. Gastric spirochaetes: 100 years of discovery before and after Kobayashi. *Keio Journal of Medicine.* December 2002;51 Suppl 2:33–37. doi:10.2302/kjm.51.supplement2_33.

8. Marshall B. Helicobacter connections. *ChemMedChem.* August 2006;1(8):783–802. doi:10.1002/cmdc.200600153.

9. Marshall B. *Helicobacter pylori:* a Nobel pursuit? *Canadian Journal of Gastroenterology and Hepatology.* November 2008;22(11):895–896. doi:10.1155/2008/459810.

10. Marshall BJ. One hundred years of discovery and rediscovery of *Helicobacter pylori* and its association with peptic ulcer disease. In: Mobley HLT, Mendz GL, Hazell SL, eds. Helicobacter pylori: *Physiology and Genetics.* ASM Press; 2001.

11. Marshall BJ, Goodwin CS, Warren JR, et al. Prospective double-blind trial of duodenal ulcer relapse after eradication of *Campylobacter pylori. The Lancet.* December 24–31, 1988;2(8626–8627):1437–1442. doi:10.1016/s0140-6736(88)90929-4.

12. Bras JM, Guerreiro RJ, Ribeiro MH, et al. G2019S dardarin substitution is a common cause of Parkinson's disease in a Portuguese cohort. *Movement Disorders.* December 2005;20(12):1653–1655. doi:10.1002/mds.20682.

13. Cookson MR, Xiromerisiou G, Singleton A. How genetics research in Parkinson's disease is enhancing understanding of the common idiopathic forms of the disease. *Current Opinion in Neurology.* December 2005;18(6):706–711. doi:10.1097/01.wco.0000186841.43505.e6.

14. Paisan-Ruiz C, Lang AE, Kawarai T, et al. LRRK2 gene in Parkinson disease: mutation analysis and case control association study. *Neurology.* September 13, 2005;65(5):696–700. doi:10.1212/01.wnl.0000167552.79769.b3.

15. Lwin A, Orvisky E, Goker-Alpan O, LaMarca ME, Sidransky E. Glucocerebrosidase mutations in subjects with parkinsonism. *Molecular Genetics and Metabolism.* January 2004;81(1):70–73. doi:10.1016/j.ymgmc.2003.11.004.

16. Sidransky E. Gaucher disease: complexity in a "simple" disorder. *Molecular Genetics and Metabolism.* September–October 2004;83(1–2):6–15. doi:10.1016/j.ymgme.2004.08.015.

17. Goker-Alpan O, Lopez G, Vithayathil J, Davis J, Hallett M, Sidransky E. The spectrum of parkinsonian manifestations associated with glucocerebrosidase mutations. *Archives of Neurology.* October 2008;65(10):1353–1357. doi:10.1001/archneur.65.10.1353.

18. Cook L, Verbrugge J, Schwantes-An TH, et al. Parkinson's disease variant detection and disclosure: PD GENEration, a North American study. *Brain*. August 1, 2024;147(8):2668–2679. doi:10.1093/brain/awae142.

19. Barreh GA, Sghaier I, Abida Y, et al. The Impact of LRRK2 G2019S on Parkinson's disease: clinical phenotype and treatment in Tunisian patients. *Journal of Movement Disorders*. July 2024;17(3):294–303. doi:10.14802/jmd.23276.

20. Kmiecik MJ, Micheletti S, Coker D, et al. Genetic analysis and natural history of Parkinson's disease due to the LRRK2 G2019S variant. *Brain*. June 3, 2024;147(6):1996–2008. doi:10.1093/brain/awae073.

21. Saunders-Pullman R, Raymond D, Elango S. LRRK2 Parkinson disease. In: Adam MP, Feldman J, Mirzaa GM, Pagon RA, Wallace SE, Amemiya A, eds. *GeneReviews®*. University of Washington, Seattle; 1993.

22. Brown EG, Goldman SM, Coffey CS, et al. Occupational pesticide exposure in Parkinson's disease related to GBA and LRRK2 variants. *Journal of Parkinson's Disease*. 2024;14(4):737–746. doi:10.3233/JPD-240015.

23. Hertz E, Chen Y, Sidransky E. Gaucher disease provides a unique window into Parkinson disease pathogenesis. *Nature Reviews Neurology*. September 2024;20(9):526–540. doi:10.1038/s41582-024-00999-z.

24. Vieira SRL, Schapira AHV. Glucocerebrosidase mutations and Parkinson disease. *Journal of Neural Transmission*. September 2022;129(9):1105–1117. doi:10.1007/s00702-022-02531-3.

25. Quintero-Espinosa DA, Jimenez-Del-Rio M, Velez-Pardo C. LRRK2 kinase inhibitor PF-06447475 protects *Drosophila melanogaster* against paraquat-induced locomotor impairment, life span reduction, and oxidative stress. *Neurochemical Research*. September 2024;49(9):2440–2452. doi:10.1007/s11064-024-04141-9.

26. Keeney MT, Rocha EM, Hoffman EK, et al. LRRK2 regulates production of reactive oxygen species in cell and animal models of Parkinson's disease. *Science Translational Medicine*. October 2, 2024;16(767):eadl3438. doi:10.1126/scitranslmed.adl3438.

27. Ilieva NM, Hoffman EK, Ghalib MA, Greenamyre JT, De Miranda BR. LRRK2 kinase inhibition protects against Parkinson's disease-associated environmental toxicants. *Neurobiology of Disease*. June 15, 2024;196:106522. doi:10.1016/j.nbd.2024.106522.

28. De Miranda BR, Castro SL, Rocha EM, Bodle CR, Johnson KE, Greenamyre JT. The industrial solvent trichloroethylene induces LRRK2 kinase activity and dopaminergic neurodegeneration in a rat model of Parkinson's disease. *Neurobiology of Disease*. June 2021;153:105312. doi:10.1016/j.nbd.2021.105312.

29. Italia S, Vivarelli S, Teodoro M, Costa C, Fenga C, Giambo F. Effects of pesticide exposure on the expression of selected genes in normal and cancer samples: identification of predictive biomarkers for risk assessment. *Environmental Toxicology and Pharmacology*. September 2024;110:104524. doi:10.1016/j.etap.2024.104524.

30. Teodoro M, Briguglio G, Fenga C, Costa C. Genetic polymorphisms as determinants of pesticide toxicity: recent advances. *Toxicology Reports*. 2019;6:564–570. doi:10.1016/j.toxrep.2019.06.004.

31. Manthripragada AD, Costello S, Cockburn MG, Bronstein JM, Ritz B. Paraoxonase 1, agricultural organophosphate exposure, and Parkinson disease. *Epidemiology*. January 2010;21(1):87–94. doi:10.1097/EDE.0b013e3181c15ec6.

32. Amin R, Darwin R, Chakraborty S, Chandran D, Chopra H, Dhama K. Bovine spongiform encephalopathy, "Mad Cow's Disease" and variant Creutzfeldt-Jakob disease in humans: a critical update. *Archives of Medical Research*. July 2023;54(5):102854. doi:10.1016/j.arcmed.2023.102854.

33. Houssin D. La vache folle: 20 ans après [Mad cow disease: 20 years after]. *La revue du praticien.* May 2018;68(5):495–500.

34. Martelli W, Trupia C, Ingravalle F, Ru G. Che fine ha fatto la mucca pazza? [What has become of the mad cow disease?]. *Epidemiologia & Prevenzione.* January–April 2022;46(1–2):23–24. doi:10.19191/EP22.1-2.P023.011.

35. Bolton DC, McKinley MP, Prusiner SB. Identification of a protein that purifies with the scrapie prion. *Science.* December 24, 1982;218(4579):1309–1311. doi:10.1126/science.6815801.

36. Diener TO, McKinley MP, Prusiner SB. Viroids and prions. *Proceedings of the National Academy of Sciences of the United States of America.* September 1982;79(17):5220–5224. doi:10.1073/pnas.79.17.5220.

37. Kasper KC, Stites DP, Bowman KA, Panitch H, Prusiner SB. Immunological studies of scrapie infection. *Journal of Neuroimmunology.* November 1982;3(3):187–201. doi:10.101 6/0165-5728(82)90022-4.

38. Prusiner SB. Research on scrapie. *The Lancet.* August 28, 1982;2(8296):494–495. doi:10.1016/s0140-6736(82)90519-0.

39. Prusiner SB. Novel proteinaceous infectious particles cause scrapie. *Science.* April 9, 1982;216(4542):136–144. doi:10.1126/science.6801762.

40. Prusiner SB, Bolton DC, Groth DF, Bowman KA, Cochran SP, McKinley MP. Further purification and characterization of scrapie prions. *Biochemistry.* December 21, 1982;21(26):6942–6950. doi:10.1021/bi00269a050.

41. Prusiner SB, Cochran SP, Groth DF, Downey DE, Bowman KA, Martinez HM. Measurement of the scrapie agent using an incubation time interval assay. *Annals of Neurology.* April 1982;11(4):353–358. doi:10.1002/ana.410110406.

42. Prusiner SB, Gajdusek C, Alpers MP. Kuru with incubation periods exceeding two decades. *Annals of Neurology.* July 1982;12(1):1–9. doi:10.1002/ana.410120102.

43. Braak H, Del Tredici K. Invited article: nervous system pathology in sporadic Parkinson disease. *Neurology.* May 13, 2008;70(20):1916–1925. doi:10.1212/01.wnl.0000312279.49272.9f.

44. Chu Y, Kordower JH. Lewy body pathology in fetal grafts. *Annals of the New York Academy of Sciences.* January 2010;1184:55–67. doi:10.1111/j.1749-6632.2009.05229.x.

45. Kordower JH, Brundin P. Lewy body pathology in long-term fetal nigral transplants: is Parkinson's disease transmitted from one neural system to another? *Neuropsychopharmacology.* January 2009;34(1):254. doi:10.1038/npp.2008.161.

46. Kordower JH, Chu Y, Hauser RA, Olanow CW, Freeman TB. Transplanted dopaminergic neurons develop PD pathologic changes: a second case report. *Movement Disorders.* December 15, 2008;23(16):2303–2306. doi:10.1002/mds.22369.

47. Hattori N. Towards the era of biological biomarkers for Parkinson disease. *Nature Reviews Neurology.* June 2024;20(6):317–318. doi:10.1038/s41582-024-00950-2.

48. Ishiguro Y, Tsunemi T, Shimada T, et al. Extracellular vesicles contain filamentous alpha-synuclein and facilitate the propagation of Parkinson's pathology. *Biochemical and Biophysical Research Communications.* April 9, 2024;703:149620. doi:10.1016/j.bbrc.2024.149620.

49. Okuzumi A, Hatano T, Matsumoto G, et al. Propagative alpha-synuclein seeds as serum biomarkers for synucleinopathies. *Nature Medicine.* June 2023;29(6):1448–1455. doi:10.1038/ s41591-023-02358-9.

50. Dorsey ER, De Miranda BR, Horsager J, Borghammer P. The body, the brain, the environment, and Parkinson's disease. *Journal of Parkinson's Disease.* 2024;14(3):363–381. doi:10.3233/ JPD-240019.

51. Borghammer P. The brain-first vs. body-first model of Parkinson's disease with comparison to alternative models. *Journal of Neural Transmission.* June 2023;130(6):737–753. doi:10.1007/ s00702-023-02633-6.

52. Olanow CW, Kordower JH. Modeling Parkinson's disease. *Annals of Neurology*. October 2009;66(4):432–436. doi:10.1002/ana.21832.

53. Beckman D, Chakrabarty P, Ott S, et al. A novel tau-based rhesus monkey model of Alzheimer's pathogenesis. *Alzheimers & Dementia*. June 2021;17(6):933–945. doi:10.1002/alz.12318.

54. Beckman D, Diniz GB, Ott S, et al. Temporal progression of tau pathology and neuroinflammation in a rhesus monkey model of Alzheimer's disease. *Alzheimer's & Dementia*. June 21, 2024. doi:10.1002/alz.13868.

55. Day JH, Della Santina CM, Maretich P, et al. HiExM: high-throughput expansion microscopy enables scalable super-resolution imaging. *bioRxiv*. September 25, 2024 [Preprint]. doi:10.1101/2023.02.07.527509.

56. Matschke J, Hartmann K, Pfefferle S, et al. Inefficient tissue immune response against MPXV in an immunocompromised mpox patient. *Journal of Medical Virology*. July 2024;96(7):e29811. doi:10.1002/jmv.29811.

57. Shin TW, Wang H, Zhang C, et al. Dense, continuous membrane labeling and expansion microscopy visualization of ultrastructure in tissues. *bioRxiv*. March 8, 2024 [Preprint]. doi:10.1101/2024.03.07.583776.

58. Valdes PA, Yu CJ, Aronson J, et al. Improved immunostaining of nanostructures and cells in human brain specimens through expansion-mediated protein decrowding. *Science Translational Medicine*. January 31, 2024;16(732):eabo0049. doi:10.1126/scitranslmed.abo0049.

59. Pai-Dhungat JV. Albert Szent-Gyorgyi: discoverer of vitamin C. *Journal of the Association of Physicians of India*. June 2015;63(6):93.

Chapter 6: The Parkinson's 25

1. Dauer W, Przedborski S. Parkinson's disease: mechanisms and models. *Neuron*. September 11, 2003;39(6):889–909. doi:10.1016/S0896-6273(03)00568-3.

2. Benefits of quitting. American Lung Association. https://www.lung.org/quit-smoking/i-want-to-quit/benefits-of-quitting. Accessed September 23, 2024.

3. Benefits of quitting smoking. Centers for Disease Control and Prevention. Updated May 15, 2024. https://www.cdc.gov/tobacco/about/benefits-of-quitting.html.

4. Spencer J. Kale, watermelon and even some organic foods pose high pesticide risk, analysis finds. *The Guardian*. April 18, 2024. https://www.theguardian.com/environment/2024/apr/18/fruits-vegetables-pesticide-consumer-reports.

5. Zhang Z-Y, Liu X-J, Hong X-Y. Effects of home preparation on pesticide residues in cabbage. *Food Control*. December 1, 2007;18(12):1484–1487. doi:10.1016/j.foodcont.2006.11.002.

6. Metcalfe-Roach A, Yu AC, Golz E, et al. MIND and Mediterranean diets associated with later onset of Parkinson's disease. *Movement Disorders*. 2021;36(4):977–984. doi:10.1002/mds.28464.

7. Alcalay RN, Gu Y, Mejia-Santana H, Cote L, Marder KS, Scarmeas N. The association between Mediterranean diet adherence and Parkinson's disease. *Movement Disorders*. 2012;27(6):771–774. doi:10.1002/mds.24918.

8. Bisaglia M. Mediterranean diet and Parkinson's disease. *International Journal of Molecular Sciences*. 2023;24(1):42.

9. Montano L, Pironti C, Pinto G, et al. Polychlorinated biphenyls (PCBs) in the environment: occupational and exposure events, effects on human health and fertility. *Toxics*. July 1, 2022;10(7):365. doi:10.3390/toxics10070365.

10. Petersen MS, Halling J, Bech S, et al. Impact of dietary exposure to food contaminants on the risk of Parkinson's disease. *NeuroToxicology*. July 1, 2008;29(4):584–590. doi:10.1016/j.neuro.2008.03.001.

11. WHO guidelines for indoor air quality: selected pollutants. World Health Organization. January 1, 2010. https://www.who.int/publications/i/item/9789289002134.

12. Hayes RB. *Dry Cleaning, Some Chlorinated Solvents and Other Industrial Chemicals*. IARC Monographs on the Evaluation of Carcinogenic Risks to Humans 63. JSTOR; 1996.

13. The latest insights for organic wine, Wine Australia. September 5, 2023. https://www.wineaustralia.com/news/market-bulletin/issue-295.

14. Xu Q, Park Y, Huang X, et al. Diabetes and risk of Parkinson's disease. *Diabetes Care*. 2011;34(4):910–915. doi:10.2337/dc10-1922.

15. Schernhammer E, Hansen J, Rugbjerg K, Wermuth L, Ritz B. Diabetes and the risk of developing Parkinson's disease in Denmark. *Diabetes Care*. 2011;34(5):1102–1108. doi:10.2337/dc10-1333.

16. Komici K, Femminella GD, Bencivenga L, Rengo G, Pagano G. Diabetes mellitus and Parkinson's disease: a systematic review and meta-analyses. *Journal of Parkinson's Disease*. 2021;11:1585–1596. doi:10.3233/JPD-212725.

17. Chohan H, Senkevich K, Patel RK, et al. Type 2 diabetes as a determinant of Parkinson's disease risk and progression. *Movement Disorders*. June 1, 2021;36(6):1420–1429. doi:10.1002/mds.28551.

18. Cheong JLY, de Pablo-Fernandez E, Foltynie T, Noyce AJ. The association between type 2 diabetes mellitus and Parkinson's disease. *Journal of Parkinson's Disease*. 2020;10:775–789. doi:10.3233/JPD-191900.

19. Ong KL, Stafford LK, McLaughlin SA, et al. Global, regional, and national burden of diabetes from 1990 to 2021, with projections of prevalence to 2050: a systematic analysis for the Global Burden of Disease Study 2021. *The Lancet*. 2023;402(10397):203–234. doi:10.1016/S0140-6736(23)01301-6.

20. Ross GW, Abbott RD, Petrovitch H, et al. Association of coffee and caffeine intake with the risk of Parkinson disease. *JAMA*. 2000;283(20):2674–2679. doi:10.1001/jama.283.20.2674.

21. Zhao Y, Lai Y, Konijnenberg H, et al. Association of coffee consumption and prediagnostic caffeine metabolites with incident Parkinson disease in a population-based cohort. *Neurology*. April 23, 2024;102(8):e209201. doi:10.1212/WNL.0000000000209201.

22. Munoz DG, Fujioka S. Caffeine and Parkinson disease. *Neurology*. 2018;90(5):205–206. doi:10.1212/WNL.0000000000004898.

23. Alavanja MC. Introduction: pesticides use and exposure extensive worldwide. *Reviews on Environmental Health*. October–December 2009;24(4):303–309. doi:10.1515/reveh.2009.24.4.303.

24. Pesticide breakdown by type, world, 1990 to 2021. Our World in Data. https://ourworldindata.org/grapher/pesticide-breakdown-by-type. Accessed September 8, 2024.

25. Tanner CM, Kamel F, Ross GW, et al. Rotenone, paraquat, and Parkinson's disease. *Environmental Health Perspectives*. 2011;119(6):866–872. doi:10.1289/chp.1002839.

26. Shrestha S, Parks CG, Umbach DM, et al. Pesticide use and incident Parkinson's disease in a cohort of farmers and their spouses. *Environmental Research*. December 1, 2020;191:110186. doi:10.1016/j.envres.2020.110186.

27. Kamel F, Tanner C, Umbach D, et al. Pesticide exposure and self-reported Parkinson's disease in the Agricultural Health Study. *American Journal of Epidemiology*. 2006;165(4):364–374. doi:10.1093/aje/kwk024.

28. Furlong M, Tanner CM, Goldman SM, et al. Protective glove use and hygiene habits modify the associations of specific pesticides with Parkinson's disease. *Environment International*. February 1, 2015;75:144–150. doi:10.1016/j.envint.2014.11.002.

29. Eberl K. Homeowner's guide to well water testing. Family Handyman. September 13, 2024. https://www.familyhandyman.com/article/homeowners-guide-to-well-water-testing.

30. Ritchie H, Spooner F, Roser M. Clean water. Our World in Data. https://ourworldindata .org/clean-water. Accessed September 8, 2024.

31. How Minnesota passed the country's first ban on trichloroethylene. Minnesota Pollution Control Agency. September 1, 2023. https://www.pca.state.mn.us/news-and-stories/tce -ban-in-effect.

32. Trichloroethylene (TCE) and water. Minnesota Department of Health. https:// www.ci.spring-park.mn.us/?SEC=B7F79193-A711-4C3F-AC50-33F1CE29B53D&DE =C8B4449A-F604-4ECF-8673-C9C12C4BAFE7.

33. Water treatment using carbon filters: GAC filter information. Minnesota Department of Health. Updated September 24, 2024. https://www.health.state.mn.us/communities /environment/hazardous/topics/gac.html.

34. Goria S, Pascal M, Corso M, Le Tertre A. Short-term exposure to air pollutants increases the risk of hospital admissions in patients with Parkinson's disease—a multicentric study on 18 French areas. *Atmospheric Environment*. November 1, 2021;264:118668. doi:10.1016/j .atmosenv.2021.118668.

35. Ham B. Study: indoor air cleaners fall short on removing volatile organic compounds. *MIT News*. October 29, 2021. https://news.mit.edu/2021/study-finds-indoor-air-cleaners -fall-short-removing-volatile-organic-compounds-1029.

36. Permethrin facts (reregistration eligibility decision [RED] fact sheet). EPA. June 2006. https://www3.epa.gov/pesticides/chem_search/reg_actions/reregistration/fs_PC-109701 _1-Jun-06.pdf.

37. Flight attendant links airline insecticide use to his Parkinson's. Beyond Pesticides. December 10, 2013. https://beyondpesticides.org/dailynewsblog/2013/12/flight-attendant-links-airline -insecticide-use-to-his-parkinsons-disease.

38. Nasuti C, Brunori G, Eusepi P, Marinelli L, Ciccocioppo R, Gabbianelli R. Early life exposure to permethrin: a progressive animal model of Parkinson's disease. *Journal of Pharmacological and Toxicological Methods*. January 1, 2017;83:80–86. doi:10.1016/j.vascn.2016.10.003.

39. Carloni M, Nasuti C, Fedeli D, et al. The impact of early life permethrin exposure on development of neurodegeneration in adulthood. *Experimental Gerontology*. January 1, 2012;47(1):60–66. doi:10.1016/j.exger.2011.10.006.

40. Smith Janssen KL. Nontoxic ways to protect your pet. National Resources Defense Council. January 22, 2016. https://www.nrdc.org/stories/nontoxic-ways-protect-your-pet.

41. Keenan J. Full guide: Safest flea and tick prevention for dogs. *Dogs Naturally Magazine*. Updated April 24, 2024. https://dogsnaturallymagazine.com/new-fda-warning-about-flea -and-tick-medications.

42. Population surrounding 1,857 Superfund remedial sites. EPA. Updated September 2020. https://www.epa.gov/sites/default/files/2015-09/documents/webpopulationrsuperfund sites9.28.15.pdf.

43. Search for Superfund sites where you live. EPA. https://www.epa.gov/superfund /search-superfund-sites-where-you-live. Accessed September 15, 2024.

44. How can I reduce my exposure and my family's exposure? Agency for Toxic Substances and Disease Registry, CDC. https://www.atsdr.cdc.gov/tox-tool/trichloroethylene/06/tce_6a _s3.html. Accessed September 19, 2024.

45. A citizen's guide to vapor intrusion mitigation. EPA. September 2012. https:// www.epa.gov/sites/default/files/2015-04/documents/a_citizens_guide_to_vapor_intrusion _mitigation_.pdf.

46. Pestano P. Dry cleaning chemicals hang around—on your clothes. Environmental Working Group. September 12, 2011. https://www.ewg.org/news-insights/news/dry-cleaning -chemicals-hang-around-your-clothes.

47. Tudi M, Daniel Ruan H, Wang L, et al. Agriculture development, pesticide application and its impact on the environment. *International Journal of Environmental Research and Public Health.* January 27, 2021;18(3):1112. doi:10.3390/ijerph18031112.

48. Pohanish RP. In: Pohanish RP, ed. *Sittig's Handbook of Pesticides and Agricultural Chemicals (Second Edition).* William Andrew Publishing; 2015:629–724. doi.org/10.1016 /B978-1-4557-3148-0.00016-9.

49. Baltazar MT, Dinis-Oliveira RJ, de Lourdes Bastos M, Tsatsakis AM, Duarte JA, Carvalho F. Pesticides exposure as etiological factors of Parkinson's disease and other neurodegenerative diseases—a mechanistic approach. *Toxicology Letters.* October 15, 2014;230(2):85–103. doi:10.1016/j.toxlet.2014.01.039.

50. Mohammadi H, Ghassemi-Barghi N, Malakshah O, Ashari S. Pyrethroid exposure and neurotoxicity: a mechanistic approach. *Archives of Industrial Hygiene and Toxicology.* 2019;70(2):74–89. doi:10.2478/aiht-2019-70-3263.

51. Singh AK, Tiwari MN, Prakash O, Singh MP. A current review of cypermethrin-induced neurotoxicity and nigrostriatal dopaminergic neurodegeneration. *Current Neuropharmacology.* March 2012;10(1):64–71. doi:10.2174/157015912799362779.

52. Stephenson J. Exposure to home pesticides linked to Parkinson disease. *JAMA.* 2000;283(23):3055–3056. doi:10.1001/jama.283.23.3055.

53. Kross BC, Burmeister LF, Ogilvie LK, Fuortes LJ, Fu CM. Proportionate mortality study of golf course superintendents. *American Journal of Industrial Medicine.* 1996;29(5):501–506.

54. Uteova A. "Botox for your lawn": the controversial use of pesticides on golf courses. *The Guardian.* August 6, 2022. https://www.theguardian.com/us-news/2022/aug/06/pesticides -golf-courses-health-problems.

55. Global golf participation reaches record levels. *Golf Course Industry.* December 14, 2021. https://www.golfcourseindustry.com/news/global-golf-participation-levels-record.

56. Faber S, Rabin A. EWG: Schools near pesticide spray zones could lose health protections. Environmental Working Group. Updated November 2, 2023. https://www .ewg.org/news-insights/news/2023/11/ewg-schools-near-pesticide-spray-zones-could-lose -health-protections.

57. Ucar T, Hall FR. Windbreaks as a pesticide drift mitigation strategy: a review. *Pest Management Science.* 2001;57(8):663–675. doi:10.1002/ps.341.

58. Zivan O, Bohbot-Raviv Y, Dubowski Y. Primary and secondary pesticide drift profiles from a peach orchard. *Chemosphere.* June 1, 2017;177:303–310. doi:10.1016/j. chemosphere.2017.03.014.

59. Imus D. Pesticides on playing fields. *Fox News.* Updated October 24, 2015. https://www .foxnews.com/health/pesticides-on-playing-fields.

60. Ingredients used in pesticide products—2,4-D. EPA. Updated February 14, 2024. https:// www.epa.gov/ingredients-used-pesticide-products/24 d.

61. The unhealthy link between football and pesticides. Pesticide-Free Cambridge. July 1, 2021. https://www.pesticidefreecambridge.org/post/the-unhealthy-link-between -football-and-pesticides.

62. The Conversation, Kaplan S. Is your kid playing soccer on a field covered in pesticides? That depends on where you live. *Fast Company.* https://www.fastcompany.com/90859065 /is-your-kid-playing-soccer-on-a-field-covered-in-pesticides-that-depends-on-where-you-live.

63. 2,4-Dichlorophenoxyacetic acid. ACS Chemistry for Life. August 27, 2012. https://www .acs.org/molecule-of-the-week/archive/d/24-dichlorophenoxyacetic-acid.html.

64. Tanner CM, Ross GW, Jewell SA, et al. Occupation and risk of parkinsonism: a multicenter case-control study. *Archives of Neurology.* September 2009;66(9):1106–1113. doi:10.1001/ archneurol.2009.195.

65. de Graaf L, Talibov M, Boulanger M, et al. Health of greenspace workers: morbidity and mortality data from the AGRICAN cohort. *Environmental Research.* 2022;212:113375.

66. Ye S, Kim H, Jeong-Choi K, et al. Parkinson's disease among firefighters: a focused review on the potential effects of exposure to toxic chemicals at the fire scene. *Korean Journal of Biological Psychiatry.* 2017;24(1):19–25.

67. Kotwani R, Clapp AN, Huggins HE, Vaou O, Hohler ADP. Assessment of Parkinson's disease symptoms and toxin exposures in firefighters: a cross-sectional survey. *Journal of Basic and Clinical Pharmacy.* 2022;13(3):172–177.

68. Gorell JM, Johnson CC, Rybicki BA, et al. Occupational exposures to metals as risk factors for Parkinson's disease. *Neurology.* March 1997;48(3):650–658. doi:10.1212/WNL.48 .3.650.

69. Attia P. *Outlive: The Science and Art of Longevity.* Harmony; 2023.

70. Ahlskog JE. Does vigorous exercise have a neuroprotective effect in Parkinson disease? *Neurology.* 2011;77(3):288–294. doi:doi:10.1212/WNL.0b013e318225ab66.

71. Müller J, Myers J. Association between physical fitness, cardiovascular risk factors, and Parkinson's disease. *European Journal of Preventive Cardiology.* September 2018;25(13):1409–1415. doi:10.1177/2047487318771168.

72. Fang X, Han D, Cheng Q, et al. Association of levels of physical activity with risk of Parkinson disease: a systematic review and meta-analysis. *JAMA Network Open.* 2018;1(5):e182421–e182421.

73. Goodwin VA, Richards SH, Taylor RS, Taylor AH, Campbell JL. The effectiveness of exercise interventions for people with Parkinson's disease: a systematic review and meta-analysis. *Movement Disorders.* 2008;23(5):631–640. doi:10.1002/mds.21922.

74. Crizzle AM, Newhouse IJ. Is physical exercise beneficial for persons with Parkinson's disease? *Clinical Journal of Sport Medicine.* September 2006;16(5):422–425. doi:10.1097/01. jsm.0000244612.55550.7d.

75. Johansson ME, Cameron IGM, Van der Kolk NM, et al. Aerobic exercise alters brain function and structure in Parkinson's disease: a randomized controlled trial. *Annals of Neurology.* 2022;91(2):203–216. doi:10.1002/ana.26291.

76. Sringean J. Sleep and circadian rhythm dysfunctions in movement disorders beyond Parkinson's disease and atypical parkinsonisms. *Current Opinion in Neurology.* August 1, 2024;37(4):414–420. doi:10.1097/WCO.0000000000001286.

77. Videnovic A, Golombek D. Circadian and sleep disorders in Parkinson's disease. *Experimental Neurology.* May 2013;243:45–56. doi:10.1016/j.expneurol.2012.08.018.

78. Lysen TS, Darweesh SKL, Ikram MK, Luik AI, Ikram MA. Sleep and risk of parkinsonism and Parkinson's disease: a population-based study. *Brain.* July 1, 2019;142(7):2013–2022. doi:10.1093/brain/awz113.

79. Postuma RB, Gagnon JF, Bertrand JA, Génier Marchand D, Montplaisir JY. Parkinson risk in idiopathic REM sleep behavior disorder: preparing for neuroprotective trials. *Neurology.* March 17, 2015;84(11):1104–1113. doi:10.1212/wnl.0000000000001364.

80. Amara AW, Chahine LM, Videnovic A. Treatment of sleep dysfunction in Parkinson's disease. *Current Treatment Options in Neurology.* July 2017;19(7):26. doi:10.1007/ s11940-017-0461-6.

81. Steele TA, St Louis EK, Videnovic A, Auger RR. Circadian rhythm sleep-wake disorders: a contemporary review of neurobiology, treatment, and dysregulation in neurodegenerative disease. *Neurotherapeutics.* January 2021;18(1):53–74. doi:10.1007/s13311-021-01031-8.

82. Videnovic A, Breen DP, Barker RA, Zee PC. The central clock in patients with Parkinson disease—reply. *JAMA Neurology.* November 2014;71(11):1456–1457. doi:10.1001/ jamaneurol.2014.2711.

83. Videnovic A, Ju YS, Arnulf I, et al. Clinical trials in REM sleep behavioural disorder: challenges and opportunities. *Journal of Neurology, Neurosurgery, and Psychiatry*. July 2020;91(7):740–749. doi:10.1136/jnnp-2020-322875.

84. Videnovic A, Noble C, Reid KJ, et al. Circadian melatonin rhythm and excessive daytime sleepiness in Parkinson disease. *JAMA Neurology*. April 2014;71(4):463–469. doi:10.1001/jamaneurol.2013.6239.

85. Zee PC, Attarian H, Videnovic A. Circadian rhythm abnormalities. *Continuum (Minneapolis, MN)*. February 2013;19(1 Sleep Disorders):132–147. doi:10.1212/01.CON.0000427209.21177.aa.

86. Jafari S, Etminan M, Aminzadeh F, Samii A. Head injury and risk of Parkinson disease: a systematic review and meta-analysis. *Movement Disorders*. August 2013;28(9):1222–1229. doi:10.1002/mds.25458.

87. Lee PC, Bordelon Y, Bronstein J, Ritz B. Traumatic brain injury, paraquat exposure, and their relationship to Parkinson disease. *Neurology*. November 13, 2012;79(20):2061–2066. doi:10.1212/WNL.0b013e3182749f28.

88. O'Connor KL, Baker MM, Dalton SL, Dompier TP, Broglio SP, Kerr ZY. Epidemiology of sport-related concussions in high school athletes: National Athletic Treatment, Injury and Outcomes Network (NATION), 2011–2012 through 2013–2014. *Journal of Athletic Training*. March 2017;52(3):175–185. doi:10.4085/1062-6050-52.1.15.

89. Marar M, McIlvain NM, Fields SK, Comstock RD. Epidemiology of concussions among United States high school athletes in 20 sports. *American Journal of Sports Medicine*. April 2012;40(4):747–755. doi:10.1177/0363546511435626.

90. Parkinson's disease and Agent Orange. US Department of Veterans Affairs. https://www.publichealth.va.gov/exposures/agentorange/conditions/parkinsonsdisease.asp. Accessed August 15, 2024.

91. Yun E. Parkinson's disease now covered under Camp Lejeune Family Member Program. US Department of Veterans Affairs. November 13, 2023. https://news.va.gov/125968/parkinsons-disease-covered-camp-lejeune-program.

92. Massaad E, Kiapour A. Long-term health outcomes of traumatic brain injury in veterans. *JAMA Network Open*. 2024;7(2):e2354546–e2354546. doi:10.1001/jamanetworkopen.2023.54546.

93. VA to expand benefits for traumatic brain injury. US Department of Veterans Affairs. Updated June 3, 2015. https://www.va.gov/healthbenefits/news/VA_to_Expand_Benefits_for_Traumatic_Brain_Injury.asp.

94. Maldonado A. Cleaning up Shaw's water. Air Force Civil Engineer Center. March 15, 2019. https://www.nellis.af.mil/News/Article/1786436/cleaning-up-shaws-water.

95. Superfund site: Plattsburgh Air Force Base, Plattsburgh, NY, Health and Environment. EPA. https://cumulis.epa.gov/supercpad/SiteProfiles/index.cfm?fuseaction=second.Healthenv&id=0202439. Accessed September 8, 2024.

96. News21 Staff, Roels C, Smith B, St. Clair A. Military bases' contamination will affect water for generations. Center for Public Integrity. August 18, 2017. https://publicintegrity.org/environment/military-bases-contamination-will-affect-water-for-generations.

Chapter 7: Amplify the Voices

1. Hack N, Akbar U, Monari EH, et al. Person-centered care in the home setting for Parkinson's disease: Operation House Call quality of care pilot study. *Parkinson's Disease*. 2015;2015:639494. doi:10.1155/2015/639494.

2. Bloem BR, Okun MS, Klein C. Parkinson's disease. *The Lancet*. June 12, 2021;397(10291):2284–2303. doi:10.1016/S0140-6736(21)00218-X.

3. Morishita T, Rahman M, Foote KD, et al. DBS candidates that fall short on a levodopa challenge test: alternative and important indications. *Neurologist*. September 2011;17(5):263–268. doi:10.1097/NRL.0b013e31822d1069.

4. Okun MS, Fernandez HH, Rodriguez RL, Foote KD. Identifying candidates for deep brain stimulation in Parkinson's disease: the role of the primary care physician. *Geriatrics*. May 2007;62(5):18–24.

5. Okun MS, Foote KD. Parkinson's disease DBS: what, when, who and why? The time has come to tailor DBS targets. *Expert Review of Neurotherapeutics*. December 2010;10(12):1847–1857. doi:10.1586/ern.10.156.

6. Okun MS, Tagliati M, Pourfar M, et al. Management of referred deep brain stimulation failures: a retrospective analysis from 2 movement disorders centers. *Archives of Neurology*. August 2005;62(8):1250–1255. doi:10.1001/archneur.62.8.noc40425.

7. Wagle Shukla A, Okun MS. Surgical treatment of Parkinson's disease: patients, targets, devices, and approaches. *Neurotherapeutics*. January 2014;11(1):47–59. doi:10.1007/s13311-013-0235-0.

8. Okun MS, Ramirez-Zamora A, Foote KD. Neuromedicine Service and Science Hub Model. *JAMA Neurology*. March 1, 2018;75(3):271–272. doi:10.1001/jamaneurol.2017.3976.

9. Wagner EH. Chronic disease management: what will it take to improve care for chronic illness? *Effective Clinical Practice*. August–September 1998;1(1):2–4.

10. Willis AW, Roberts E, Beck JC, et al. Incidence of Parkinson disease in North America. *npj Parkinson's Disease*. December 15, 2022;8(1):170. doi:10.1038/s41531-022-00410-y.

11. Dorsey ER, Bloem BR. The Parkinson pandemic—a call to action. *JAMA Neurology*. January 1, 2018;75(1):9–10. doi:10.1001/jamaneurol.2017.3299.

12. Dorsey ER, Sherer T, Okun MS, Bloem BR. The emerging evidence of the Parkinson pandemic. *Journal of Parkinson's Disease*. 2018;8(s1):S3–S8. doi:10.3233/JPD-181474.

13. Chamberlin S, Mphande M, Phiri K, Kalande P, Dovel K. How HIV clients find their way back to the ART clinic: a qualitative study of disengagement and re-engagement with HIV care in Malawi. *AIDS and Behavior*. March 2022;26(3):674–685. doi:10.1007/s10461-021-03427-1.

14. Galli M, Borderi M, Viale P. HIV policy in Italy and recommendations across the HIV care continuum. *Infezioni in medicina*. March 1, 2020;28(1):17–28.

15. Jacob Arriola KR, Ellis A, Webb-Girard A, et al. Designing integrated interventions to improve nutrition and WASH behaviors in Kenya. *Pilot and Feasibility Studies*. 2020;6:10. doi:10.1186/s40814-020-0555-x.

16. Johnson M, Samarina A, Xi H, et al. Barriers to access to care reported by women living with HIV across 27 countries. *AIDS Care*. 2015;27(10):1220–1230. doi:10.1080/09540121.2015.1046416.

17. Morgan-Siebe JP. A social work plan to promote HIV testing: a social marketing approach. *Social Work in Health Care*. March 2017;56(3):141–154. doi:10.1080/00981389.2016.1265626.

18. Parker A, Johnson-Motoyama M, Mariscal ES, Guilamo-Ramos V, Reynoso E, Fernandez C. Novel service delivery approach to address reproductive health disparities within immigrant Latino communities in geographic hot spots: an implementation study. *Health and Social Work*. August 1, 2020;45(3):155–163. doi:10.1093/hsw/hlaa014.

19. All-cause mortality after antiretroviral therapy initiation in HIV-positive women from Europe, sub-Saharan Africa and the Americas. *AIDS*. February 1, 2020;34(2):277–289. doi:10.1097/QAD.0000000000002399.

20. de Sousa ACL, Eleuterio TA, Coutinho JVA, Guimaraes RM. Assessing antiretroviral therapy success in HIV/AIDS morbidity and mortality trends in Brazil, 1990–2017: an interrupted

time series study. *International Journal of STD and AIDS*. February 2021;32(2):127–134. doi:10.1177/0956462420952989.

21. Ji Y, Wang Z, Shen J, et al. Trends and characteristics of all-cause mortality among HIV-infected inpatients during the HAART era (2006–2015) in Shanghai, China. *BioScience Trends*. March 22, 2017;11(1):62–68. doi:10.5582/bst.2016.01195.

22. Johnson LF, May MT, Dorrington RE, et al. Estimating the impact of antiretroviral treatment on adult mortality trends in South Africa: a mathematical modelling study. *PLOS Medicine*. December 2017;14(12):e1002468. doi:10.1371/journal.pmed.1002468.

23. Mor Z, Sheffer R, Chemtob D. Causes of death and mortality trends of all individuals reported with HIV/AIDS in Israel, 1985–2010. *Journal of Public Health (Oxford)*. March 1, 2018;40(1):56–64. doi:10.1093/pubmed/fdx039.

24. Saavedra A, Campinha-Bacote N, Hajjar M, et al. Causes of death and factors associated with early mortality of HIV-infected adults admitted to Korle-Bu Teaching Hospital. *Pan African Medical Journal*. 2017;27:48. doi:10.11604/pamj.2017.27.48.8917.

25. Smiley CL, Rebeiro PF, Cesar C, et al. Estimated life expectancy gains with antiretroviral therapy among adults with HIV in Latin America and the Caribbean: a multisite retrospective cohort study. *The Lancet HIV*. May 2021;8(5):e266–e273. doi:10.1016/S2352-3018(20)30358-1.

26. Koenig R. Global health. South Africa bolsters HIV/AIDS plan, but obstacles remain. *Science*. December 1, 2006;314(5804):1378–1379. doi:10.1126/science.314.5804.1378.

27. Leeper SC, Reddi A. United States global health policy: HIV/AIDS, maternal and child health, and the President's Emergency Plan for AIDS Relief (PEPFAR). *AIDS*. September 10, 2010;24(14):2145–2149. doi:10.1097/QAD.0b013e32833cbb41.

28. Matheson R, Brion S, Sharma A, et al. Realizing the promise of the global plan: engaging communities and promoting the health and human rights of women living with HIV. *Journal of Acquired Immune Deficiency Syndromes*. May 1, 2017;75 Suppl 1:S86–S93. doi:10.1097/QAI.0000000000001330.

29. Mendelson M, Matsoso MP. The World Health Organization Global Action Plan for antimicrobial resistance. *South African Medical Journal*. April 6, 2015;105(5):325. doi:10.7196/samj.9644.

30. Bogetofte H, Alamyar A, Blaabjerg M, Meyer M. Levodopa therapy for Parkinson's disease: history, current status and perspectives. *CNS & Neurological Disorders—Drug Targets*. 2020;19(8):572–583. doi:10.2174/1871527319666200722153156.

31. Fahn S. The history of dopamine and levodopa in the treatment of Parkinson's disease. *Movement Disorders*. 2008;23 Suppl 3:S497–S508. doi:10.1002/mds.22028.

32. Goetz CG. The history of Parkinson's disease: early clinical descriptions and neurological therapies. *Cold Spring Harbor Perspectives in Medicine*. September 2011;1(1):a008862. doi:10.1101/cshperspect.a008862.

33. Goetz CG, Chmura TA, Lanska DJ. Seminal figures in the history of movement disorders: Sydenham, Parkinson, and Charcot: part 6 of the MDS-sponsored History of Movement Disorders exhibit, Barcelona, June 2000. *Movement Disorders*. May 2001;16(3):537–540. doi:10.1002/mds.1113.

34. Goldman JG, Goetz CG. History of Parkinson's disease. *Handbook of Clinical Neurology*. 2007;83:107–128. doi:10.1016/S0072-9752(07)83005-3.

35. Hoehn MM. The natural history of Parkinson's disease in the pre-levodopa and post-levodopa eras. *Neurologic Clinics*. May 1992;10(2):331–339.

36. Li S, Le W. Milestones of Parkinson's disease research: 200 years of history and beyond. *Neuroscience Bulletin*. October 2017;33(5):598–602. doi:10.1007/s12264-017-0178-2.

37. Mulhearn RJ. The history of James Parkinson and his disease. *Australian and New Zealand Journal of Medicine*. May 1971;1 Suppl 1:1–6. doi:10.1111/j.1445-5994.1971.tb 02558.x.

38. Zheng GQ. Therapeutic history of Parkinson's disease in Chinese medical treatises. *Journal of Alternative and Complementary Medicine*. November 2009;15(11):1223–1230. doi:10.1089/ acm.2009.0101.

39. Azmi H, Walter BL, Brooks A, Richard IH, Amodeo K, Okun MS. Editorial: hospitalization and Parkinson's disease: safety, quality and outcomes. *Frontiers in Aging Neuroscience*. 2024;16:1398947. doi:10.3389/fnagi.2024.1398947.

40. Chou KL, Zamudio J, Schmidt P, et al. Hospitalization in Parkinson disease: a survey of National Parkinson Foundation centers. *Parkinsonism & Related Disorders*. July 2011;17(6):440–445. doi:10.1016/j.parkreldis.2011.03.002.

41. Hassan A, Wu SS, Schmidt P, et al. High rates and the risk factors for emergency room visits and hospitalization in Parkinson's disease. *Parkinsonism & Related Disorders*. November 2013;19(11):949–954. doi:10.1016/j.parkreldis.2013.06.006.

42. Shahgholi L, De Jesus S, Wu SS, et al. Hospitalization and rehospitalization in Parkinson disease patients: data from the National Parkinson Foundation Centers of Excellence. *PLOS One*. 2017;12(7):e0180425. doi:10.1371/journal.pone.0180425.

43. Zeldenrust F, Lidstone S, Wu S, et al. Variations in hospitalization rates across Parkinson's Foundation Centers of Excellence. *Parkinsonism & Related Disorders*. December 2020;81:123–128. doi:10.1016/j.parkreldis.2020.09.006.

44. Akbar U, He Y, Dai Y, et al. Weight loss and impact on quality of life in Parkinson's disease. *PLOS One*. 2015;10(5):e0124541. doi:10.1371/journal.pone.0124541.

45. Ma K, Xiong N, Shen Y, et al. Weight loss and malnutrition in patients with Parkinson's disease: current knowledge and future prospects. *Frontiers in Aging Neuroscience*. 2018;10:1. doi:10.3389/fnagi.2018.00001.

46. Martino T, Melchionda D, Tonti P, et al. Weight loss and decubitus duodenal ulcer in Parkinson's disease treated with levodopa-carbidopa intestinal gel infusion. *Journal of Neural Transmission*. December 2016;123(12):1395–1398. doi:10.1007/s00702-016-1618-2.

47. Uc EY, Struck LK, Rodnitzky RL, Zimmerman B, Dobson J, Evans WJ. Predictors of weight loss in Parkinson's disease. *Movement Disorders*. July 2006;21(7):930–936. doi:10.1002/ mds.20837.

48. Wills AM, Li R, Perez A, Ren X, Boyd J. Predictors of weight loss in early treated Parkinson's disease from the NET-PD LS-1 cohort. *Journal of Neurology*. August 2017;264(8):1746–1753. doi:10.1007/s00415-017-8562-4.

49. Yoon SY, Heo SJ, Lee HJ, et al. Initial BMI and weight loss over time predict mortality in Parkinson disease. *Journal of American Medical Directors Association*. October 2022;23(10):1719 e1–1719 e7. doi:10.1016/j.jamda.2022.07.015.

50. Byun J, Post RH, Frost CJ, Self A, Glenn AB, Gren LH. Assessing the approach to HIV case management. *Social Work in Public Health*. 2019;34(4):307–317. doi:10.1080/19371918.201 9.1606751.

51. Gomez Sanchez MC. Intervencion de la enfermera gestora de casos durante el ingreso hospitalario de pacientes con infeccion VIH [Intervention of the case management nurse in hospital admissions of patients with HIV infection]. *Revista española de salud pública*. June 2011;85(3):237–244. doi:10.1590/S1135-57272011000300002.

52. Johnson S. Case management concerns for HIV-infected adolescents. *HIV Clinical Trials*. Spring 2012;24(2):14.

53. Ko NY, Lai YY, Liu HY, et al. Impact of the nurse-led case management program with retention in care on mortality among people with HIV-1 infection: a prospective cohort

study. *International Journal of Nursing Studies*. June 2012;49(6):656–663. doi:10.1016/j.ijnurstu.2012.01.004.

54. Marseille EA, Kevany S, Ahmed I, et al. Case management to improve adherence for HIV-infected patients receiving antiretroviral therapy in Ethiopia: a micro-costing study. *Cost Effectiveness and Resource Allocation*. December 20, 2011;9:18. doi:10.1186/1478-7547-9-18.

55. Steiner C, MacKellar D, Cham HJ, et al. Community-wide HIV testing, linkage case management, and defaulter tracing in Bukoba, Tanzania: pre-intervention and post-intervention, population-based survey evaluation. *The Lancet HIV*. October 2020;7(10):e699–e710. doi:10.1016/S2352-3018(20)30199-5.

56. Willis S, Castel AD, Ahmed T, Olejemeh C, Frison L, Kharfen M. Linkage, engagement, and viral suppression rates among HIV-infected persons receiving care at medical case management programs in Washington, DC. *Journal of Acquired Immune Deficiency Syndromes*. November 1, 2013;64 Suppl 1(0 1):S33–S41. doi:10.1097/QAI.0b013e3182a99b67.

57. Wilson MG, Husbands W, Makoroka L, et al. Counselling, case management and health promotion for people living with HIV/AIDS: an overview of systematic reviews. *AIDS and Behavior*. June 2013;17(5):1612–1625. doi:10.1007/s10461-012-0283-1.

58. Doucet S, Luke A, Anthonisen G, et al. Patient navigation programs for people with dementia, their caregivers, and members of their care team: a scoping review protocol. *JBI Evidence Synthesis*. January 1, 2022;20(1):270–276. doi:10.11124/JBIES-21-00049.

59. Doucet S, Luke A, Splane J, Azar R. Patient navigation as an approach to improve the integration of care: the case of NaviCare/SoinsNavi. *International Journal of Integrated Care*. November 15, 2019;19(4):7. doi:10.5334/ijic.4648.

60. Kelly KJ, Doucet S, Luke A. Exploring the roles, functions, and background of patient navigators and case managers: a scoping review. *International Journal of Nursing Studies*. October 2019;98:27–47. doi:10.1016/j.ijnurstu.2019.05.016.

61. Luke A, Luck KE, Doucet S. Experiences of caregivers as clients of a patient navigation program for children and youth with complex care needs: a qualitative descriptive study. *International Journal of Integrated Care*. November 10, 2020;20(4):10. doi:10.5334/ijic.5451.

62. Robinson-White S, Conroy B, Slavish KH, Rosenzweig M. Patient navigation in breast cancer: a systematic review. *Cancer Nursing*. March–April 2010;33(2):127–140. doi:10.1097/NCC.0b013e3181c40401.

63. Glick JL, Andrinopoulos KM, Theall KP, Kendall C. "Tiptoeing around the system": alternative healthcare navigation among gender minorities in New Orleans. *Transgender Health*. 2018;3(1):118–126. doi:10.1089/trgh.2018.0015.

64. Roland KB, Milliken EL, Rohan EA, et al. Use of community health workers and patient navigators to improve cancer outcomes among patients served by federally qualified health centers: a systematic literature review. *Health Equity*. 2017;1(1):61–76. doi:10.1089/heq.2017.0001.

65. Kline RM, Rocque GB, Rohan EA, et al. Patient navigation in cancer: the business case to support clinical needs. *Journal of Oncology Practice*. November 2019;15(11):585–590. doi:10.1200/JOP.19.00230.

66. Reid AE, Doucet S, Luke A. Exploring the role of lay and professional patient navigators in Canada. *Journal of Health Services Research Policy*. October 2020;25(4):229–237. doi:10.1177/1355819620911679.

67. Bloem BR, Munneke M. Revolutionising management of chronic disease: the Parkinson-Net approach. *BMJ*. March 19, 2014;348:g1838. doi:10.1136/bmj.g1838.

68. Bloem BR, Rompen L, Vries NM, Klink A, Munneke M, Jeurissen P. ParkinsonNet: a low-cost health care innovation with a systems approach from the Netherlands. *Health Affairs (Millwood)*. November 2017;36(11):1987–1996. doi:10.1377/hlthaff.2017.0832.

69. Bloem BR, Ypinga JHL, Willis A, et al. Using medical claims analyses to understand interventions for Parkinson patients. *Journal of Parkinson's Disease.* 2018;8(1):45–58. doi:10.3233/JPD-171277.

70. Canoy M, Faber MJ, Munneke M, Oortwijn W, Nijkrake MJ, Bloem BR. Hidden treasures and secret pitfalls: application of the capability approach to ParkinsonNet. *Journal of Parkinson's Disease.* 2015;5(3):575–580. doi:10.3233/JPD-150612.

71. Keus SH, Nijkrake MJ, Borm GF, et al. The ParkinsonNet trial: design and baseline characteristics. *Movement Disorders.* May 15, 2010;25(7):830–837. doi:10.1002/mds.22815.

72. Keus SH, Oude Nijhuis LB, Nijkrake MJ, Bloem BR, Munneke M. Improving community healthcare for patients with Parkinson's disease: the Dutch model. *Parkinson's Disease.* 2012;2012:543426. doi:10.1155/2012/543426.

73. Munneke M, Nijkrake MJ, Keus SH, et al. Efficacy of community-based physiotherapy networks for patients with Parkinson's disease: a cluster-randomised trial. *The Lancet Neurology.* January 2010;9(1):46–54. doi:10.1016/S1474-4422(09)70327-8.

74. Nijkrake MJ, Keus SH, Overeem S, et al. The ParkinsonNet concept: development, implementation and initial experience. *Movement Disorders.* May 15, 2010;25(7):823–829. doi:10.1002/mds.22813.

75. Rompen L, de Vries NM, Munneke M, et al. Introduction of network-based healthcare at Kaiser Permanente. *Journal of Parkinson's Disease.* 2020;10(1):207–212. doi:10.3233/JPD-191620.

76. Sturkenboom IH, Graff MJ, Hendriks JC, et al. Efficacy of occupational therapy for patients with Parkinson's disease: a randomised controlled trial. *The Lancet Neurology.* June 2014;13(6):557–566. doi:10.1016/S1474-4422(14)70055-9.

77. Talebi AH, Ypinga JHL, De Vries NM, et al. Specialized versus generic allied health therapy and the risk of Parkinson's disease complications. *Movement Disorders.* February 2023;38(2):223–231. doi:10.1002/mds.29274.

78. van der Eijk M, Bloem BR, Nijhuis FA, et al. Multidisciplinary collaboration in professional networks for PD: a mixed-method analysis. *Journal of Parkinson's Disease.* 2015;5(4):937–945. doi:10.3233/JPD-150673.

79. van der Eijk M, Faber MJ, Aarts JW, Kremer JA, Munneke M, Bloem BR. Using online health communities to deliver patient-centered care to people with chronic conditions. *Journal of Medical Internet Research.* June 25, 2013;15(6):e115. doi:10.2196/jmir.2476.

80. van Nimwegen M, Speelman AD, Hofman-van Rossum EJ, et al. Physical inactivity in Parkinson's disease. *Journal of Neurology.* December 2011;258(12):2214–2221. doi:10.1007/s00415-011-6097-7.

81. van Nimwegen M, Speelman AD, Overeem S, et al. Promotion of physical activity and fitness in sedentary patients with Parkinson's disease: randomised controlled trial. *BMJ.* March 1, 2013;346:f576. doi:10.1136/bmj.f576.

82. Wensing M, van der Eijk M, Koetsenruijter J, Bloem BR, Munneke M, Faber M. Connectedness of healthcare professionals involved in the treatment of patients with Parkinson's disease: a social networks study. *Implementation Science.* July 3, 2011;6:67. doi:10.1186/1748-5908-6-67.

83. Ypinga JHL, de Vries NM, Boonen L, et al. Effectiveness and costs of specialised physiotherapy given via ParkinsonNet: a retrospective analysis of medical claims data. *The Lancet Neurology.* February 2018;17(2):153–161. doi:10.1016/S1474-4422(17)30406-4.

84. Martinez-Martin P, Skorvanek M, Henriksen T, et al. Impact of advanced Parkinson's disease on caregivers: an international real-world study. *Journal of Neurology.* April 2023;270(4):2162–2173. doi:10.1007/s00415-022-11546-5.

85. Schiess N, Cataldi R, Okun MS, et al. Six action steps to address global disparities in Parkinson disease: a World Health Organization priority. *JAMA Neurology.* September 1, 2022;79(9):929–936. doi:10.1001/jamaneurol.2022.1783.

86. Mosley PE, Moodie R, Dissanayaka N. Caregiver burden in Parkinson disease: a critical review of recent literature. *Journal of Geriatric Psychiatry and Neurology*. September 2017;30(5):235–252. doi:10.1177/0891988717720302.

87. Oguh O, Kwasny M, Carter J, Stell B, Simuni T. Caregiver strain in Parkinson's disease: national Parkinson Foundation Quality Initiative study. *Parkinsonism & Related Disorders*. November 2013;19(11):975–979. doi:10.1016/j.parkreldis.2013.06.015.

88. Santos-Garcia D, de la Fuente-Fernandez R. Factors contributing to caregivers' stress and burden in Parkinson's disease. *Acta Neurologica Scandinavica*. April 2015;131(4):203–210. doi:10.1111/ane.12305.

89. Abendroth M. Development and initial validation of a Parkinson's disease caregiver strain risk screen. *Journal of Nursing Measurement*. 2015;23(1):4–21. doi:10.1891/1061-3749.23.1.4.

90. Geerlings AD, Kapelle WM, Sederel CJ, et al. Caregiver burden in Parkinson's disease: a mixed-methods study. *BMC Medicine*. July 10, 2023;21(1):247. doi:10.1186/s12916-023-02933-4.

91. Tan SB, Williams AF, Tan EK, Clark RB, Morris ME. Parkinson's disease caregiver strain in Singapore. *Frontiers in Neurology*. 2020;11:455. doi:10.3389/fneur.2020.00455.

92. De Jesus S, Daya A, Blumberger L, et al. Prevalence of late-stage Parkinson's disease in the US healthcare system: insights from TriNetX. *Movement Disorders*. September 2024;39(9):1592–1601. doi:10.1002/mds.29900.

93. Kluger BM, Katz M, Galifianakis NB, et al. Patient and family outcomes of community neurologist palliative education and telehealth support in Parkinson disease. *JAMA Neurology*. January 1, 2024;81(1):39–49. doi:10.1001/jamaneurol.2023.4260.

94. Kluger BM, Miyasaki J, Katz M, et al. Comparison of integrated outpatient palliative care with standard care in patients with Parkinson disease and related disorders: a randomized clinical trial. *JAMA Neurology*. May 1, 2020;77(5):551–560. doi:10.1001/jamaneurol.2019.4992.

95. Kluger BM, Pantilat S, Miyasaki J. Palliative care in Parkinson disease—is it beneficial for all?—reply. *JAMA Neurology*. November 1, 2020;77(11):1450–1451. doi:10.1001/jamaneurol.2020.3215.

96. Ahn S, Springer K, Gibson JS. Social withdrawal in Parkinson's disease: a scoping review. *Geriatric Nursing*. November–December 2022;48:258–268. doi:10.1016/j.gerinurse.2022.10.010.

97. Carolan K. "It just makes you more vulnerable as an employee": understanding the effects of disability stigma on employment in Parkinson's disease. *Chronic Illness*. December 2024;20(4):655–668. doi:10.1177/17423953231185386.

98. de la Rosa T, Scorza FA. Contextualizing stigma in Parkinson's disease research. *Clinics (São Paulo)*. 2024;79:100425. doi:10.1016/j.clinsp.2024.100425.

99. Dobreva I, Thomas J, Marr A, et al. Improving conversations about Parkinson's dementia. *Movement Disorders Clinical Practice*. July 2024;11(7):814–824. doi:10.1002/mdc3.14054.

100. Logan BA, Neargarder S, Kinger SB, Larum AK, Salazar RD, Cronin-Golomb A. Self-perceived stigma in Parkinson's disease in an online sample: comparison with in-person sample, role of anxiety, and relative utility of four measures of stigma perception. *Applied Neuropsychology: Adult*. March 5, 2024:1–10. doi:10.1080/23279095.2024.2321578.

101. Mastel-Smith B, Hermanns M, Melendez J, et al. "I got laughed at for the shuffle noise I make": Parkinson's disease and stigma. *Research and Theory for Nursing Practice*. August 21, 2024;38(3):321–338. doi:10.1891/RTNP-2024-0015.

102. Stopic V, Jost ST, Baldermann JC, et al. Parkinson's Disease Stigma Questionnaire (PDStigmaQuest): development and pilot study of a questionnaire for stigma in patients with idiopathic Parkinson's disease. *Journal of Parkinson's Disease*. 2023;13(5):829–839. doi:10.3233/JPD-230071.

103. Subramanian I. What you need to know about stigma in Parkinson's disease. Parkinson Secrets. October 12, 2023. https://www.parkinsonsecrets.com/blog/what-you-need-to-know-about-stigma-in-parkinsons-disease.

104. Zhang J, Hu W, Chen H, Meng F, Li L, Okun MS. Implementation of a novel Bluetooth technology for remote deep brain stimulation programming: the pre- and post-Covid-19 Beijing experience. *Movement Disorders.* June 2020;35(6):909–910. doi:10.1002/mds.28098.

105. Bloem BR, Dorsey ER, Okun MS. The coronavirus disease 2019 crisis as catalyst for telemedicine for chronic neurological disorders. *JAMA Neurology.* August 1, 2020;77(8):927–928. doi:10.1001/jamaneurol.2020.1452.

106. Dorsey ER, Bloem BR, Okun MS. A new day: the role of telemedicine in reshaping care for persons with movement disorders. *Movement Disorders.* November 2020;35(11):1897–1902. doi:10.1002/mds.28296.

107. Dorsey ER, Okun MS, Bloem BR. Care, convenience, comfort, confidentiality, and contagion: the 5 C's that will shape the future of telemedicine. *Journal of Parkinson's Disease.* 2020;10(3):893–897. doi:10.3233/JPD-202109.

108. Hubble JP. Interactive video conferencing and Parkinson's disease. *Kansas Medicine.* December 1992;93(12):351–352.

109. Hubble JP, Pahwa R, Michalek DK, Thomas C, Koller WC. Interactive video conferencing: a means of providing interim care to Parkinson's disease patients. *Movement Disorders.* July 1993;8(3):380–382. doi:10.1002/mds.870080326.

110. Yang W, Hamilton JL, Kopil C, et al. Current and projected future economic burden of Parkinson's disease in the U.S. *npj Parkinson's Disease.* July 9, 2020;6(1):15. doi:10.1038/s41531-020-0117-1.

111. Okun MS. U.S. tax credits to promote practical proactive preventative care for Parkinson's disease. *Journal of Parkinson's Disease.* 2024;14(2):221–226. doi:10.3233/JPD-240046.

112. Carter JH, Lyons KS, Lindauer A, Malcom J. Pre-death grief in Parkinson's caregivers: a pilot survey-based study. *Parkinsonism & Related Disorders.* December 2012;18 Suppl 3:S15–S18. doi:10.1016/j.parkreldis.2012.06.015.

113. Carter JH, Stewart BJ, Archbold PG, et al. Living with a person who has Parkinson's disease: the spouse's perspective by stage of disease. Parkinson's Study Group. *Movement Disorders.* January 1998;13(1):20–28. doi:10.1002/mds.870130108.

114. Carter JH, Stewart BJ, Lyons KS, Archbold PG. Do motor and nonmotor symptoms in PD patients predict caregiver strain and depression? *Movement Disorders.* July 15, 2008;23(9):1211–1216. doi:10.1002/mds.21686.

115. Drouot M. Prise en charge dietetique du patient parkinsonien: une necessite a chaque etape du systeme digestif [Dietary management of the Parkinson's patient: a necessity at every stage of the digestive system]. *Soins.* March 2024;69(883):26–28. doi:10.1016/j.soin.2023.12.021.

116. Evatt ML. Nutritional therapies in Parkinson's disease. *Current Treat Options in Neurology.* May 2007;9(3):198–204. doi:10.1007/BF02938409.

117. Flanagan R, Rusch C, Lithander FE, Subramanian I. The missing piece of the puzzle—the key role of the dietitian in the management of Parkinson's disease. *Parkinsonism & Related Disorders.* April 2024;121:106021. doi:10.1016/j.parkreldis.2024.106021.

118. Schindler A, Pizzorni N, Cereda E, et al. Consensus on the treatment of dysphagia in Parkinson's disease. *Journal of the Neurological Sciences.* November 15, 2021;430:120008. doi:10.1016/j.jns.2021.120008.

119. Hirayama M, Nishiwaki H, Hamaguchi T, Ohno K. Gastrointestinal disorders in Parkinson's disease and other Lewy body diseases. *npj Parkinson's Disease.* May 5, 2023;9(1):71. doi:10.1038/s41531-023-00511-2.

120. Pasricha TS, Guerrero-Lopez IL, Kuo B. Management of gastrointestinal symptoms in Parkinson's disease: a comprehensive review of clinical presentation, workup, and treatment. *Journal of Clinical Gastroenterology*. March 1, 2024;58(3):211–220. doi:10.1097/MCG.0000000000001961.

121. Raeder V, Batzu L, Untucht R, et al. The Gut Dysmotility Questionnaire for Parkinson's disease: insights into development and pretest studies. *Frontiers in Neurology*. 2023;14:1149604. doi:10.3389/fneur.2023.1149604.

122. Safarpour D, Stover N, Shprecher DR, et al. Consensus practice recommendations for management of gastrointestinal dysfunction in Parkinson disease. *Parkinsonism & Related Disorders*. July 2024;124:106982. doi:10.1016/j.parkreldis.2024.106982.

123. Yuan XY, Chen YS, Liu Z. Relationship among Parkinson's disease, constipation, microbes, and microbiological therapy. *World Journal of Gastroenterology*. January 21, 2024;30(3):225–237. doi:10.3748/wjg.v30.i3.225.

124. Bhattacharya RK, Dubinsky RM, Lai SM, Dubinsky H. Is there an increased risk of hip fracture in Parkinson's disease? A nationwide inpatient sample. *Movement Disorders*. September 15, 2012;27(11):1440–1443. doi:10.1002/mds.25073.

125. Hosseinzadeh A, Khalili M, Sedighi B, Iranpour S, Haghdoost AA. Parkinson's disease and risk of hip fracture: systematic review and meta-analysis. *Acta Neurologica Belgica*. June 2018;118(2):201–210. doi:10.1007/s13760-018-0932-x.

126. Huyke-Hernandez FA, Parashos SA, Schroder LK, Switzer JA. Hip fracture care in Parkinson disease: a retrospective analysis of 1,239 patients. *Geriatric Orthopaedic Surgery & Rehabilitation*. 2022;13:21514593221118225. doi:10.1177/21514593221118225.

127. Lisk R, Watters H, Yeong K. Hip fracture outcomes in patients with Parkinson's disease. *Clinical Medicine (London)*. June 2017;17 Suppl 3:s20. doi:10.7861/clinmedicine.17-3-s20.

128. Nam JS, Kim YW, Shin J, Chang JS, Yoon SY. Hip fracture in patients with Parkinson's disease and related mortality: a population-based study in Korea. *Gerontology*. 2021;67(5):544–553. doi:10.1159/000513730.

129. Cassani E, Cilia R, Laguna J, et al. *Mucuna pruriens* for Parkinson's disease: low-cost preparation method, laboratory measures and pharmacokinetics profile. *Journal of the Neurological Sciences*. June 15, 2016;365:175–180. doi:10.1016/j.jns.2016.04.001.

130. Caronni S, Del Sorbo F, Barichella M, et al. *Mucuna pruriens* to treat Parkinson's disease in low-income countries: recommendations and practical guidelines from the farmer to clinical trials. Paving the way for future use in clinical practice. *Parkinsonism & Related Disorders*. July 2024;124:106983. doi:10.1016/j.parkreldis.2024.106983.

131. Cilia R, Dekker MCJ, Cubo E, Agoriwo MW. Delivery of allied health therapies to people with Parkinson's disease in Africa. *Journal of Parkinson's Disease*. 2024;14(s1):S227–S239. doi:10.3233/JPD-230262.

Chapter 8: Navigate the First Frontiers of New Treatments

1. Cotzias GC, Papavasiliou PS. Autoimmunity in patients treated with levodopa. *JAMA*. February 17, 1969;207(7):1353–1354.

2. Cotzias GC. Levodopa in the treatment of parkinsonism. *JAMA*. December 27, 1971;218(13):1903–1908.

3. Cotzias GC, Papavasiliou PS, Steck A, Duby S. Parkinsonism and levodopa. *Clinical Pharmacology & Therapeutics*. March–April 1971;12(2):319–322. doi:10.1002/cpt1971122part2319.

4. Papavasiliou PS, Cotzias GC, Duby SE, Steck AJ, Fehling C, Bell MA. Levodopa in parkinsonism: potentiation of central effects with a peripheral inhibitor. *New England Journal of Medicine*. January 6, 1972;286(1):8–14. doi:10.1056/NEJM197201062860102.

5. DeLong MR. Activity of basal ganglia neurons during movement. *Brain Research*. May 12, 1972;40(1):127–135. doi:10.1016/0006-8993(72)90118-7.

6. DeLong MR. Putamen: activity of single units during slow and rapid arm movements. *Science*. March 23, 1973;179(4079):1240–1242. doi:10.1126/science.179.4079.1240.

7. DeLong MR. [Neuronal activity in the basal ganglia of the behaving monkey: insights into function and pathophysiology of clinical disorders]. *Rinsho Shinkeigaku*. December 1982;22(12):1084–1086.

8. DeLong MR. The neurophysiologic basis of abnormal movements in basal ganglia disorders. *Neurobehavioral Toxicology and Teratology*. November–December 1983;5(6):611–616.

9. Alexander GE, DeLong MR, Strick PL. Parallel organization of functionally segregated circuits linking basal ganglia and cortex. *Annual Review of Neuroscience*. 1986;9:357–381. doi:10.1146/annurev.ne.09.030186.002041.

10. Alexander GE, Crutcher MD, DeLong MR. Basal ganglia-thalamocortical circuits: parallel substrates for motor, oculomotor, "prefrontal" and "limbic" functions. *Progress in Brain Research*. 1990;85:119–146.

11. DeLong MR, Benabid AL. Discovery of high-frequency deep brain stimulation for treatment of Parkinson disease: 2014 Lasker Award. *JAMA*. September 17, 2014;312(11):1093–1094. doi:10.1001/jama.2014.11132.

12. Langston JW. MPTP: insights into the etiology of Parkinson's disease. *European Neurology*. 1987;26 Suppl 1:2–10. doi:10.1159/000116349.

13. Langston JW. Busqueda de la causa de la enfermedad de Parkinson [Search for the cause of Parkinson's disease]. *Archivos de neurobiologiá (Madrid)*. November–December 1991;54(6):264–271.

14. Langston JW. The MPTP story. *Journal of Parkinson's Disease*. 2017;7(s1):S11–S19. doi:10.3233/JPD-179006.

15. Langston JW, Ballard P, Tetrud JW, Irwin I. Chronic parkinsonism in humans due to a product of meperidine-analog synthesis. *Science*. February 25, 1983;219(4587):979–980. doi:10.1126/science.6823561.

16. Langston JW, Ballard PA, Jr. Parkinson's disease in a chemist working with 1-methyl-4-phenyl-1,2,3,6-tetrahydropyridine. *New England Journal of Medicine*. August 4, 1983;309(5):310. doi:10.1056/nejm198308043090511.

17. Tetrud JW, Langston JW. MPTP-induced parkinsonism as a model for Parkinson's disease. *Acta Neurologica Scandinavica. Supplementum*. 1989;126:35–40. doi:10.1111/j.1600-0404.1989.tb01780.x.

18. Polymeropoulos MH, Higgins JJ, Golbe LI, et al. Mapping of a gene for Parkinson's disease to chromosome 4q21-q23. *Science*. November 15, 1996;274(5290):1197–1199. doi:10.1126/science.274.5290.1197.

19. Nussbaum RL, Polymeropoulos MH. Genetics of Parkinson's disease. *Human Molecular Genetics*. 1997;6(10):1687–1691. doi:10.1093/hmg/6.10.1687.

20. Beach TG, White CL, Hamilton RL, et al. Evaluation of alpha-synuclein immunohistochemical methods used by invited experts. *Acta Neuropathologica*. September 2008;116(3):277–288. doi:10.1007/s00401-008-0409-8.

21. Adler CH, Dugger BN, Hinni ML, et al. Submandibular gland needle biopsy for the diagnosis of Parkinson disease. *Neurology*. March 11, 2014;82(10):858–864. doi:10.1212/WNL.0000000000000204.

22. Beach TG, Carew J, Serrano G, et al. Phosphorylated alpha-synuclein-immunoreactive retinal neuronal elements in Parkinson's disease subjects. *Neuroscience Letters*. June 13, 2014;571:34–38. doi:10.1016/j.neulet.2014.04.027.

23. Beach TG, Adler CH, Serrano G, et al. Prevalence of submandibular gland synucleinopathy in Parkinson's disease, dementia with Lewy bodies and other Lewy body disorders. *Journal of Parkinson's Disease*. 2016;6(1):153–163. doi:10.3233/JPD-150680.

24. Beach TG, Corbille AG, Letournel F, et al. Multicenter assessment of immunohistochemical methods for pathological alpha-synuclein in sigmoid colon of autopsied Parkinson's disease and control subjects. *Journal of Parkinson's Disease*. October 19, 2016;6(4):761–770. doi:10.3233/JPD-160888.

25. Adler CH, Beach TG, Shill HA, et al. GBA mutations in Parkinson disease: earlier death but similar neuropathological features. *European Journal of Neurology*. November 2017;24(11):1363–1368. doi:10.1111/ene.13395.

26. Adler CH, Dugger BN, Hentz JG, et al. Peripheral synucleinopathy in early Parkinson's disease: submandibular gland needle biopsy findings. *Movement Disorders*. May 2017;32(5):722–723. doi:10.1002/mds.27044.

27. Beach TG, Serrano GE, Kremer T, et al. Immunohistochemical method and histopathology judging for the systemic synuclein sampling study (S4). *Journal of Neuropathology & Experimental Neurology*. September 1, 2018;77(9):793–802. doi:10.1093/jnen/nly056.

28. Adler CH, Beach TG, Zhang N, et al. Unified staging system for Lewy body disorders: clinicopathologic correlations and comparison to Braak staging. *Journal of Neuropathology & Experimental Neurology*. October 1, 2019;78(10):891–899. doi:10.1093/jnen/nlz080.

29. Beach TG, Adler CH, Sue LI, et al. Vagus nerve and stomach synucleinopathy in Parkinson's disease, incidental Lewy body disease, and normal elderly subjects: evidence against the "body-first" hypothesis. *Journal of Parkinson's Disease*. 2021;11(4):1833–1843. doi:10.3233/JPD-212733.

30. Beach TG, Russell A, Sue LI, et al. Increased risk of autopsy-proven pneumonia with sex, season and neurodegenerative disease. *medRxiv*. January 8, 2021 [Preprint]. doi:10.1101/2021.01.07.21249410.

31. Adler CH, Serrano GE, Shill HA, et al. Symmetry of synuclein density in autopsied Parkinson's disease submandibular glands. *Neuroscience Letters*. March 10, 2024;825:137702. doi:10.1016/j.neulet.2024.137702.

32. Weiner WJ. There is no Parkinson disease. *Archives of Neurology*. June 2008;65(6):705–708. doi:10.1001/archneur.65.6.705.

33. Okubadejo NU, Okun MS, Jankovic J. Tapping the brakes on new Parkinson disease biological staging. *JAMA Neurology*. August 1, 2024;81(8):789–790. doi:10.1001/jamaneurol.2024.2054.

34. Greene BR, Premoli I, McManus K, McGrath D, Caulfield B. Predicting fall counts using wearable sensors: a novel digital biomarker for Parkinson's disease. *Sensors (Basel)*. December 22, 2021;22(1):54. doi:10.3390/s22010054.

35. Diao JA, Raza MM, Venkatesh KP, Kvedar JC. Watching Parkinson's disease with wrist-based sensors. *npj Digital Medicine*. June 13, 2022;5(1):73. doi:10.1038/s41746-022-00619-4.

36. Chen C, Kowahl NR, Rainaldi E, et al. Wrist-worn sensor-based measurements for drug effect detection with small samples in people with Lewy body dementia. *Parkinsonism & Related Disorders*. April 2023;109:105355. doi:10.1016/j.parkreldis.2023.105355.

37. Schalkamp AK, Peall KJ, Harrison NA, Sandor C. Wearable movement-tracking data identify Parkinson's disease years before clinical diagnosis. *Nature Medicine*. August 2023;29(8):2048–2056. doi:10.1038/s41591-023-02440-2.

38. Sharma M, Mishra RK, Hall AJ, et al. Remote at-home wearable-based gait assessments in progressive supranuclear palsy compared to Parkinson's disease. *BMC Neurology*. December 11, 2023;23(1):434. doi:10.1186/s12883-023-03466-2.

39. Tsakanikas V, Ntanis A, Rigas G, et al. Evaluating gait impairment in Parkinson's disease from instrumented insole and IMU sensor data. *Sensors (Basel)*. April 12, 2023;23(8):3902. doi:10.3390/s23083902.

40. Battista L, Romaniello A. A new wrist-worn tool supporting the diagnosis of parkinsonian motor syndromes. *Sensors (Basel)*. March 19, 2024;24(6):1965. doi:10.3390/s24061965.

41. Goncalves HR, Branquinho A, Pinto J, Rodrigues AM, Santos CP. Digital biomarkers of mobility and quality of life in Parkinson's disease based on a wearable motion analysis LAB. *Computer Methods and Programs in Biomedicine*. February 2024;244:107967. doi:10.1016/j.cmpb.2023.107967.

42. Illner V, Novotny M, Kouba T, et al. Smartphone voice calls provide early biomarkers of parkinsonism in rapid eye movement sleep behavior disorder. *Movement Disorders*. October 2024;39(10):1752–1762. doi:10.1002/mds.29921.

43. Janssen Daalen JM, van den Bergh R, Prins EM, et al. Digital biomarkers for non-motor symptoms in Parkinson's disease: the state of the art. *npj Digital Medicine*. July 11, 2024;7(1):186. doi:10.1038/s41746-024-01144-2.

44. Kamo H, Oyama G, Yamasaki Y, Nagayama T, Nawashiro R, Hattori N. A proof of concept: digital diary using 24-hour monitoring using wearable device for patients with Parkinson's disease in nursing homes. *Frontiers in Neurology*. 2024;15:1356042. doi:10.3389/fneur.2024.1356042.

45. Salaorni F, Bonardi G, Schena F, Tinazzi M, Gandolfi M. Wearable devices for gait and posture monitoring via telemedicine in people with movement disorders and multiple sclerosis: a systematic review. *Expert Review of Medical Devices*. January–February 2024;21(1–2):121–140. doi:10.1080/17434440.2023.2298342.

46. Sjaelland NS, Gramkow MH, Hasselbalch SG, Frederiksen KS. Digital biomarkers for the assessment of non-cognitive symptoms in patients with dementia with Lewy bodies: a systematic review. *Journal of Alzheimer's Disease*. 2024;100(2):431–451. doi:10.3233/JAD-240327.

47. Wu X, Ma L, Wei P, et al. Wearable sensor devices can automatically identify the on-off status of patients with Parkinson's disease through an interpretable machine learning model. *Frontiers in Neurology*. 2024;15:1387477. doi:10.3389/fneur.2024.1387477.

48. Zhang F, Mithani K, Breitbart S, et al. Actigraph-based quantification of sleep in children with dystonia undergoing deep brain stimulation. *Neurosurgical Focus*. June 2024;56(6):E17. doi:10.3171/2024.3.FOCUS2462.

49. Zhang W, Ling Y, Chen Z, et al. Wearable sensor-based quantitative gait analysis in Parkinson's disease patients with different motor subtypes. *npj Digital Medicine*. June 26, 2024;7(1):169. doi:10.1038/s41746-024-01163-z.

50. Srivastava G, Singh K, Tiwari MN, Singh MP. Proteomics in Parkinson's disease: current trends, translational snags and future possibilities. *Expert Review of Proteomics*. February 2010;7(1):127–139. doi:10.1586/epr.09.91.

51. Chahine LM, Stern MB, Chen-Plotkin A. Blood-based biomarkers for Parkinson's disease. *Parkinsonism & Related Disorders*. January 2014;20 Suppl 1:S99–S103. doi:10.1016/S1353-8020(13)70025-7.

52. Chen-Plotkin AS, Albin R, Alcalay R, et al. Finding useful biomarkers for Parkinson's disease. *Science Translational Medicine*. August 15, 2018;10(454):eaam6003. doi:10.1126/scitranslmed.aam6003.

53. Posavi M, Diaz-Ortiz M, Liu B, et al. Characterization of Parkinson's disease using blood-based biomarkers: a multicohort proteomic analysis. *PLOS Medicine*. October 2019;16(10):e1002931. doi:10.1371/journal.pmed.1002931.

54. Del Campo M, Vermunt L, Peeters CFW, et al. CSF proteome profiling reveals biomarkers to discriminate dementia with Lewy bodies from Alzheimer's disease. *Nature Communications*. September 13, 2023;14(1):5635. doi:10.1038/s41467-023-41122-y.

55. Shantaraman A, Dammer EB, Ugochukwu O, et al. Network proteomics of the Lewy body dementia brain reveals presynaptic signatures distinct from Alzheimer's disease. *Molecular Neurodegeneration*. August 6, 2024;19(1):60. doi:10.1186/s13024-024-00749-1.

56. Hällqvist J, Bartl M, Dakna M, et al. Plasma proteomics identify biomarkers predicting Parkinson's disease up to 7 years before symptom onset. *Nature Communications*. 2024;15(1):4759. doi:10.1038/s41467-024-48961-3.

57. Su C, Hou Y, Xu J, et al. Identification of Parkinson's disease PACE subtypes and repurposing treatments through integrative analyses of multimodal data. *npj Digital Medicine*. July 9, 2024;7(1):184. doi:10.1038/s41746-024-01175-9.

58. Cirnaru MD, Marte A, Belluzzi E, et al. LRRK2 kinase activity regulates synaptic vesicle trafficking and neurotransmitter release through modulation of LRRK2 macro-molecular complex. *Frontiers in Molecular Neuroscience*. 2014;7:49. doi:10.3389/fnmol.2014.00049.

59. Melrose HL. LRRK2 and ubiquitination: implications for kinase inhibitor therapy. *Biochemical Journal*. September 15, 2015;470(3):e21–e24. doi:10.1042/BJ20150785.

60. Berwick DC, Javaheri B, Wetzel A, et al. Pathogenic LRRK2 variants are gain-of-function mutations that enhance LRRK2-mediated repression of beta-catenin signaling. *Molecular Neurodegeneration*. January 19, 2017;12(1):9. doi:10.1186/s13024-017-0153-4.

61. Fuji RN, Flagella M, Baca M, et al. Effect of selective LRRK2 kinase inhibition on nonhuman primate lung. *Science Translational Medicine*. February 4, 2015;7(273):273ra15. doi:10.1126/scitranslmed.aaa3634.

62. Qin Q, Zhi LT, Li XT, Yue ZY, Li GZ, Zhang H. Effects of LRRK2 inhibitors on nigrostriatal dopaminergic neurotransmission. *CNS Neuroscience & Therapeutics*. February 2017;23(2):162–173. doi:10.1111/cns.12660.

63. Tasegian A, Singh F, Ganley IG, Reith AD, Alessi DR. Impact of type II LRRK2 inhibitors on signaling and mitophagy. *Biochemical Journal*. October 15, 2021;478(19):3555–3573. doi:10.1042/BCJ20210375.

64. Volta M, Melrose H. LRRK2 mouse models: dissecting the behavior, striatal neurochemistry and neurophysiology of PD pathogenesis. *Biochemical Society Transactions*. February 8, 2017;45(1):113–122. doi:10.1042/BST20160238.

65. Migdalska-Richards A, Ko WKD, Li Q, Bezard E, Schapira AHV. Oral ambroxol increases brain glucocerebrosidase activity in a nonhuman primate. *Synapse*. July 2017;71(7):e21967. doi:10.1002/syn.21967.

66. Magalhaes J, Gegg ME, Migdalska-Richards A, Schapira AH. Effects of ambroxol on the autophagy-lysosome pathway and mitochondria in primary cortical neurons. *Scientific Reports*. January 23, 2018;8(1):1385. doi:10.1038/s41598-018-19479-8.

67. Mullin S, Smith L, Lee K, et al. Ambroxol for the treatment of patients with Parkinson disease with and without glucocerebrosidase gene mutations: a nonrandomized, noncontrolled trial. *JAMA Neurology*. April 1, 2020;77(4):427–434. doi:10.1001/jamaneurol.2019.4611.

68. Yang SY, Gegg M, Chau D, Schapira A. Glucocerebrosidase activity, cathepsin D and monomeric alpha-synuclein interactions in a stem cell derived neuronal model of a PD associated GBA1 mutation. *Neurobiology of Disease*. February 2020;134:104620. doi:10.1016/j.nbd.2019.104620.

69. Vieira SRL, Schapira AHV. Glucocerebrosidase mutations: a paradigm for neurodegeneration pathways. *Free Radical Biology and Medicine*. November 1, 2021;175:42–55. doi:10.1016/j.freeradbiomed.2021.08.230.

70. Yang SY, Taanman JW, Gegg M, Schapira AHV. Ambroxol reverses tau and alpha-synuclein accumulation in a cholinergic N370S GBA1 mutation model. *Human Molecular Genetics.* July 21, 2022;31(14):2396–2405. doi:10.1093/hmg/ddac038.

71. Menozzi E, Toffoli M, Schapira AHV. Targeting the GBA1 pathway to slow Parkinson disease: insights into clinical aspects, pathogenic mechanisms and new therapeutic avenues. *Pharmacology & Therapeutics.* June 2023;246:108419. doi:10.1016/j.pharmthera.2023.108419.

72. Dash D, Mestre TA. Therapeutic update on Huntington's disease: symptomatic treatments and emerging disease-modifying therapies. *Neurotherapeutics.* October 2020;17(4):1645–1659. doi:10.1007/s13311-020-00891-w.

73. Durr A. Therapie par ARN anti-sens dans la maladie de Huntington—un immense espoir et beaucoup d'inconnues [Anti-sense oligonucleotides RNA therapy in Huntington disease: a great promise and many unknowns]. *Médical sciences (Paris).* November 2019;35(11):834–836. doi:10.1051/medsci/2019165.

74. Imbimbo BP, Triaca V, Imbimbo C, Nistico R. Investigational treatments for neurodegenerative diseases caused by inheritance of gene mutations: lessons from recent clinical trials. *Neural Regeneration Research.* August 2023;18(8):1679–1683. doi:10.4103/1673-5374.363185.

75. Tabrizi SJ, Leavitt BR, Landwehrmeyer GB, et al. Targeting huntingtin expression in patients with Huntington's disease. *New England Journal of Medicine.* June 13, 2019;380(24):2307–2316. doi:10.1056/NEJMoa1900907.

76. Friedman JH. In early Parkinson disease, daily subcutaneous lixisenatide reduced motor disability progression at 12 mo. *Annals of Internal Medicine.* September 2024;177(9):JC100. doi:10.7326/ANNALS-24-01662-JC.

77. Holscher C. Glucagon-like peptide-1 class drugs show clear protective effects in Parkinson's and Alzheimer's disease clinical trials: a revolution in the making? *Neuropharmacology.* August 1, 2024;253:109952. doi:10.1016/j.neuropharm.2024.109952.

78. Irfan H, Muneer SU, Maheshwari AB, Kumar N, Iftikhar S. Lixisenatide in early Parkinson's disease: efficacy, safety, and future directions: a correspondence. *Neurosurgical Review.* May 24, 2024;47(1):232. doi:10.1007/s10143-024-02475-0.

79. Kalinderi K, Papaliagkas V, Fidani L. GLP-1 receptor agonists: a new treatment in Parkinson's disease. *International Journal of Molecular Sciences.* March 29, 2024;25(7):3812. doi:10.3390/ijms25073812.

80. Meissner WG, Remy P, Giordana C, et al. Trial of lixisenatide in early Parkinson's disease. *New England Journal of Medicine.* April 4, 2024;390(13):1176–1185. doi:10.1056/NEJMoa2312323.

81. Rozani V, Bezimianski MG, Azuri J, Bitan M, Peretz C. Anti-diabetic drug use and reduced risk of Parkinson's disease: a community-based cohort study. *Parkinsonism & Related Disorders.* September 6, 2024;128:107132. doi:10.1016/j.parkreldis.2024.107132.

82. Vijiaratnam, N, et al. (2025). Exenatide once a week versus placebo as a potential disease-modifying treatment for people with Parkinson's disease in the UK: a phase 3, multicentre, double-blind, parallel-group, randomised, placebo-controlled trial. *The Lancet* 405(10479): 627–636.

83. Boucherie DM, Duarte GS, Machado T, et al. Parkinson's disease drug development since 1999: a story of repurposing and relative success. *Journal of Parkinson's Disease.* 2021;11(2):421–429. doi:10.3233/JPD-202184.

84. Tanner CM, Ostrem JL. Parkinson's disease. *New England Journal of Medicine.* August 1, 2024;391(5):442–452. doi:10.1056/NEJMra2401857.

85. Fanty L, Yu J, Chen N, et al. The current state, challenges, and future directions of deep brain stimulation for obsessive compulsive disorder. *Expert Review of Medical Devices.* July–December 2023;20(10):829–842. doi:10.1080/17434440.2023.2252732.

86. Frey J, Cagle J, Johnson KA, et al. Past, present, and future of deep brain stimulation: hardware, software, imaging, physiology and novel approaches. *Frontiers in Neurology.* 2022;13:825178. doi:10.3389/fneur.2022.825178.

87. Johnson KA, Dosenbach NUF, Gordon EM, et al. Proceedings of the 11th Annual Deep Brain Stimulation Think Tank: pushing the forefront of neuromodulation with functional network mapping, biomarkers for adaptive DBS, bioethical dilemmas, AI-guided neuromodulation, and translational advancements. *Frontiers in Human Neuroscience.* 2024;18:1320806. doi:10.3389/fnhum.2024.1320806.

88. Arcot Desai S, Afzal MF, Barry W, et al. Expert and deep learning model identification of iEEG seizures and seizure onset times. *Frontiers in Neuroscience.* 2023;17:1156838. doi:10.3389/fnins.2023.1156838.

89. Chiang S, Khambhati AN, Tcheng TK, et al. State-dependent effects of responsive neurostimulation depend on seizure localization. *Brain.* July 25, 2024:awae240. doi:10.1093/brain/awae240.

90. Denison T, Morrell MJ. Neuromodulation in 2035: the Neurology Future Forecasting Series. *Neurology.* January 11, 2022;98(2):65–72. doi:10.1212/WNL.0000000000013061.

91. Jarosiewicz B, Morrell M. The RNS system: brain-responsive neurostimulation for the treatment of epilepsy. *Expert Review of Medical Devices.* February 2021;18(2):129–138. doi:10.1080/17434440.2019.1683445.

92. Jobst BC, Kapur R, Barkley GL, et al. Brain-responsive neurostimulation in patients with medically intractable seizures arising from eloquent and other neocortical areas. *Epilepsia.* June 2017;58(6):1005–1014. doi:10.1111/epi.13739.

93. Nair DR, Laxer KD, Weber PB, et al. Nine-year prospective efficacy and safety of brain-responsive neurostimulation for focal epilepsy. *Neurology.* September 1, 2020;95(9):e1244–e1256. doi:10.1212/WNL.0000000000010154.

94. Sun FT, Arcot Desai S, Tcheng TK, Morrell MJ. Changes in the electrocorticogram after implantation of intracranial electrodes in humans: the implant effect. *Clinical Neurophysiology.* March 2018;129(3):676–686. doi:10.1016/j.clinph.2017.10.036.

95. Warren AEL, Butson CR, Hook MP, et al. Targeting thalamocortical circuits for closed-loop stimulation in Lennox-Gastaut syndrome. *Brain Communications.* 2024;6(3):fcae161. doi:10.1093/braincomms/fcae161.

96. Gittis AH, Yttri EA. Translating insights from optogenetics to therapies for Parkinson's disease. *Current Opinion in Biomedical Engineering.* December 2018;8:14–19. doi:10.1016/j.cobme.2018.08.008.

97. Luscher C, Pascoli V, Creed M. Optogenetic dissection of neural circuitry: from synaptic causalities to blue prints for novel treatments of behavioral diseases. *Current Opinion in Neurobiology.* December 2015;35:95–100. doi:10.1016/j.conb.2015.07.005.

98. Luscher C, Pollak P. Optogenetically inspired deep brain stimulation: linking basic with clinical research. *Swiss Medical Weekly.* 2016;146:w14278. doi:10.4414/smw.2016.14278.

99. Murphy C, Matikainen-Ankney B, Chang YH, Copits B, Creed MC. Optogenetically-inspired neuromodulation: translating basic discoveries into therapeutic strategies. *International Review of Neurobiology.* 2021;159:187–219. doi:10.1016/bs.irn.2021.06.002.

100. Vedam-Mai V, Deisseroth K, Giordano J, et al. Proceedings of the Eighth Annual Deep Brain Stimulation Think Tank: advances in optogenetics, ethical issues affecting DBS research, neuromodulatory approaches for depression, adaptive neurostimulation, and emerging DBS technologies. *Frontiers in Human Neuroscience.* 2021;15:644593. doi:10.3389/fnhum.2021.644593.

101. Eisinger RS, Cernera S, Gittis A, Gunduz A, Okun MS. A review of basal ganglia circuits and physiology: application to deep brain stimulation. *Parkinsonism & Related Disorders.* February 2019;59:9–20. doi:10.1016/j.parkreldis.2019.01.009.

102. Gittis A. Probing new targets for movement disorders. *Science*. August 3, 2018;361(6401):462. doi:10.1126/science.aau4916.

103. Gittis AH, Sillitoe RV. Circuit-specific deep brain stimulation provides insights into movement control. *Annual Review of Neuroscience*. August 2024;47(1):63–83. doi:10.1146/annurev-neuro-092823-104810.

104. Kariv S, Choi JW, Mirpour K, et al. Pilot study of acute behavioral effects of pallidal burst stimulation in Parkinson's disease. *Movement Disorders*. July 15, 2024;39(10):1873–1877. doi:10.1002/mds.29928.

105. Bower KL, Noecker AM, Frankemolle-Gilbert AM, McIntyre CC. Model-based analysis of pathway recruitment during subthalamic deep brain stimulation. *Neuromodulation*. April 2024;27(3):455–463. doi:10.1016/j.neurom.2023.02.084.

106. Hitti FL, Widge AS, Riva-Posse P, et al. Future directions in psychiatric neurosurgery: proceedings of the 2022 American Society for Stereotactic and Functional Neurosurgery meeting on surgical neuromodulation for psychiatric disorders. *Brain Stimulation*. May–June 2023;16(3):867–878. doi:10.1016/j.brs.2023.05.011.

107. Noecker AM, Mlakar J, Petersen MV, Griswold MA, McIntyre CC. Holographic visualization for stereotactic neurosurgery research. *Brain Stimulation*. March–April 2023;16(2):411–414. doi:10.1016/j.brs.2023.02.001.

108. Al Awadhi A, Tyrand R, Horn A, et al. Electrophysiological confrontation of Lead-DBS-based electrode localizations in patients with Parkinson's disease undergoing deep brain stimulation. *Neuroimage: Clinical*. 2022;34:102971. doi:10.1016/j.nicl.2022.102971.

109. Neudorfer C, Butenko K, Oxenford S, et al. Lead-DBS v3.0: mapping deep brain stimulation effects to local anatomy and global networks. *Neuroimage*. March 2023;268:119862. doi:10.1016/j.neuroimage.2023.119862.

110. Oxenford S, Roediger J, Neudorfer C, et al. Lead-OR: a multimodal platform for deep brain stimulation surgery. *Elife*. May 20, 2022;11:e72929. doi:10.7554/eLife.72929.

111. Yearley AG, Chua M, Horn A, Cosgrove GR, Rolston JD. Deep brain stimulation lead localization variability comparing intraoperative MRI versus postoperative computed tomography. *Operative Neurosurgery (Hagerstown)*. November 1, 2023;25(5):441–448. doi:10.1227/ons.0000000000000849.

112. Abbas A, Hassan MA, Shaheen RS, et al. Safety and efficacy of unilateral focused ultrasound pallidotomy on motor complications in Parkinson's disease (PD): a systematic review and meta-analysis. *Neurological Sciences*. October 2024;45(10):4687–4698. doi:10.1007/s10072-024-07617-2.

113. Cosgrove GR, Lipsman N, Lozano AM, et al. Magnetic resonance imaging-guided focused ultrasound thalamotomy for essential tremor: 5-year follow-up results. *Journal of Neurosurgery*. April 1, 2023;138(4):1028–1033. doi:10.3171/2022.6.JNS212483.

114. Elias WJ. A trial of focused ultrasound thalamotomy for essential tremor. *New England Journal of Medicine*. December 1, 2016;375(22):2202–2203. doi:10.1056/NEJMc1612210.

115. Krishna V, Fishman PS, Eisenberg HM, et al. Trial of globus pallidus focused ultrasound ablation in Parkinson's disease. *New England Journal of Medicine*. February 23, 2023;388(8):683–693. doi:10.1056/NEJMoa2202721.

116. Martinez-Fernandez R, Natera-Villalba E, Manez Miro JU, et al. Prospective long-term follow-up of focused ultrasound unilateral subthalamotomy for Parkinson disease. *Neurology*. March 28, 2023;100(13):e1395–e1405. doi:10.1212/WNL.0000000000206771.

117. Aubignat M, Tir M. Continuous subcutaneous foslevodopa-foscarbidopa in Parkinson's disease: a mini-review of current scope and future outlook. *Movement Disorders Clinical Practice*. October 2024;11(10):1188–1194. doi:10.1002/mdc3.14161.

118. Dean MN, Standaert DG. Levodopa infusion therapies for Parkinson disease. *Current Opinion in Neurology.* August 1, 2024;37(4):409–413. doi:10.1097/WCO.0000000000001277.

119. Fung VSC, Aldred J, Arroyo MP, et al. Continuous subcutaneous foslevodopa/foscarbidopa infusion for the treatment of motor fluctuations in Parkinson's disease: considerations for initiation and maintenance. *Clinical Parkinsonism & Related Disorders.* 2024;10:100239. doi:10.1016/j.prdoa.2024.100239.

120. Poplawska-Domaszewicz K, Batzu L, Falup-Pecurariu C, Chaudhuri KR. Subcutaneous levodopa: a new engine for the vintage molecule. *Neurology Therapy.* August 2024;13(4):1055–1068. doi:10.1007/s40120-024-00635-4.

121. Rozankovic PB, Johansson A, Peter K, Milanov I, Odin P. Monotherapy with infusion therapies—useful or not? *Journal of Neural Transmission.* July 5, 2024;doi:10.1007/s00702-024-02801-2.

122. Schroter N, Sajonz BEA, Jost WH, Rijntjes M, Coenen VA, Groppa S. Advanced therapies in Parkinson's disease: an individualized approach to their indication. *Journal of Neural Transmission.* April 13, 2024;131:1285–1293. doi:10.1007/s00702-024-02773-3.

123. Espay AJ, Stocchi F, Pahwa R, et al. Safety and efficacy of continuous subcutaneous levodopa-carbidopa infusion (ND0612) for Parkinson's disease with motor fluctuations (BouNDless): a phase 3, randomised, double-blind, double-dummy, multicentre trial. *The Lancet Neurology.* May 2024;23(5):465–476. doi:10.1016/S1474-4422(24)00052-8.

124. Henriksen T, Katzenschlager R, Bhidayasiri R, Staines H, Lockhart D, Lees A. Practical use of apomorphine infusion in Parkinson's disease: lessons from the TOLEDO study and clinical experience. *Journal of Neural Transmission.* November 2023;130(11):1475–1484. doi:10.1007/s00702-023-02686-7.

125. Reyniers JA. Germ-free life applied to nutrition studies. *Lobund Reports.* November 1946;(1):87–120.

126. Reyniers JA. The production and use of germ-free animals in experimental biology and medicine. *American Journal of Veterinary Research.* July 1957;18(68):678–687.

127. Reyniers JA, Sacksteder MR. Apparatus and method for shipping germ-free and disease-free animals via public transportation. *Applied Microbiology.* March 1958;6(2):146–152. doi:10.1128/am.6.2.146-152.1958.

128. Reyniers JA, Trexler PC, Ervin RF. Rearing germ-free albino rats. *Lobund Reports.* November 1946;(1):1–84.

129. Reyniers JA, Trexler PC, Ervin R., et al. A complete life-cycle in the "germ-free" bantam chicken. *Nature.* 1949;163:67–68. doi:10.1038/163067a0.

130. Sampson TR. Fecal microbiome transplants for Parkinson disease. *JAMA Neurology.* September 1, 2024;81(9):911–913. doi:10.1001/jamaneurol.2024.2293.

131. Scheperjans F, Levo R, Bosch B, et al. Fecal microbiota transplantation for treatment of Parkinson disease: a randomized clinical trial. *JAMA Neurology.* 2024;81(9):925–938. doi:10.1001/jamaneurol.2024.2305.

132. Blackmer-Reynolds LD, Sampson TR. The gut-brain axis goes viral. *Cell Host & Microbe.* March 9, 2022;30(3):283–285. doi:10.1016/j.chom.2022.02.013.

133. Fields CT, Sampson TR, Bruce-Keller AJ, Kiraly DD, Hsiao EY, de Vries GJ. Defining dysbiosis in disorders of movement and motivation. *Journal of Neuroscience.* October 31, 2018;38(44):9414–9422. doi:10.1523/JNEUROSCI.1672-18.2018.

134. Hamilton AM, Blackmer-Reynolds L, Li Y, et al. Diet-microbiome interactions promote enteric nervous system resilience following spinal cord injury. *bioRxiv.* June 8, 2024 [Preprint]. doi:10.1101/2024.06.06.597793.

135. Sampson T. The impact of indigenous microbes on Parkinson's disease. *Neurobiology of Disease.* February 2020;135:104426. doi:10.1016/j.nbd.2019.03.014.

136. Sampson T. Microbial amyloids in neurodegenerative amyloid diseases. *FEBS Journal.* December 2, 2023. doi:10.1111/febs.17023.

137. Sampson TR, Challis C, Jain N, et al. A gut bacterial amyloid promotes alpha-synuclein aggregation and motor impairment in mice. *Elife.* February 11, 2020;9:e53111. doi:10.7554/eLife.53111.

138. Barker RA, Barrett J, Mason SL, Bjorklund A. Fetal dopaminergic transplantation trials and the future of neural grafting in Parkinson's disease. *The Lancet Neurology.* January 2013;12(1):84–91. doi:10.1016/S1474-4422(12)70295-8.

139. Barker RA, Bjorklund A. Animal models of Parkinson's disease: are they useful or not? *Journal of Parkinson's Disease.* 2020;10(4):1335–1342. doi:10.3233/JPD-202200.

140. Barker RA, Bjorklund A. Restorative cell and gene therapies for Parkinson's disease. *Handbook of Clinical Neurology.* 2023;193:211–226. doi:10.1016/B978-0-323-85555-6.00012-6.

141. Barker RA, Bjorklund A, Frucht SJ, Svendsen CN. Stem cell–derived dopamine neurons: will they replace DBS as the leading neurosurgical treatment for Parkinson's disease? *Journal of Parkinson's Disease.* 2021;11(3):909–917. doi:10.3233/JPD-219008.

142. Barker RA, Bjorklund A, Gash DM, et al. GDNF and Parkinson's disease: where next? A summary from a recent workshop. *Journal of Parkinson's Disease.* 2020;10(3):875–891. doi:10.3233/JPD-202004.

143. Barker RA, Bjorklund A, Parmar M. The history and status of dopamine cell therapies for Parkinson's disease. *Bioessays.* July 26, 2024:e2400118. doi:10.1002/bies.202400118.

144. Barker RA, TRANSEURO Consortium. Designing stem-cell-based dopamine cell replacement trials for Parkinson's disease. *Nature Medicine.* July 2019;25(7):1045–1053. doi:10.1038/s41591-019-0507-2.

145. Bjorklund A, Barker RA. The basal forebrain cholinergic system as target for cell replacement therapy in Parkinson's disease. *Brain.* June 3, 2024;147(6):1937–1952. doi:10.1093/brain/awae026.

146. Bjorklund A, Dunnett SB, Brundin P, et al. Neural transplantation for the treatment of Parkinson's disease. *The Lancet Neurology.* July 2003;2(7):437–445. doi:10.1016/s1474-4422(03)00442-3.

147. Kirkeby A, Nelander J, Hoban DB, et al. Preclinical quality, safety, and efficacy of a human embryonic stem cell–derived product for the treatment of Parkinson's disease, STEM-PD. *Cell Stem Cell.* October 5, 2023;30(10):1299–1314 e9. doi:10.1016/j.stem.2023.08.014.

148. Centers for Disease Control and Prevention. CDC's 60th anniversary. Director's perspective—William H. Foege, M.D., M.P.H., 1977–1983. *Morbidity and Mortality Weekly Report.* October 6, 2006;55(39):1071–1074.

149. Foege WH. Confronting emerging infections: lessons from the smallpox eradication campaign. *Emerging Infectious Diseases.* July–September 1998;4(3):412–413. doi:10.3201/eid0403.980318.

150. Foege WH, Lane JM. End of routine smallpox vaccination in childhood. *Annals of Internal Medicine.* February 1972;76(2):324–326. doi:10.7326/0003-4819-76-2-324.

151. Foege WH, Millar JD, Henderson DA. Smallpox eradication in West and Central Africa. *Bulletin of the World Health Organization.* 1975;52(2):209–222.

152. Foege WH, Millar JD, Lane JM. Selective epidemiologic control in smallpox eradication. *American Journal of Epidemiology.* October 1971;94(4):311–315. doi:10.1093/oxfordjournals.aje.a121325.

153. Millar JD, Foege WH. Status of eradication of smallpox (and control of measles) in West and Central Africa. *Journal of Infectious Diseases.* December 1969;120(6):725–732. doi:10.1093/infdis/120.6.725.

154. Fleming SM, Davis A, Simons E. Targeting alpha-synuclein via the immune system in Parkinson's disease: current vaccine therapies. *Neuropharmacology*. January 1, 2022;202:108870. doi:10.1016/j.neuropharm.2021.108870.

155. Knecht L, Folke J, Dodel R, Ross JA, Albus A. Alpha-synuclein immunization strategies for synucleinopathies in clinical studies: a biological perspective. *Neurotherapeutics*. September 2022;19(5):1489–1502. doi:10.1007/s13311-022-01288-7.

156. Saleh M, Markovic M, Olson KE, Gendelman HE, Mosley RL. Therapeutic strategies for immune transformation in Parkinson's disease. *Journal of Parkinson's Disease*. 2022;12(s1):S201–S222. doi:10.3233/JPD-223278.

157. Schneeberger A, Tierney L, Mandler M. Active immunization therapies for Parkinson's disease and multiple system atrophy. *Movement Disorders*. February 2016;31(2):214–224. doi:10.1002/mds.26377.

158. Stott SRW, Wyse RK, Brundin P. Novel approaches to counter protein aggregation pathology in Parkinson's disease. *Progress in Brain Research*. 2020;252:451–492. doi:10.1016/bs.pbr.2019.10.007.

159. Chu WT, Hall J, Gurrala A, et al. Evaluation of an adoptive cellular therapy–based vaccine in a transgenic mouse model of alpha-synucleinopathy. *ACS Chemical Neuroscience*. January 18, 2023;14(2):235–245. doi:10.1021/acschemneuro.2c00539.

160. Elkouzi A, Vedam-Mai V, Eisinger RS, Okun MS. Emerging therapies in Parkinson disease—repurposed drugs and new approaches. *Nature Reviews Neurology*. April 2019;15(4):204–223. doi:10.1038/s41582-019-0155-7.

161. Gill EL, Koelmel JP, Meke L, et al. Ultrahigh-performance liquid chromatography–high-resolution mass spectrometry metabolomics and lipidomics study of stool from transgenic Parkinson's disease mice following immunotherapy. *Journal of Proteome Research*. January 3, 2020;19(1):424–431. doi:10.1021/acs.jproteome.9b00605.

162. Lang AE, Siderowf AD, Macklin EA, et al. Trial of Cinpanemab in early Parkinson's disease. *New England Journal of Medicine*. August 4, 2022;387(5):408–420. doi:10.1056/NEJMoa2203395.

163. Pagano G, Taylor KI, Anzures-Cabrera J, et al. Trial of Prasinezumab in early-stage Parkinson's disease. *New England Journal of Medicine*. August 4, 2022;387(5):421–432. doi:10.1056/NEJMoa2202867.

164. Whone A. Monoclonal antibody therapy in Parkinson's disease—the end? *New England Journal of Medicine*. August 4, 2022;387(5):466–467. doi:10.1056/NEJMe2207681.

165. Piller C. Challenged papers underpin several drugs. *Science*. September 26, 2024; 385(6716):1410. doi:10.1126/science.adt3536.

166. Espay AJ, Herrup K, Kepp KP, Daly T. The proteinopenia hypothesis: loss of Abeta(42) and the onset of Alzheimer's disease. *Ageing Research Reviews*. December 2023;92:102112. doi:10.1016/j.arr.2023.102112.

167. Ezzat K, Sturchio A, Espay AJ. The shift to a proteinopenia paradigm in neurodegeneration. *Handbook of Clinical Neurology*. 2023;193:23–32. doi:10.1016/B978-0-323-85555-6.00001-1.

Chapter 9: Navigate the Final Frontier

1. Roberts WS, Price S, Wu M, Parmar MS. Emerging gene therapies for Alzheimer's and Parkinson's diseases: an overview of clinical trials and promising candidates. *Cureus*. August 2024;16(8):e67037. doi:10.7759/cureus.67037.

2. Allen GF, Land JM, Heales SJ. A new perspective on the treatment of aromatic L-amino acid decarboxylase deficiency. *Molecular Genetics and Metabolism*. May 2009;97(1):6–14. doi:10.1016/j.ymgme.2009.01.010.

3. Bankiewicz KS, Forsayeth J, Eberling JL, et al. Long-term clinical improvement in MPTP-lesioned primates after gene therapy with AAV-hAADC. *Molecular Therapy*. October 2006;14(4):564–570. doi:10.1016/j.ymthe.2006.05.005.

4. Christine CW, Bankiewicz KS, Van Laar AD, et al. Magnetic resonance imaging-guided phase 1 trial of putaminal AADC gene therapy for Parkinson's disease. *Annals of Neurology*. May 2019;85(5):704–714. doi:10.1002/ana.25450.

5. Mittermeyer G, Christine CW, Rosenbluth KH, et al. Long-term evaluation of a phase 1 study of AADC gene therapy for Parkinson's disease. *Human Gene Therapy*. April 2012;23(4):377–381. doi:10.1089/hum.2011.220.

6. Pearson TS, Gilbert L, Opladen T, et al. AADC deficiency from infancy to adulthood: symptoms and developmental outcome in an international cohort of 63 patients. *Journal of Inherited Metabolic Disease*. September 2020;43(5):1121–1130. doi:10.1002/jimd.12247.

7. Feigin A, Kaplitt MG, Tang C, et al. Modulation of metabolic brain networks after subthalamic gene therapy for Parkinson's disease. *Proceedings of the National Academy of Sciences of the United States of America*. December 4, 2007;104(49):19559–19564. doi:10.1073/pnas.0706006104.

8. Kaplitt MG, Feigin A, Tang C, et al. Safety and tolerability of gene therapy with an adeno-associated virus (AAV) borne GAD gene for Parkinson's disease: an open label, phase I trial. *The Lancet*. June 23, 2007;369(9579):2097–2105. doi:10.1016/S0140-6736(07)60982-9.

9. Drager NM, Sattler SM, Huang CT, et al. A CRISPRi/a platform in human iPSC-derived microglia uncovers regulators of disease states. *Nature Neuroscience*. September 2022;25(9):1149–1162. doi:10.1038/s41593-022-01131-4.

10. Sachdev A, Gill K, Sckaff M, et al. Reversal of C9orf72 mutation-induced transcriptional dysregulation and pathology in cultured human neurons by allele-specific excision. *Proceedings of the National Academy of Sciences of the United States of America*. April 23, 2024;121(17):e2307814121. doi:10.1073/pnas.2307814121.

11. Salomonsson SE, Clelland CD. Building CRISPR gene therapies for the central nervous system: a review. *JAMA Neurology*. March 1, 2024;81(3):283–290. doi:10.1001/jamaneurol.2023.4983.

12. Banks J. The gene editing juggernaut is picking up speed. *IEEE Pulse*. September–October 2023;14(5):23–26. doi:10.1109/MPULS.2023.3344054.

13. Barrangou R. Nobel dreams come true for Doudna and Charpentier. *CRISPR Journal*. October 2020;3(5):317–318. doi:10.1089/crispr.2020.29109.rba.

14. Bhattacharjee R, Das Roy L, Choudhury A. Understanding on CRISPR/Cas9 mediated cutting-edge approaches for cancer therapeutics. *Discover Oncology*. June 8, 2022;13(1):45. doi:10.1007/s12672-022-00509-x.

15. Bosley KS, Botchan M, Bredenoord AL, et al. CRISPR germline engineering—the community speaks. *Nature Biotechnology*. May 2015;33(5):478–486. doi:10.1038/nbt.3227.

16. Derry WB. CRISPR: development of a technology and its applications. *FEBS Journal*. January 2021;288(2):358–359. doi:10.1111/febs.15621.

17. Doudna JA, Charpentier E. The new frontier of genome engineering with CRISPR-Cas9. *Science*. November 28, 2014;346(6213):1258096. doi:10.1126/science.1258096.

18. Farhud DD, Zarif-Yeganeh M. CRISPR pioneers win 2020 Nobel Prize for Chemistry. *Iranian Journal of Public Health*. December 2020;49(12):2235–2239. doi:10.18502/ijph.v49i12.4800.

19. Gaudelli NM, Komor AC. Celebrating Rosalind Franklin's centennial with a Nobel win for Doudna and Charpentier. *Molecular Therapy*. December 2, 2020;28(12):2519–2520. doi:10.1016/j.ymthe.2020.11.013.

20. Gostimskaya I. CRISPR-Cas9: a history of its discovery and ethical considerations of its use in genome editing. *Biochemistry (Moscow)*. August 2022;87(8):777–788. doi:10.1134/S0006297922080090.

21. Ozkan J. Jennifer A. Doudna and Emmanuelle Charpentier. *European Heart Journal*. June 7, 2021;42(22):2143–2145. doi:10.1093/eurheartj/ehaa1054.

22. Pan S, Zhang H. CRISPR-Cas9系统的发现 [Discovery in CRISPR-Cas9 system]. *Zhong Nan Da Xue Xue Bao Yi Xue Ban*. December 28, 2021;46(12):1392–1402. doi:10.11817/j.issn.1672-7347.2021.210169.

23. Wolthuis RMF, van de Vrugt HJ, Cornel MC. Genetische reparatie met CRISPR in de kliniek [CRISPR gene therapy enters the clinic: the future starts now]. *Nederlands Tijdschrift voor Geneeskunde*. August 30, 2021;165.

24. Zhang H, Qin C, An C, et al. Application of the CRISPR/Cas9-based gene editing technique in basic research, diagnosis, and therapy of cancer. *Molecular Cancer*. October 1, 2021;20(1):126. doi:10.1186/s12943-021-01431-6.

25. Baltimore D, Berg P, Botchan M, et al. Biotechnology. A prudent path forward for genomic engineering and germline gene modification. *Science*. April 3, 2015;348(6230):36–38. doi:10.1126/science.aab1028.

26. Doudna JA. The promise and challenge of therapeutic genome editing. *Nature*. February 2020;578(7794):229–236. doi:10.1038/s41586-020-1978-5.

27. Brouillette M. You can edit a pig, but it will still be a pig. *Scientific American*. March 2016;314(3):A22. doi:10.1038/scientificamerican0316-22b.

28. Horwitz JP. Design of some nucleic acid antimetabolites: expectations and reality. *Investigational New Drugs*. April 1989;7(1):51–57. doi:10.1007/BF00178191.

29. Palomino E, Meltsner BR, Kessel D, Horwitz JP. Synthesis and in vitro evaluation of some modified 4-thiopyrimidine nucleosides for prevention or reversal of AIDS-associated neurological disorders. *Journal of Medicinal Chemistry*. January 1990;33(1):258–263. doi:10.1021/jm00163a043.

30. Colson ER, Horwitz RI, Bia FJ, Viscoli CM. Zidovudine (AZT) for treatment of patients infected with human immunodeficiency virus type 1. An evaluation of effectiveness in clinical practice. *Archives of Internal Medicine*. April 1991;151(4):709–713.

31. Gilden D. Honing the immune attack on HIV. *GMHC Treatment Issues*. December 1996;10(12):8–11.

32. Gilden D. Outrunning HIV to protect immune defenses. *GMHC Treatment Issues*. November 1996;10(11):1–5.

33. Frei E, III, Holland JF, Schneiderman MA, et al. A comparative study of two regimens of combination chemotherapy in acute leukemia. *Blood*. December 1958;13(12):1126–1148.

34. Freireich EJ, Gehan EA, Sulman D, Boggs DR, Frei E, III. The effect of chemotherapy on acute leukemia in the human. *Journal of Chronic Diseases*. December 1961;14:593 608. doi:10.1016/0021-9681(61)90118-7.

35. Freireich EJ. A symposium on cancer chemotherapy. IV. Acute leukemia. *Medical Annals of the District of Columbia*. December 1962;31:675–682.

36. Freireich EJ, Frei E, II. Recent advances in acute leukemia. *Progress in Hematology*. 1964;4:187–202.

37. Guillard A. Le "déclin" des parkinsoniens traités par la L-dopa [The deterioration of patients with parkinsonism treated with L-dopa]. *Nouvelle presse medicale*. October 18, 1975;4(35):2503–2506.

38. Marttila RJ, Rinne UK, Siirtola T, Sonninen V. Mortality of patients with Parkinson's disease treated with levodopa. *Journal of Neurology*. October 7, 1977;216(3):147–153. doi:10.1007/BF00313615.

39. Shaw KM, Lees AJ, Stern GM. The impact of treatment with levodopa on Parkinson's disease. *Quarterly Journal of Medicine.* 1980;49(195):283–293.

40. Diamond SG, Markham CH, Hoehn MM, McDowell FH, Muenter MD. Multi-center study of Parkinson mortality with early versus later dopa treatment. *Annals of Neurology.* July 1987;22(1):8–12. doi:10.1002/ana.410220105.

41. Mortality in DATATOP: a multicenter trial in early Parkinson's disease. Parkinson Study Group. *Annals of Neurology.* March 1998;43(3):318–325. doi:10.1002/ana.410430309.

42. Ishihara LS, Cheesbrough A, Brayne C, Schrag A. Estimated life expectancy of Parkinson's patients compared with the UK population. *Journal of Neurology, Neurosurgery, and Psychiatry.* December 2007;78(12):1304–1309. doi:10.1136/jnnp.2006.100107.

43. Forsaa EB, Larsen JP, Wentzel-Larsen T, Alves G. What predicts mortality in Parkinson disease? a prospective population-based long-term study. *Neurology.* October 5, 2010;75(14):1270–1276. doi:10.1212/WNL.0b013e3181f61311.

44. Green AR, Haddad PM, Aronson JK. Marketing medicines: charting the rise of modern therapeutics through a systematic review of adverts in UK medical journals (1950–1980). *British Journal of Clinical Pharmacology.* August 2018;84(8):1668–1685. doi:10.1111/bcp.13549.

45. Airan R. Neuromodulation with nanoparticles. *Science.* August 4, 2017;357(6350):465. doi:10.1126/science.aao1200.

46. Airan RD, Meyer RA, Ellens NP, et al. Noninvasive targeted transcranial neuromodulation via focused ultrasound gated drug release from nanoemulsions. *Nano Letters.* February 8, 2017;17(2):652–659. doi:10.1021/acs.nanolett.6b03517.

47. Wang JB, Di Ianni T, Vyas DB, et al. Focused ultrasound for noninvasive, focal pharmacologic neurointervention. *Frontiers in Neuroscience.* 2020;14:675. doi:10.3389/fnins.2020.00675.

48. Zhong Q, Yoon BC, Aryal M, et al. Polymeric perfluorocarbon nanoemulsions are ultrasound-activated wireless drug infusion catheters. *Biomaterials.* June 2019;206:73–86. doi:10.1016/j.biomaterials.2019.03.021.

49. Burns J, Buck AC, D'Souza S, Dube A, Bardien S. Nanophytomedicines as therapeutic agents for Parkinson's disease. *ACS Omega.* November 14, 2023;8(45):42045–42061. doi:10.1021/acsomega.3c04862.

50. Pardridge WM. Treatment of Parkinson's disease with biologics that penetrate the blood-brain barrier via receptor-mediated transport. *Frontiers in Aging Neuroscience.* 2023;15:1276376. doi:10.3389/fnagi.2023.1276376.

51. Sardoiwala MN, Biswal L, Choudhury SR. Immunomodulator-derived nanoparticles induce neuroprotection and regulatory T cell action to alleviate parkinsonism. *ACS Applied Materials & Interfaces.* July 31, 2024;16(30):38880–38892. doi:10.1021/acsami.3c18226.

52. Shaikh MAJ, Kumar G, Bagiyal P, et al. Enhancing drug bioavailability for Parkinson's disease: the promise of chitosan delivery mechanisms. *Annales pharmaceutiques françaises.* July 30, 2024:S0003-4509(24)00107-X. doi:10.1016/j.pharma.2024.07.008.

53. Tapia-Arellano A, Cabrera P, Cortes-Adasme E, Riveros A, Hassan N, Kogan MJ. Tau- and alpha-synuclein-targeted gold nanoparticles: applications, opportunities, and future outlooks in the diagnosis and therapy of neurodegenerative diseases. *Journal of Nanobiotechnology.* May 13, 2024;22(1):248. doi:10.1186/s12951-024-02526-0.

54. Wu X, Yuan R, Xu Y, et al. Functionalized lipid nanoparticles modulate the blood-brain barrier and eliminate alpha-synuclein to repair dopamine neurons. *Asian Journal of Pharmaceutical Sciences.* April 2024;19(2):100904. doi:10.1016/j.ajps.2024.100904.

55. Busch C. *The Serendipity Mindset: The Art and Science of Creating Good Luck.* Riverhead Books; 2020.

56. Hubsher G, Haider M, Okun MS. Amantadine: the journey from fighting flu to treating Parkinson disease. *Neurology.* April 3, 2012;78(14):1096–1099. doi:10.1212/WNL.0b013e31824e8f0d.

57. Young RR. Robert S. Schwab, MD. 1903–1972. *Archives of Neurology.* September 1972;27(3):271–272. doi:10.1001/archneur.1972.00490150079012.

58. Schwab RS, England AC, Jr. Amantadine HCL (Symmetrel) and its relation to levo-dopa in the treatment of Parkinson's disease. *Transactions of the American Neurological Association.* 1969;94:85–90.

59. Schwab RS, England AC, Jr., Poskanzer DC, Young RR. Amantadine in the treatment of Parkinson's disease. *JAMA.* May 19, 1969;208(7):1168–1170.

60. Schwab RS, Poskanzer DC, England AC, Jr., Young RR. Amantadine in Parkinson's disease. Review of more than two years' experience. *JAMA.* November 13, 1972;222(7):792–795. doi:10.1001/jama.222.7.792.

61. Schwab RS, Young RR. Non-resting tremor in Parkinson's disease. *Transactions of the American Neurological Association.* 1971;96:305–307.

62. da Silva-Junior FP, Braga-Neto P, Sueli Monte F, de Bruin VM. Amantadine reduces the duration of levodopa-induced dyskinesia: a randomized, double-blind, placebo-controlled study. *Parkinsonism & Related Disorders.* November 2005;11(7):449–452. doi:10.1016/j.parkreldis.2005.05.008.

63. deVries T, Dentiste A, Handiwala L, Jacobs D. Bioavailability and pharmacokinetics of once-daily amantadine extended-release tablets in healthy volunteers: results from three randomized, crossover, open-label, phase 1 studies. *Neurology and Therapy.* December 2019;8(2):449–460. doi:10.1007/s40120-019-0144-1.

64. Oertel W, Eggert K, Pahwa R, et al. Randomized, placebo-controlled trial of ADS-5102 (amantadine) extended-release capsules for levodopa-induced dyskinesia in Parkinson's disease (EASE LID 3). *Movement Disorders.* December 2017;32(12):1701–1709. doi:10.1002/mds.27131.

65. Pahwa R, Tanner CM, Hauser RA, et al. ADS-5102 (amantadine) extended-release capsules for levodopa-induced dyskinesia in Parkinson disease (EASE LID Study): a randomized clinical trial. *JAMA Neurology.* August 1, 2017;74(8):941–949. doi:10.1001/jamaneurol.2017.0943.

66. Rascol O, Tonges L, deVries T, et al. Immediate-release/extended-release amantadine (OS320) to treat Parkinson's disease with levodopa-induced dyskinesia: analysis of the randomized, controlled ALLAY-LID studies. *Parkinsonism & Related Disorders.* March 2022;96:65–73. doi:10.1016/j.parkreldis.2022.01.022.

67. Sawada H, Oeda T, Kuno S, et al. Amantadine for dyskinesias in Parkinson's disease: a randomized controlled trial. *PLOS One.* December 31, 2010;5(12):e15298. doi:10.1371/journal.pone.0015298.

68. Stocchi F, Rascol O, Destee A, et al. AFQ056 in Parkinson patients with levodopa-induced dyskinesia: 13-week, randomized, dose-finding study. *Movement Disorders.* November 2013;28(13):1838–1846. doi:10.1002/mds.25561.

Chapter 10: The PLAN

1. H.R. 2365—118th Congress: Dr. Emmanuel Bilirakis and Honorable Jennifer Wexton National Plan to End Parkinson's Act. GovTrack.us. https://www.govtrack.us/congress/bills/118/hr2365.

2. Alvord K. Congresswoman and mom of 2 speaks candidly about her incurable brain disease: "I'm too young for this" (exclusive). *People.* May 9, 2024.

3. Klaus P. The devil is in the details—only what get measured gets managed. In: *Measuring Customer Experience: How to Develop and Execute the Most Profitable Customer Experience Strategies.* Palgrave Macmillan UK; 2015:81–101.

4. Marras C, Beck JC, Bower JH, et al. Prevalence of Parkinson's disease across North America. *npj Parkinson's Disease*. July 10, 2018;4(1):21. doi:10.1038/s41531-018-0058-0.

5. Schoenberg BS, Anderson DW, Haerer AF. Prevalence of Parkinson's disease in the biracial population of Copiah County, Mississippi. *Neurology*. 1985;35(6):841–841. doi:10.1212/WNL.35.6.841.

6. Savica R, Grossardt BR, Bower JH, Ahlskog JE, Rocca WA. Time trends in the incidence of Parkinson disease. *JAMA Neurology*. 2016;73(8):981–989. doi:10.1001/jamaneurol.2016.0947.

7. Darweesh SKL, Koudstaal PJ, Stricker BH, Hofman A, Ikram MA. Trends in the incidence of Parkinson disease in the general population: the Rotterdam Study. *American Journal of Epidemiology*. 2016;183(11):1018–1026. doi:10.1093/aje/kwv271.

8. Chlorpyrifos. EPA. https://www.epa.gov/ingredients-used-pesticide-products/chlorpyrifos. Accessed August 22, 2024.

9. Guillen A. Chemical rule delayed by Trump's regulatory freeze. *PoliticoPro*. January 27, 2025. https://subscriber.politicopro.com/article/2025/01/chemical-rule-delayed-by-trumps-regulatory-freeze-00200701.

10. McCord CP. Toxicity of trichloroethylene. *Journal of the American Medical Association*. 1932;99(5):409–409. doi:10.1001/jama.1932.02740570055030.

11. Aerotron-100: a direct TCE replacement. Reliance Specialty Products, Inc. https://relspec.com/replace-tce?gad_source=1&gclid=EAIaIQobChMIhK_iksiniQMVtjUIBR0q-AXSEAAYAyAAEgIU-vD_BwE. Accessed October 15, 2024.

12. Choosing the right alternative to trichloroethylene or perchloroethylene. Enviro Tech International, Inc. https://envirotechint.com/choosing-the-right-alternative-to-trichloroethylene-or-perchloroethylene. Accessed October 15, 2024.

13. Martuzzi M, Tickner JA, Organization WH. *The Precautionary Principle: Protecting Public Health, the Environment and the Future of Our Children*. World Health Organization. Regional Office for Europe; 2004.

14. Wingspread statement on the precautionary principle. SEHN. August 5, 2013. https://www.sehn.org/sehn/wingspread-conference-on-the-precautionary-principle.

15. Tickner JA, Raffensperger C, and Myers N. *The Precautionary Principle in Action: A Handbook*. Science and Environmental Health Network; 1999.

16. Hardmon T, Libert R, dirs. *Semper Fi: Always Faithful*. Wider Film Projects; 2011.

17. What is the current state of agriculture in the US? USA Facts. Updated February 24, 2023. https://usafacts.org/topics/agriculture.

18. Module V section D: the economics of organic agriculture. Center for Integrated Agricultural Systems. https://cias.wisc.edu/curriculum-new/module-v/module-v-section-d. Accessed September 18, 2024.

19. Federal farm subsidies: what the data says. USA Facts. Updated October 5, 2023. https://usafacts.org/topics/agriculture.

20. Estimated annual agricultural pesticide use, 2018. US Geological Survey. https://water.usgs.gov/nawqa/pnsp/usage/maps/show_map.php?year=2018&map=PARAQUAT&hilo=L. Accessed August 22, 2024.

21. Organic Agriculture Program. National Institute of Food and Agriculture. https://www.nifa.usda.gov/grants/programs/organic-agriculture-program. Accessed October 24, 2024.

22. Gillam C, Uteuova A. Secret files suggest chemical giant feared weedkiller's link to Parkinson's disease. *The Guardian*. October 20, 2022. https://www.theguardian.com/us-news/2022/oct/20/syngenta-weedkiller-pesticide-parkinsons-disease-paraquat-documents.

23. Beckley-Jackson L. Don't drink the water: the Camp Lejeune water contamination incident. *DttP*. 2016;44(4):4–9.

24. Superfund site: Hopewell Precision, Hopewell Junction, NY, cleanup activities. EPA. Updated August 9, 2024. https://cumulis.epa.gov/supercpad/SiteProfiles/index.cfm ?fuseaction=second.cleanup&id=0201588.

25. Hopewell Precision area contamination. New York State Department of Health. https:// www.health.ny.gov/environmental/investigations/hopewell/public_health_assessment.htm. Accessed September 28, 2024.

26. Stock S, Paredes D. Concern for Mountain View toxic plume expanded. *NBC Bay Area*. February 23, 2013. https://www.nbcbayarea.com/news/local/questions-about-toxic-testing -at-moffett-field/2047771.

27. DeBolt D, Sheyner G. Local company's toxic plume map causes alarm. *Mountain View Voice*. May 5, 2014. https://www.mv-voice.com/news/2014/05/22/local-companys-toxic-plume -map-causes-alarm.

28. Remedy proposed for Brownfield site contamination: public comment period announced. New York State Department of Environmental Conservation. June 2022. https://extapps.dec .ny.gov/data/DecDocs/C224287/Fact%20Sheet.BCP.C224287.2022-06-07.FS%231_RAWP _comment%20period-final-English.pdf.

29. McKinley J. His home sits alongside America's first Superfund site. No one told him. *New York Times*. June 12, 2023. https://www.nytimes.com/2023/06/12/nyregion /love-canal-toxic-homes.html.

30. Toxic release inventory. New York State Department of Environmental Conservation. https://dec.ny.gov/environmental-protection/waste-management/toxic-release-inventory. Accessed September 28, 2024.

31. Rechtschaffen C. CPR perspective: the public right to know. Center for Progressive Reform. March 1, 2003. https://progressivereform.org/publications/perspright.

32. Suwol R. Mother knows best. California Safe Schools. https://www.calisafe.org/news _release19.html. Accessed September 28, 2024.

33. California Safe Schools. LA Unified School District parents gain right to know of toxic exposure: parents must request written notice of pesticide application. CorpWatch. October 18, 2002. https://www.corpwatch.org/article/la-unified-school-district-parents-gain-right-know -toxic-exposure.

34. Whelan C. Local pesticide concerns lead to positive changes in public schools. *CBS News*. April 2, 2015. https://www.cbsnews.com/losangeles/news/local-pesticide-concerns -lead-to-positive-changes-in-public-schools.

35. Mithers CL. Danger in the schoolyard. California Safe Schools. May 2000. https://www .calisafe.org/danger_rep.htm.

36. Healthy Schools Act (HSA). California Environmental Protection Agency. https://www .cdpr.ca.gov/docs/schoolipm/school_ipm_law/hsa_faq.pdf. Accessed September 24, 2024.

37. Best practices for reducing near-road pollution exposure at schools. EPA. November 2015. https://19january2017snapshot.epa.gov/sites/production/files/2015-10/documents/ochp_2015 _near_road_pollution_booklet_v16_508.pdf.

38. Barboza T. Freeway pollution travels farther than we thought. Here's how to protect yourself. *Los Angeles Times*. December 30, 2017. https://www.latimes.com/local/california/la -me-freeway-pollution-what-you-can-do-20171230-htmlstory.html.

39. Rowangould GM. A census of the US near-roadway population: public health and envi-ronmental justice considerations. *Transportation Research Part D: Transport and Environment*. December 1, 2013;25:59–67. doi:10.1016/j.trd.2013.08.003.

40. Ritz B, Lee P-C, Hansen J, et al. Traffic-related air pollution and Parkinson's disease in Denmark: a case-control study. *Environmental Health Perspectives*. 2016;124(3):351–356. doi:10.1289/ehp.1409313.

41. Jo S, Kim Y-J, Park KW, et al. Association of NO$_2$ and other air pollution exposures with the risk of Parkinson disease. *JAMA Neurology.* 2021;78(7):800–808.

42. Lee PC, Liu LL, Sun Y, et al. Traffic-related air pollution increased the risk of Parkinson's disease in Taiwan: a nationwide study. *Environment International.* November 2016;96:75–81. doi:10.1016/j.envint.2016.08.017.

43. Hu CY, Fang Y, Li FL, et al. Association between ambient air pollution and Parkinson's disease: systematic review and meta-analysis. *Environmental Research.* January 2019;168:448–459. doi:10.1016/j.envres.2018.10.008.

44. Christensen GM, Li Z, Liang D, et al. Association of PM$_{2.5}$ exposure and Alzheimer disease pathology in brain bank donors—effect modification by APOE genotype. *Neurology.* 2024;102(5):e209162.

45. Tham R, Schikowski T. The role of traffic-related air pollution on neurodegenerative diseases in older people: an epidemiological perspective. *Journal of Alzheimer's Disease.* 2021;79(3):949–959. doi:10.3233/jad-200813.

46. Oudin A, Forsberg B, Adolfsson AN, et al. Traffic-related air pollution and dementia incidence in northern Sweden: a longitudinal study. *Environmental Health Perspectives.* 2016;124(3):306–312. doi:10.1289/ehp.1408322.

47. Jbaily A, Zhou X, Liu J, et al. Air pollution exposure disparities across US population and income groups. *Nature.* January 1, 2022;601(7892):228–233. doi:10.1038/s41586-021-04190-y.

48. Matz CJ, Egyed M, Hocking R, Seenundun S, Charman N, Edmonds N. Human health effects of traffic-related air pollution (TRAP): a scoping review protocol. *Systematic Reviews.* August 29, 2019;8(1):223. doi:10.1186/s13643-019-1106-5.

49. Su JG, Apte JS, Lipsitt J, et al. Populations potentially exposed to traffic-related air pollution in seven world cities. *Environment International.* May 1, 2015;78:82–89. doi:10.1016/j.envint.2014.12.007.

50. White O. What is an "organic" golf course, and why aren't there more of them? *Golf.* July 29, 2021. https://golf.com/travel/courses/organic-golf-course-pesticide-complications.

51. Form 990 return of organization exempt from income tax. Michael J Fox Foundation. 2021. https://www.michaeljfox.org/sites/default/files/media/document/2021%20990%20MJFF%20-%20Public%20Disclosure.pdf.

52. Form 990 return of organization exempt from income tax. Parkinson's Foundation. 2021. https://www.parkinson.org/sites/default/files/documents/PF-IRS-990-2021.pdf.

53. Dorsey ER, Thompson JP, Frasier M, et al. Funding of Parkinson research from industry and US federal and foundation sources. *Movement Disorders.* April 15, 2009;24(5):731–737. doi:10.1002/mds.22446.

54. Moses H, III, Matheson DH, Cairns-Smith S, George BP, Palisch C, Dorsey ER. The anatomy of medical research: US and international comparisons. *JAMA.* January 13, 2015;313(2):174–189. doi:10.1001/jama.2014.15939.

55. Estimates of funding for various research, condition, and disease categories (RCDC). NIH RePORT. May 14, 2024. https://report.nih.gov/funding/categorical-spending.

56. Frank R. Sales of $100 million homes set to double this year as trophy properties recover. *CNBC.* July 26, 2024. https://www.cnbc.com/2024/07/26/sales-of-100-million-homes-set-to-double-this-year.html.

57. Zap C. What does a record-setting $210M mansion sale mean for the Malibu real estate market? Realtor. June 21, 2024. https://www.realtor.com/news/trends/record-setting-210m-mansion-malibu-california-insights.

58. Wexton and Bilirakis introduce bipartisan HEALTHY BRAINS Act to advance research into neurodegenerative diseases risks. Wexton.house.gov. August 5, 2024. https://wexton.house.gov/news/documentsingle.aspx?DocumentID=956.

59. H.R.9233—HEALTHY BRAINS Act of 2024. Congress.gov. https://www.congress.gov /bill/118th-congress/house-bill/9233. Accessed September 19, 2024.

60. Bloem BR, Okun MS, Klein C. Parkinson's disease. *The Lancet.* June 12, 2021;397(10291):2284–2303. doi:10.1016/S0140-6736(21)00218-X.

61. Gledo I, Pranjic N, Drljević K, Prasko S, Drljevic I, Brzeziński P. Female breast cancer in relation to exposure to medical iatrogenic diagnostic radiation during life. *Contemporary Oncology.* 2012;16(6):551–556. doi:10.5114/wo.2012.32489.

62. De Miranda BR, Goldman SM, Miller GW, Greenamyre JT, Dorsey ER. Preventing Parkinson's disease: an environmental agenda. *Journal of Parkinson's Disease.* 2022;12(1):45–68. doi:10.3233/jpd-212922.

63. Bruder C, Bulliard J-L, Germann S, et al. Estimating lifetime and 10-year risk of lung cancer. *Preventive Medicine Reports.* 2018;11:125–130.

64. Brown EG, Goldman SM, Coffey CS, et al. Occupational pesticide exposure in Parkinson's disease related to GBA and LRRK2 variants. *Journal of Parkinson's Disease.* 2024;14(4):737–746. doi:10.3233/JPD-240015.

65. Biomonitoring—lead. EPA. https://www.epa.gov/americaschildrenenvironment /biomonitoring-lead. Accessed September 28, 2024.

66. Domonoske C. The world has finally stopped using leaded gasoline. Algeria used the last stockpile. NPR. August 30, 2021. https://www.npr.org/2021/08/30/1031429212/the-world -has-finally-stopped-using-leaded-gasoline-algeria-used-the-last-stockp.

67. Protect your family from sources of lead. EPA. June 10, 2024. https://www.epa.gov/lead /protect-your-family-sources-lead.

68. Brugnone F, Perbellini L, Giuliari C, Cerpelloni M, Soave M. Blood and urine concentrations of chemical pollutants in the general population. *Medicina del lavoro.* September–October 1994;85(5):370–389.

69. Dorsey ER, Willis AW. Caring for the majority. *Movement Disorders.* 2013;28(3):261–262.

70. Fothergill-Misbah N, Hooker J, Kwasa J, Walker R. Access to medicines for Parkinson's disease in Kenya: a qualitative exploration. *Movement Disorders Clinical Practice.* November 2024;11(11):1373–1378. doi:10.1002/mdc3.14192.

71. Schiess N, Cataldi R, Okun MS, et al. Six action steps to address global disparities in Parkinson disease: a World Health Organization priority. *JAMA Neurology.* September 1, 2022;79(9):929–936. doi:10.1001/jamaneurol.2022.1783.

72. Okubadejo NU, Ojo OO, Wahab KW, et al. A nationwide survey of Parkinson's disease medicines availability and affordability in Nigeria. *Movement Disorders Clinical Practice.* January 2019;6(1):27–33. doi:10.1002/mdc3.12682.

73. Mokaya J, Dotchin CL, Gray WK, Hooker J, Walker RW. The accessibility of Parkinson's disease medication in Kenya: results of a national survey. *Movement Disorders Clinical Practice.* July–August 2016;3(4):376–381. doi:10.1002/mdc3.12294.

74. Dave S, Peter T, Fogarty C, Karatzas N, Belinsky N, Pant Pai N. Which community-based HIV initiatives are effective in achieving UNAIDS 90-90-90 targets? A systematic review and meta-analysis of evidence (2007–2018). *PLOS One.* 2019;14(7):e0219826. doi:10.1371/journal. pone.0219826.

75. Inzaule SC, Ondoa P, Peter T, et al. Affordable HIV drug-resistance testing for monitoring of antiretroviral therapy in sub-Saharan Africa. *The Lancet Infectious Diseases.* November 2016;16(11):e267–e275. doi:10.1016/S1473-3099(16)30118-9.

76. Khan S, Spiegelman D, Walsh F, et al. Early access to antiretroviral therapy versus standard of care among HIV-positive participants in Eswatini in the public health sector: the MaxART stepped-wedge randomized controlled trial. *Journal of International AIDS Society.* September 2020;23(9):e25610. doi:10.1002/jia2.25610.

77. Penazzato M, Townsend CL, Sam-Agudu NA, et al. Advancing the prevention and treatment of HIV in children: priorities for research and development. *The Lancet HIV*. September 2022;9(9):e658–e666. doi:10.1016/S2352-3018(22)00101-1.

78. Stevens WS, Gous NM, MacLeod WB, et al. Multidisciplinary point-of-care testing in South African primary health care clinics accelerates HIV ART initiation but does not alter retention in care. *Journal of Acquired Immune Deficiency Syndromes*. September 1, 2017;76(1):65–73. doi:10.1097/QAI.0000000000001456.

79. Cassani E, Cilia R, Laguna J, et al. *Mucuna pruriens* for Parkinson's disease: low-cost preparation method, laboratory measures and pharmacokinetics profile. *Journal of the Neurological Sciences*. June 15, 2016;365:175–180. doi:10.1016/j.jns.2016.04.001.

80. Bose S, Dun C, Zhang GQ, Walsh C, Makary MA, Hicks CW. Medicare beneficiaries in disadvantaged neighborhoods increased telemedicine use during the Covid-19 pandemic. *Health Affairs*. 2022;41(5):635–642.

81. Aamodt WW, Willis AW, Dahodwala N. Racial and ethnic disparities in Parkinson disease. *Neurology Clinical Practice*. 2023;13(2):e200138. doi:10.1212/CPJ.0000000000200138.

82. Willis AW, Schootman M, Evanoff BA, Perlmutter JS, Racette BA. Neurologist care in Parkinson disease: a utilization, outcomes, and survival study. *Neurology*. August 30, 2011;77(9):851–857. doi:10.1212/WNL.0b013e31822c9123.

83. Qi S, Yin P, Wang L, et al. Prevalence of Parkinson's disease: a community-based study in China. *Movement Disorders*. December 2021;36(12):2940–2944. doi:10.1002/mds.28762.

84. Dorsey ER, Elbaz A, Nichols E, et al. Global, regional, and national burden of Parkinson's disease, 1990–2016: a systematic analysis for the Global Burden of Disease Study 2016. *The Lancet Neurology*. 2018;17(11):939–953. doi:10.1016/S1474-4422(18)30295-3.

85. Li G, Ma J, Cui S, et al. Parkinson's disease in China: a forty-year growing track of bedside work. *Translational Neurodegeneration*. July 31, 2019;8(1):22. doi:10.1186/s40035-019-0162-z.

86. Hermanns M. The invisible and visible stigmatization of Parkinson's disease. *Journal of the American Association of Nurse Practitioners*. 2013;25(10):563–566. doi:10.1111/1745-7599.12008.

87. de la Rosa T, Scorza FA. Stigma in Parkinson's disease: placing it outside the body. *Clinics (Sao Paulo)*. 2022;77:100008. doi:10.1016/j.clinsp.2022.100008.

88. Ahn S, Springer K, Gibson JS. Social withdrawal in Parkinson's disease: a scoping review. *Geriatric Nursing*. November–December 2022;48:258–268. doi:10.1016/j.gerinurse.2022.10.010.

89. Carolan K. "It just makes you more vulnerable as an employee": understanding the effects of disability stigma on employment in Parkinson's disease. *Chronic Illness*. December 2024;20(4):655–668. doi:10.1177/17423953231185386.

90. de la Rosa T, Scorza FA. Contextualizing stigma in Parkinson's disease research. *Clinics (São Paulo)*. 2024;79:100425. doi:10.1016/j.clinsp.2024.100425.

91. Dobreva I, Thomas J, Marr A, et al. Improving conversations about Parkinson's dementia. *Movement Disorders Clinical Practice*. July 2024;11(7):814–824. doi:10.1002/mdc3.14054.

92. Logan BA, Neargarder S, Kinger SB, Larum AK, Salazar RD, Cronin-Golomb A. Self-perceived stigma in Parkinson's disease in an online sample: comparison with in-person sample, role of anxiety, and relative utility of four measures of stigma perception. *Applied Neuropsychology: Adult*. March 5, 2024:1–10. doi:10.1080/23279095.2024.2321578.

93. Mastel-Smith B, Hermanns M, Melendez J, et al. "I got laughed at for the shuffle noise I make": Parkinson's disease and stigma. *Research and Theory for Nursing Practice*. August 21, 2024;38(3):321–338. doi:10.1891/RTNP-2024-0015.

94. Stopic V, Jost ST, Baldermann JC, et al. Parkinson's Disease Stigma Questionnaire (PDStigmaQuest): development and pilot study of a questionnaire for stigma in patients with idiopathic Parkinson's disease. *Journal of Parkinson's Disease*. 2023;13(5):829–839. doi:10.3233/JPD-230071.

95. Parkinson's Africa. https://www.parkinsonsafrica.org. Accessed October 15, 2024.

96. Thomas O. From our founder, Omotola Thomas. Parkinson's Africa. https://www.parkinsonsafrica.org/about-us/our-history. Accessed September 15, 2024.

97. Stecher B. Interview with African Parkinson's Advocate Omotola Thomas. *Journal of Parkinson's Disease*. March 31, 2019. https://www.journalofparkinsonsdisease.com/blog/tomorrow/interview-african-parkinsons-advocate-omotola-thomas.

98. Team P. "Shrinking—a therapist newly diagnosed with Parkinson's." Parky. January 25, 2024. https://parkynow.com/shrinking.

99. Olz McCoy DP, Natasha Fothergill-Misbah. *Shaking Hands with the Devil*. 2023. https://shakinghandsfilm.com.

100. Program announcement for the Department of Defense, Defense Health Program. Department of Defense—Congressionally Directed Medical Research Programs. https://cdmrp.health.mil/funding/pa/HT942524PRPEIRA_GG.pdf. Accessed September 19, 2024.

101. Champion a critical budget boost for veterans' Parkinson's care. Michael J. Fox Foundation. Updated August 28, 2023. https://www.michaeljfox.org/news/champion-critical-budget-boost-veterans-parkinsons-care.

102. Espay AJ, Morgante F, Merola A, et al. Levodopa-induced dyskinesia in Parkinson disease: current and evolving concepts. *Annals of Neurology*. December 1, 2018;84(6):797–811. doi:10.1002/ana.25364.

103. 90-90-90: an ambitious treatment target to help end the AIDS epidemic. UNAIDS. October 2014. https://www.unaids.org/sites/default/files/media_asset/90-90-90_en.pdf.

104. 90-90-90: treatment for all. UNAIDS. https://www.unaids.org/en/resources/909090. Accessed August 30, 2024.

105. Levi J, Raymond A, Pozniak A, Vernazza P, Kohler P, Hill A. Can the UNAIDS 90-90-90 target be achieved? A systematic analysis of national HIV treatment cascades. *BMJ Global Health*. 2016;1(2):e000010. doi:10.1136/bmjgh-2015-000010.

106. US Burden of Disease Collaborators, Mokdad AH, Ballestros K, et al. The state of US health, 1990–2016: burden of diseases, injuries, and risk factors among US states. *JAMA*. 2018;319(14):1444–1472. doi:10.1001/jama.2018.0158.

107. Dattani S, Rodes-Guirao L, Ritchie H, Ortiz-Ospina E, Roser M. Life expectancy. Our World in Data. 2023. https://ourworldindata.org/life-expectancy.

108. Roser M, Ritchie H. HIV/AIDS. Our World in Data. November 2014. https://ourworldindata.org/hiv-aids.

109. Global HIV & AIDS statistics—fact sheet. UNAIDS. Updated August 2, 2024. https://www.unaids.org/en/resources/fact-sheet.

110. Greve P, Van Zoonen P. Organochlorine pesticides and PCBs in tissues from Dutch citizens (1968–1986). *International Journal of Environmental Analytical Chemistry*. 1990;38(2):265–277.

111. Klein C, Westenberger A. Genetics of Parkinson's disease. *Cold Spring Harbor Perspectives in Medicine*. January 2012;2(1):a008888. doi:10.1101/cshperspect.a008888.

112. How Minnesota passed the country's first ban on trichloroethylene. Minnesota Pollution Control Agency. 2023. https://www.pca.state.mn.us/news-and-stories/tce-ban-in-effect.

113. Murray CJ, Aravkin AY, Zheng P, et al. Global burden of 87 risk factors in 204 countries and territories, 1990–2019: a systematic analysis for the Global Burden of Disease Study 2019. *The Lancet*. 2020;396(10258):1223–1249.

114. Fink A, Pavlou MAS, Roomp K, Schneider JG. Declining trends in the incidence of Parkinson's disease: a cohort study in Germany. *Journal of Parkinson's Disease*. 2025;15(1):182–188. doi:10.1177/1877718x241306132.

115. Zhang Z, Yan X, Jones KC, et al. Pesticide risk constraints to achieving Sustainable Development Goals in China based on national modeling. *npj Clean Water*. November 3, 2022;5(1):59. doi:10.1038/s41545-022-00202-0.

116. Textor C. Pesticide consumption volume in China from 1990 to 2018. Statista. January 3, 2024. https://www.statista.com/statistics/863620/pesticide-consumption-volume-in -china.

117. Trichloroethylene market. Fact.MR. https://www.factmr.com/report/3701/trichloro ethylene-market. Accessed July 24, 2024.

118. Dorsey ER, Zafar M, Lettenberger SE, et al. Trichloroethylene: an invisible cause of Parkinson's disease? *Journal of Parkinson's Disease*. 2023;13(2):203–218. doi:10.3233/JPD-225047.

119. Urasa SJ, Dekker MCJ, Howlett WP, Mwezi RJ, Dorsey ER, Bloem BR. Parkinson's disease in sub-Saharan Africa: pesticides as a double-edged sword. *Journal of Parkinson's Disease*. 2024;14(3):437–449. doi:10.3233/jpd-230409.

120. Zhong J, Zhang X, Gui K, et al. Reconstructing 6-hourly PM2.5 datasets from 1960 to 2020 in China. *Earth System Science Data*. 2022;14(7):3197–3211. doi:10.5194/ essd-14-3197-2022.

121. Pesticide usage by country 2024. World Population Review https://worldpopulationreview .com/country-rankings/pesticide-usage-by-country. Accessed September 13, 2024.

122. Wang X, Chi Y, Li F. Exploring China stepping into the dawn of chemical pesticide-free agriculture in 2050. *Frontiers in Plant Science*. 2022;13:942117. doi:10.3389/fpls.2022.942117.

123. Huang Y. China's battle against air pollution: an update. Council on Foreign Relations. April 24, 2024. https://www.cfr.org/blog/chinas-battle-against-air-pollution-update.

124. Sharma A, Kumar V, Shahzad B, et al. Worldwide pesticide usage and its impacts on ecosystem. *SN Applied Sciences*. 2019;1:1–16.

125. Ritchie H, Roser M. Air pollution. Our World in Data. 2017. https://ourworldindata .org/air-pollution.

126. Dorsey ER, De Miranda BR, Horsager J, Borghammer P. The body, the brain, the environment, and Parkinson's disease. *Journal of Parkinson's Disease*. 2024;14(3):363–381. doi:10.3233/JPD-240019.

127. Anaduaka EG, Uchendu NO, Asomadu RO, Ezugwu AL, Okeke ES, Chidike Ezeorba TP. Widespread use of toxic agrochemicals and pesticides for agricultural products storage in Africa and developing countries: possible panacea for ecotoxicology and health implications. *Heliyon*. April 2023;9(4):e15173. doi:10.1016/j.heliyon.2023.e15173.

128. Westcott N. *Youthquake: Why African Demography Should Matter to the World*. Oxford University Press UK; 2022.

129. Zúñiga-Venegas LA, Hyland C, Muñoz-Quezada MT, et al. Health effects of pesticide exposure in Latin American and the Caribbean populations: a scoping review. *Environmental Health Perspectives*. September 2022;130(9):96002. doi:10.1289/ehp9934.

130. Isaifan RJ. Air pollution burden of disease over highly populated states in the Middle East. *Frontiers in Public Health*. 2022;10:1002707. doi:10.3389/fpubh.2022.1002707.

131. NAPA—National Alzheimer's Project Act. Office of the Assistant Secretary for Planning and Evaluation. https://aspe.hhs.gov/collaborations-committees-advisory-groups/napa. Accessed October 15, 2024.

132. Kaiser J. The Alzheimer's gamble: NIH tries to turn billions in new funding into treatment for deadly brain disease. *Science*. August 30, 2018. https://www.science.org/content/article /alzheimer-s-gamble-nih-tries-turn-billions-new-funding-treatment-deadly-brain-disease.

133. Edward de Bono—lateral thinking. Strategies for Influence. https://strategiesfor influence.com/edward-de-bono-lateral-thinking. Accessed September 17, 2024.

134. Spooner F. The global malaria death rate increased for the first time in 20 years due to Covid-19. Our World in Data. Updated July 8, 2024. https://ourworldindata.org/data-insights /the-global-malaria-death-rate-increased-for-the-first-time-in-20-years-due-to-covid-19.

135. Fleck A. Global number of TB deaths is declining again. Statista. November 7, 2023. https://www.statista.com/chart/31215/worldwide-number-of-deaths-caused-by-tuberculosis.

136. 2020 Alzheimer's disease facts and figures. Alzheimer's Association International Conference. March 2020. https://aaic.alz.org/downloads2020/2020_Facts_and_Figures_Fact _Sheet.pdf.

137. Wong W. Economic burden of Alzheimer disease and managed care considerations. *American Journal of Managed Care.* August 2020;26(8 Suppl):S177–S183. doi:10.37765/ ajmc.2020.88482.

138. Yang W, Hamilton JL, Kopil C, et al. Current and projected future economic burden of Parkinson's disease in the U.S. *npj Parkinson's Disease.* July 9, 2020;6(1):15. doi:10.1038/ s41531-020-0117-1.

139. Categorical spending. NIH RePORT. May 14, 2024. https://report.nih.gov/funding /categorical-spending#.

140. Our research strategy. Michael J. Fox Foundation. https://www.michaeljfox.org /our-research-strategy. Accessed September 20, 2024.

141. The Michael J. Fox Foundation for Parkinson's Research, consolidated financial statements, December 31, 2021 and 2020. Michael J. Fox Foundation. https://www.michaeljfox.org /sites/default/files/media/document/2021%20Audited%20Consolidated%20Financial%20 Statements%20FINAL.pdf. Accessed September 23, 2024.

142. Trichloroethylene and perchloroethylene market insights, 2027. Transparency Market Research. November 2019. https://www.transparencymarketresearch.com/trichloroethylene -and-perchloroethylene-market.html.

143. von Ehrenstein OS, Ling C, Cui X, et al. Prenatal and infant exposure to ambient pesticides and autism spectrum disorder in children: population based case-control study. *BMJ.* 2019;364:l1962. doi:10.1136/bmj.l1962.

144. Trichloroethylene—ToxFAQs™. Agency for Toxic Substances and Disease Registry, CDC. June 2019. https://www.atsdr.cdc.gov/toxfaqs/tfacts19.pdf.

145. Rauh V, Arunajadai S, Horton M, et al. Seven-year neurodevelopmental scores and prenatal exposure to chlorpyrifos, a common agricultural pesticide. *Environmental Health Perspectives.* August 2011;119(8):1196–1201. doi:10.1289/ehp.1003160.

146. Rauh VA, Garfinkel R, Perera FP, et al. Impact of prenatal chlorpyrifos exposure on neurodevelopment in the first 3 years of life among inner-city children. *Pediatrics.* December 2006;118(6):e1845–e1859. doi:10.1542/peds.2006-0338.

147. Rauh VA, Perera FP, Horton MK, et al. Brain anomalies in children exposed prenatally to a common organophosphate pesticide. *Proceedings of the National Academy of Sciences of the United States of America.* May 15, 2012;109(20):7871–7876. doi:10.1073/pnas.1203396109.

148. Malek AM, Barchowsky A, Bowser R, Youk A, Talbott EO. Pesticide exposure as a risk factor for amyotrophic lateral sclerosis: a meta-analysis of epidemiological studies: pesticide exposure as a risk factor for ALS. *Environmental Research.* August 1, 2012;117:112–119. doi:10.1016/j. envres.2012.06.007.

149. Su F-C, Goutman SA, Chernyak S, et al. Association of environmental toxins with amyotrophic lateral sclerosis. *JAMA Neurology.* 2016;73(7):803–811. doi:10.1001/ jamaneurol.2016.0594.

150. Yu Y, Su F-C, Callaghan BC, Goutman SA, Batterman SA, Feldman EL. Environmental risk factors and amyotrophic lateral sclerosis (ALS): a case-control study of ALS in Michigan. *PLOS One.* 2014;9(6):e101186. doi:10.1371/journal.pone.0101186.

151. Bove FJ, Ruckart PZ, Maslia M, Larson TC. Evaluation of mortality among Marines and navy personnel exposed to contaminated drinking water at USMC base Camp Lejeune: a retrospective cohort study. *Environmental Health*. February 19, 2014;13(1):10. doi:10.1186/1476-069X-13-10.

152. Heineman EF, Cocco P, Gómez MR, et al. Occupational exposure to chlorinated aliphatic hydrocarbons and risk of astrocytic brain cancer. *American Journal of Industrial Medicine*. August 1, 1994;26(2):155–169. doi:10.1002/ajim.4700260203.

153. DeBolt D. TCE causes cancer, other health woes, EPA says. Palo Alto Online. October 7, 2011. https://www.paloaltoonline.com/news/2011/10/07/tce-causes-cancer-other -health-problems-epa-says.

154. Bowman S. EPA announces plan for cleaning up remaining cancer-causing contamination in Franklin. *IndyStar*. June 6, 2022. https://www.indystar.com/story/news environment/2022/06/06/epa-cancer-causing-contamination-franklin-trichloroethylene -tetrachloroethylene/7489997001.

155. Steinmetz JD, Seeher KM, Schiess N, et al. Global, regional, and national burden of disorders affecting the nervous system, 1990–2021: a systematic analysis for the Global Burden of Disease Study 2021. *The Lancet Neurology*. 2024;23(4):344–381. doi:10.1016/ S1474-4422(24)00038-3.

156. Hyde L. *The Gift: Creativity and the Artist in the Modern World*. Vintage; 2009.

INDEX

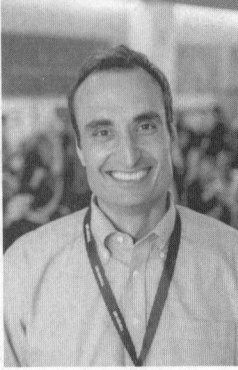

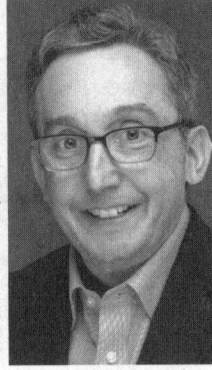

Ray Dorsey is the director of the Center for the Brain & the Environment at the Atria Health and Research Institute. The center's mission is to identify the root causes of brain diseases from autism to Alzheimer's so that we can *prevent* them.

Ray is also a professor of neurology (part-time) at the University of Rochester where he previously directed the Center for Health + Technology. He also chaired the international Huntington Study Group, led the movement disorders division at Johns Hopkins, and consulted for McKinsey & Company.

Michael S. Okun is an internationally renowned neurologist, translational scientist, and thought leader in movement disorders and neuromodulation. He is the cofounder and Director of the Norman Fixel Institute for Neurological Diseases and has led numerous NIH- and foundation-funded studies advancing brain circuit therapeutics. The author of more than 600 peer-reviewed publications, Dr. Okun's research has shaped clinical practice guidelines and expanded the understanding of Parkinson's disease pathophysiology and treatment. He is widely recognized for integrating patient-centered care with cutting-edge neuroscience to drive global innovation in the field.

In 2015, the White House recognized both Ray and Michael as a "Champions for Change" for Parkinson's disease.